Family Medicine

A Guidebook for Practitioners of the Art

Second Edition

David B. Shires, M.B., Ch.B., M.P.H., C.C.F.P., F.C.F.P.

Professor
Department of Family Medicine
Dalhousie University
Halifax, Nova Scotia
Canada

Brian K. Hennen, M.A., M.D., C.C.F.P., F.C.F.P.

Professor and Head
Department of Family Medicine
Dalhousie University
Halifax, Nova Scotia
Canada

Donald I. Rice, M.D., F.C.F.P.

Honorary President and Former Executive Director
College of Family Physicians of Canada
Toronto, Ontario
Canada

McGraw-Hill Book Company

New York   St. Louis   San Francisco   Auckland   Bogotá   Hamburg
Lisbon   London   Madrid   Mexico   Milan   Montreal
New Delhi   Panama   Paris   San Juan   São Paulo   Singapore   Sydney
Tokyo   Toronto

To three families
who contributed much to this book
through their patience,
understanding, support, and love

This book was set in Baskerville by Compset, Inc.
The editors were Beth Kaufman Barry and Julia L. White;
the cover was designed by Edward R. Schultheis;
the production supervisor was Thomas J. LoPinto.
Arcata Graphics/Halliday was printer and binder.

ISBN 0-07-056921-5

FAMILY MEDICINE
A Guidebook for Practitioners of the Art

3 4 5 6 7 8 9 0   HALHAL   8 9

Library of Congress Cataloging in Publication Data

Shires, David B.
  Family medicine.

  Includes bibliographies and index.
  1. Family medicine.   I. Hennen, Brian K.   II. Rice, Donald I.   III. Title. [DNLM: 1. Family Practice.
WB 110 S558f]
R729.5.G4S5   1987   610   86-7423
ISBN 0-07-056921-5

Contents

1

PRIMARY CARE TO THE FAMILY

2 COMMON PROBLEMS

3 FACILITATING HEALTH MAINTENANCE

4 PATIENT MANAGEMENT

5 TEAM FUNCTION

6 RESEARCH AND TEACHING SKILLS

7 OFFICE MANAGEMENT

8 THE COMPLETE APPROACH

List of Contributors

G. C. duBOIS
Department of Family Medicine
Dalhousie University
Halifax, Nova Scotia
Canada

N. H. HANSEN, M.D., C.C.F.P., F.C.F.P.
Department of Family Medicine
Dalhousie University
Halifax, Nova Scotia
Canada

B. K. HENNEN, M.D., C.C.F.P., F.C.F.P.
Department of Family Medicine
Dalhousie University
Halifax, Nova Scotia
Canada

B. PRIME-WALKER, B.Sc.N.
Department of Family Medicine
Dalhousie University
Halifax, Nova Scotia
Canada

R. W. PUTNAM, M.D., C.C.F.P.
Division of Continuing Medical Education
Dalhousie University
Halifax, Nova Scotia
Canada

C. S. REDDEN
Formerly, Office of the Dean of Medicine
Dalhousie University
Halifax, Nova Scotia
Canada

B. SEITZ, M.A.
Clinical Psychologist
Brooklyn, New York

G. MacDOUGALL, M.S.W.
Children's Aid Agency
Halifax, Nova Scotia
Canada

H. C. STILL, M.B., B. Ch., C.C.F.P.,
   F.C.F.P.
Department of Family Medicine
Dalhousie University
Halifax, Nova Scotia
Canada

M. K. LAURENCE, M.S.W., Ph.D.
Faculty of Social Work
Wilfrid Laurier University
Waterloo, Ontario
Canada

S. DYER, B.S.
Department of Family Medicine
Dalhousie University
Halifax, Nova Scotia
Canada

R. MacLACHLAN, M.D., C.C.F.P.
Department of Family Medicine
Dalhousie University
Halifax, Nova Scotia
Canada

D. I. RICE, M.D., F.C.F.P.
Honorary President and Former Executive
   Director
College of Family Physicians of Canada
Toronto, Ontario
Canada

S. URQUHART, R.N.
Department of Family Medicine
Dalhousie University
Halifax, Nova Scotia
Canada

A. E. MacLEOD, D.D.S.
Dental Practitioner
Cape Breton
Nova Scotia
Canada

M. NIXON, M.D., C.C.F.P.
Department of Family Medicine
St. John Regional Hospital
St. John, New Brunswick
Canada

M. R. SEITZ, Ph.D.
Department of Speech
Brooklyn College of the City University of
   New York
Brooklyn, New York

S. SHERWIN, Ph.D.
Department of Philosophy
Dalhousie University
Halifax, Nova Scotia
Canada

D. B. SHIRES, M.B., Ch.B., M.P.H.,
   C.C.F.P., F.C.F.P.
Department of Family Medicine
Dalhousie University
Halifax, Nova Scotia
Canada

L. MUZZERALL, B.N., R.N.
Department of Family Medicine
Dalhousie University
Halifax, Nova Scotia
Canada

D. CURTIS, M.A.
Clinical Psychologist
Halifax, Nova Scotia
Canada

D. C. BROWN, M.D., C.C.F.P., F.C.F.P.
Department of Family Medicine
Dalhousie University
Halifax, Nova Scotia
Canada

D. GASS, M.D., C.C.F.P.
Department of Family Medicine
Dalhousie University
Halifax, Nova Scotia
Canada

P. N. STERN, PH.D., R.N.
School of Nursing
Dalhousie University
Halifax, Nova Scotia
Canada

F. CROMBIE, M.D., C.C.F.P.
Department of Family Medicine
Dalhousie University
Halifax, Nova Scotia
Canada

Foreword

D. I. Rice, M.D.

The first residency training programs in family medicine leading to a higher qualification—certification in family medicine (Canada) and board certification in family practice (United States)—were introduced in North America in the mid-1960s. Since that time, thousands of family physicians have taken this additional training and have acquired the appropriate qualifications.

Despite this significant development, there still exists a degree of resistance to the concept of specific graduate training for family physicians, particularly among medical students and the established medical community, notably older and more experienced general practitioners. A number of medical specialists and other health professionals have difficulty acknowledging a major objective of this additional training: the acceptance of the family physician as the major provider of primary health care. While this attitude is subject to speculation, legitimate resistance to the concept of specialty training for family physicians results from a continuing limited knowledge on the part of many individuals as to what the discipline of family medicine is all about.

An objective of *Family Medicine: A Guidebook for Practitioners of the Art* is to make a contribution to the better understanding of this new and rapidly developing medical discipline. Three new terms have been added to the medical literature as a result of these new developments in medical education: *family medicine, family practice,* and *family physician.*

FAMILY MEDICINE: THE DISCIPLINE

Unlike general practice, family medicine is not a collection of bits and pieces of established specialty disciplines but encompasses a distinct body of knowledge appropriate to the needs of a changing society. While having its roots in general practice and maintaining a relation to the scientific aspects of the traditional specialties, family medicine is centered on the family as the basic social unit. The discipline is health-oriented as well as disease-oriented; it emphasizes the importance of disease prevention and health maintenance as well as curative medicine.

FAMILY PRACTICE: THE ART

The modus operandi by which the body of knowledge that is encompassed in the discipline of family medicine is dispensed to the community is properly called family practice. It is more than the provision of episodic care to the individual. It is primary, or first-contact, care; it is continuing ongoing care; and it is comprehensive care that is not limited by age, sex, or medical problems. Family practice encompasses ambulatory care, home care, and appropriate hospital care; it acknowledges the importance of practice management and establishes a pattern of practice designed to ensure efficient and cost-effective patient care.

FAMILY PHYSICIAN: THE PRACTITIONER

An individual physician who "practices" family medicine is not a generalist but a family physician. Trained in breadth and in the appropriate depth in related specialties, the family physician is not a minispecialist in these specialties but one who relates to specialists and other health professionals in a primary-care and consulting relationship that is designed to ensure optimal patient care.

The authors of *Family Medicine: A Guidebook for Practitioners of the Art* are sensitive to the different needs among the audience to whom this book is directed. For the medical student destined to a career in family medicine, it provides a comprehensive yet succinct and practical overview of the art and science of family medicine. For the established general practitioner, it provides an opportunity, and indeed a challenge, to better understand and accept how a general practice may be modified in order to ensure improved patient care and enrich professional satisfaction. For the family physician who has had the benefit of formal training in family medicine and is engaged in family practice or academic family medicine, this updated and revised textbook will provide an important reference in a program of continuing medical education. For other health professionals with an interest and responsibility in the discipline of family medicine, it will provide a better understanding of the principles on which the discipline is based and the application of those principles to the needs of a constantly changing society.

The authors have also been mindful of the rapid development of family medicine at an international level. While the content of this book is the result of experience in the teaching and practice of family medicine within the context of North American medicine, the book in general, and in particular the Part that deals with common health problems, has application to the needs of family physicians and improved patient care the world over.

I feel privileged to be associated with this second edition of *Family Medicine: A Guidebook for Practitioners of the Art* and commend it to you for your reading and learning pleasure.

Preface

This is a book about caring for people. It reflects the philosophy of family medicine we try to practice, summarizing our clinical and pedagogical experiences and those of our colleagues.

We are pleased to welcome Donald Rice as a principal author of this second edition. Dr. Rice's work in family medicine is world renowned, and his contribution to making this edition a working guide to the art of family medicine has proved invaluable.

Of special note is the fact that all the contributors have worked within the Metro Halifax–Dalhousie University setting in conjunction with us; thus the book reflects a unity of experience and mutual understanding not often seen in a multiple-author work. However, the viewpoints and opinions stem from a variety of sources, reflecting a worldwide range of understanding in the literature on family medicine and preventing the book from being a parochial document.

We have tried to blend the art of family medicine and the applications of medical and social sciences into a book for the medical student, the resident, and the practicing physician. We address the appropriate role of the family physician in the provision of primary health care in the context of family and community. For the second edition we have updated all chapters and added several new parts.

In Part 1, we define and describe the role of the family physician as a provider of primary care, stressing the concepts of responsibility for continuity of care, the family as a unit of care, anticipatory guidance, and the family as a prime resource for solving problems of health. In addition, we have added chapters on chronic handicaps, child abuse, and understanding families as a prelude to counseling.

In Part 2, we consider the family physician in the role of problem solver and provide a diagnostic and management approach to some of the common health problems presented to family physicians, using these problems to exemplify principles in family practice.

In Part 3, we review family medicine beyond the physician's office wall. Focusing initially on environmental factors that influence health and borrowing knowledge from epidemiology, we make a case for identification of health risks as a means of promoting health. This involves influencing lifestyle habits in individuals as well as lifelong health maintenance. This part concludes with a description of how the family physician can help patients maintain health through lifestyle and specific programs such as Bodycheck.

Patient management is the subject of Part 4. This part explores patient attitudes toward self-care and shows how these attitudes affect compliance with therapy. This part provides practical advice as well as guidance in seeking additional resources and concludes with an outline of therapeutics and the problems of prescribing. For the second edition, we have added a chapter on transcultural health and included a chapter on patient education.

In Part 5, under the general heading of "Team Function," we describe the many problems which a family physician may have difficulty handling alone. We suggest a strong role for the family practice nurse in providing continuing health care and outline methods by which this can be accomplished. The chapter "Consulting Wisely" focuses initially on guidelines for consulting other physicians and then considers other team members who share in the provision of primary care.

In Part 6, we discuss research and education as inherent parts of family medicine.

As the manager of a medical practice, the physician is always faced with business, legal, financial, and management problems. In Part 7, some solutions to these problems are offered by experienced business management consultants. The authors of these chapters share some personal management skills that we can use to good advantage. A new addition to the second edition is a chapter on computer applications in practice.

In Part 8, we explore ethical issues in family medicine and discuss what it means to be a family physician in terms of the moral responsibilities of medical practice. We conclude with a summary of what we call the whole-person approach and the future of family medicine.

We hope that this approach to family medicine will add to the body of knowledge and influence attitudes in a way that will make all of us better family practitioners.

ACKNOWLEDGMENTS

In addition to thanking those who helped prepare the first edition of this book, we would like to thank the persons whose efforts made possible the production of the second edition. The generation of the book was greatly encouraged by the moral and financial support of the College of Family Physicians of Canada.

First, we would like to thank McGraw-Hill through the person of Beth Kaufman Barry, our editor, for her encouragement and support and for putting up with all our requests for more time.

Molly Wolf, our editorial and research assistant, showed unfailing energy in keeping us going and making it possible for us to complete the work.

Bill Owen and Sheila Plant of the Dalhousie Kellogg Library reviewed hundreds of bibliographic references.

Ingrid Ring, Anne Hardman, Clare Mosher, Della Reid, Muriel Dunn, Caroline Bologna, Carolyn Hicks, Renee Davis, and Jessie MacDonald worked tirelessly on entering and reentering revised versions of the manuscript and still were able to smile at the end of it.

Dr. Mary MacCara, of the School of Clinical Pharmacy, reviewed all the sections of the book dealing with pharmacology and gave us many constructive suggestions. We would also like to thank Dr. Alexander Reid of Newcastle (Australia) for his critical reading of the first edition and his suggestions for revision. Our colleagues, especially at the Dalhousie Family Medicine Centre, and patients, students, and residents put up with our preoccupations while writing the book. Drs. Ian McWhinney, Keith Hodgkin, Nathan Epstein, John Geyman, David Marsland, Maurice Wood, and Fitzhugh Mayo lead those whose published works have formed the basis of our understanding of family medicine.

To all these and others we are grateful. The final editing and any resulting errors are, of course, our responsibility alone.

David B. Shires
Brian K. Hennen
Donald I. Rice

Part One

Primary Care to the Family

Chapter 1

Continuity of Care

B. K. Hennen, M.D.

The essence of family medicine is continuity of care. Continuity of care means much more than caring for the same patient over a long period of time. It also involves organizing the provision of care and therefore includes the family physician's relationships with other health professionals who are called upon for advice or help.

The primary function of the family physician is to help families manage current illnesses and to show them how to prevent, or at least reduce, the likelihood of further illness. The family physician must accomplish this function in the framework of an increasingly complex social system characterized by rapid technological advances. The physician must also take account of changing patterns of illness and changing expectations about health.

All family physicians feel a strong commitment to provide a personal kind of care, a commitment that includes the promise to guide the patient through the complexities of health care services. When they have difficulty meeting this commitment, for example, when they lose direct contact with patients who are hospitalized, practitioners are acutely aware of the break in continuity and generally consider it a deficit of the system.[1]

Commitment to continuity

An independent businessman in his middle fifties was admitted to a special care unit in a tertiary care hospital for aortic valve replacement. On entering the milieu of complex technology (monitors, gadgets, etc.) and suffering a relative loss of autonomy and privacy, he became uncooperative, and refused surgery if he had to return to the special care unit. A psychiatrist was consulted but was rejected outright with much verbal abuse. The surgeon, about to refuse to operate, suggested as a last resort that the nurse phone the patient's family doctor (who, after 48 hours, had not yet been notified of the patient's admission). The family doctor came in, sat with the patient for a half hour, listened to his anxieties and worries, reviewed the reasons why surgery was indicated, and explained the necessity for the intensive care milieu. The patient was reassured and better informed and subsequently underwent a successful operation.

Components of continuity

Continuity of care is the quintessence of family medicine, permeating every aspect: first contact, longitudinal responsibility, integration of care, and the concept of the family as the unit of care.[2]

Providing first-contact medical care means being closest to the patient. Initially, it means that one is the first doctor whom the patient contacts when sick. But from then on it involves the responsibility of being the personal advocate, protector, interpreter, and care integrator for the patient no matter where he or she is required to be—at home, in a hospital, or in a nursing home. When one problem is resolved, the doctor must be available to help with the next one.

When continuity ends

As McWhinney has emphasized, the patient's relationship with the family physician is not limited by the duration of illness.[3] It ends when the patient or doctor elects to end it, when either party dies, or when the doctor ceases to practice. Otherwise, care should continue to be available either directly from the doctor or from deputized colleagues.

Advantages of continuity

Continuity of care has been the subject of many studies, and ways of measuring it are being refined.[4] Some of the advantages noted include better compliance with prescribed medications,[5] less likelihood of patient delay in seeking necessary help,[6] increased patient and doctor satisfaction,[7,8] better disclosure of behavioral problems,[8] and lower costs as a result of performing fewer laboratory tests.[9,10] Some authors have reported no advantage.[11]

Continuity of care has four dimensions: chronological, geographical, interdisciplinary, and interpersonal.[12]

Chronological continuity

1 The *chronological* dimension includes those aspects of care that relate to human growth and development, whether of the individual or of the family. This leads to the family physician's commitment to offer care to persons from infancy to old age in the context of their family attachments or in the absence of such at-

tachments. The chronological dimension also applies to the natural history of illness and the manner in which family physicians use repeated observations over time as a diagnostic and management tool. Such long-term observations also serve as a basis for the scientific study of medicine, leading to new knowledge in the field.

2 The *geographical* dimension refers to the provision of primary care, whether it be in the home, the physician's office, the acute care hospital, the chronic care hospital, the rehabilitation institution, the nursing home, or the community resource center. The important thing is for the family physician to be the closest physician to the patient throughout the patient's contacts within the health system. Nowhere, even in the tertiary care or highly specialized unit, should the patient lóse contact with the family physician.

Geographical continuity

3 The *interdisciplinary* dimension refers to those aspects of care which cross the lines between the traditional clinical disciplines. For example, a patient with chronic osteoarthritis develops a recurrent urinary tract infection and becomes depressed. The arthritis remains static, the episodes of urinary infection respond quickly to management, and the depression responds gradually to supportive psychotherapy. The patient's spouse has phobic anxiety and migraine and will also require care. In caring for a patient, the family physician may have to manage diseases of several body systems (each at a different stage), support the patient in dealing with problems of living which may or may not be related to the diseases, and manage a comparable constellation of illness in other family members. The physician must also coordinate these activities without interrupting more than necessary the usual family functioning.

Interdisciplinary continuity

4 The *interpersonal* dimension of care continuity contains three elements: (*a*) doctor-patient relationships, (*b*) family relationships, and (*c*) interprofessional relationships. The first element involves the establishment of rapport and mutual trust, or, as Carmichael described it, "that tenured relationship" which gets you out of bed at night.[13] As an example of the second element, consider a woman who fears liquor because of her father's drunkenness. Her adolescent son drinks in response to her prohibitive attitude. The family physician must understand both patients' reactions. The third element involves having trusted associates you can rely on: the surgeon who will come because he or she knows you do not ask for help without cause; the social worker who returns your call promptly because you do likewise; the admissions clerk who can usually secure you a bed because you stop in personally to explain your patient's needs; the associates, professional and nonprofessional, who work in your office every day and develop continued understanding of and familiarity with each other's strengths, weaknesses, and idiosyncrasies.

Interpersonal continuity

Cementing these interprofessional relationships involves the skillful use of continuity of information, which relies to a great ex-

The medical record

tent on the written record. The proper record system records acute episodes and ensures their follow-up; records the progress of the chronic illness; records the multifaceted problems of physical, social, and psychological illness; and draws together information about the various family members.

Continuity in action

Each of these dimensions of continuity can be translated into specific actions, including the following:

Applying the Denver Developmental Screening Test[14] to infants

Anticipating specific stress periods in the life cycle of the family

Considering why the patient came with that symptom at that time

Ensuring appropriate follow-up for the acute illness

Planning ahead with the patient who has a chronic illness

Guiding the patient's course from the house call into the hospital then the nursing home, and back home

Coping with a patient with multiple complaints and a poor family situation

Responding to the tug of responsibility when the malingerer's spouse calls to say he or she cannot cope anymore

Anticipating the new father's reluctance to hold the crying baby and showing him that the baby will not break if he picks it up

Recording accurately on the patient's record the natural history of the illness

Making use of the family record to ask about a child's hearing while the mother is in for her Pap smear

Bringing continuity together

Very often we apply different combinations of these dimensions at the same time. Perhaps the best example is that of caring for a family in which one member has a fatal illness. We care for the person, specifically treat the patient's (often multisystem) disease, deal with the fact that the patient is dying, and care for the family before and after the death.

These are the dimensions of continuity which are to be found throughout the family physician's activities. The understanding of families, the skills of anticipation and prevention, the awareness of how people decide to seek the doctor's help when they are sick, and, finally, the ability to discriminate clinically which patients need which services in the health care system are all part of caring for patients continuously—the family physician's job.

REFERENCES

1 J. Weston Smith, "Pros of the General Practitioner in Hospital," *Update,* **9:**743–749, 1974.

2 J. J. Alpert and E. G. Charney, *The Education of Physicians for Primary Care*, Department of Health, Education and Welfare, Bureau of Health Services Research, DHEW Publication (HRA) 74–3113, 1973.

3 I. R. McWhinney, "Continuity of Care in Family Practice. Part 2: Implication of Continuity," *Journal of Family Practice*, **2**:373–374, 1975.

4 M. A. Godkin and C. A. Rice, "A Measure of Continuity of Care for Physicians in Practice," *Family Medicine*, **16**(4):136–140, 1984.

5 P. R. A. Ettlinger and G. K. Freeman, "General Practice Compliance Study: Is It Worth It Being a Personal Doctor?" *British Medical Journal*, **282**:1192–1193, 1981.

6 P. G. May and R. Kaelbling, "The Family Doctor as a Current Source of Continual Comprehensive Medical Care," *Ohio State Medical Journal*, **67**:1007–1013, 1971.

7 M. B. Sussman et al., *The Walking Patient: A Study in Outpatient Care*, Western Reserve University Press, Cleveland, 1967.

8 M. M. Becker et al., "A Field Experiment to Evaluate Various Outcomes of Continuity of Physician Care," *American Journal of Public Health*, **64**:1062–1070, 1974.

9 J. Alpert et al., "Attitudes and Satisfaction of Low-Income Families Receiving Comprehensive Health Care," *American Journal of Public Health*, **60**:499–506, 1970.

10 M. C. Heagarty et al., "Some Comparative Costs in Comprehensive versus Fragmented Pediatric Care," *Pediatrics*, **46**:596–603, 1970.

11 L. Gordis and M. Markowitz, "Evaluation of the Effectiveness of Comprehensive and Continuous Pediatric Care," *Pediatrics*, **48**:766–776, 1971.

12 B. K. Hennen, "Continuity of Care in Family Practice. Part 1: Dimensions of Continuity," *Journal of Family Practice*, **2**:371–372, 1975.

13 L. P. Carmichael, "Family Medicine Workshop," *Presentation to the Society of Teachers of Family Medicine*, Miami, Fla., January 1969.

14 W. K. Frankenburg and J. B. Dodds, The Denver Developmental Screening Test. Copyright by Mead Johnson Laboratories, January 1969.

Chapter 2

Family Structure and Function

B. K. Hennen, M.D.

Families have both structure and function. Family members are assigned roles specific to some function within the family. At first glance, the family group does not seem to be based on an efficient model, but strengths of affection and duty tend to compensate for the apparent awkwardness of its organization.

STRUCTURE AND FUNCTION

Definition of family

To understand families better we can look at them in terms of structure and function. Although a family can be defined in many ways (for example, two related persons living together for 6 months; one parent and a child; any mixture of parents, children, and siblings living together), for the purpose of this discussion it will be defined as a married man and woman with or without children and with or without living parents. The couple and children are often referred to as the *nuclear family*. If we include the couple's parents and other relatives, we are referring to the *extended family*.

Alternate families

A substantial number of people live in social units that do not fit this definition. The functions accomplished are often the same, and the structures are often similar; common-law marriages, single-parent families, homosexual unions, and communes are examples. In these families, the problems and solutions may be similar to those found in the traditional family. When the family form differs from the traditional structures, the difference may require additional consideration in regard to the provision of health care.

Small groups have their own dynamics, which depend primarily on interpersonal communications. The family is a special kind of small group, one which has inherent strengths because of inherited and developmental commonalities, affectional ties, and societal expectations that it should operate in certain ways. Family membership implies a lifelong involvement with no option to leave; one can never totally deny one's parents, siblings, or children.

Some physical and psychological attributes are genetically influenced, so family members often have similar attributes. Living in the same home, sharing social activities, having similar schooling, and experiencing the same successes and failures give family members a common background in which they can comfortably develop. Families also develop their own attitudes toward discipline, sexuality, communication, privacy, and so on. The family gives its members a sense of belonging as well as affection, companionship, and security. It is also a source for advice and help.

Shared attributes

Society expects families to have a sense of responsibility toward their members (the police return a drunken teenager to her parents; the doctor phones an elderly widower's children to ask them to assume his care). Society also protects the rights of family membership (child guardianship and custody decisions favor legal and natural parents; adoptive parents tend to be chosen from those who come from the same religious background as the child's original family).

Society's expectations of family

Compared with other small groups, however, the family has many built-in problems, which Martinson amplifies in *Family in Society*.[1] This writer points out that members differ markedly in age, many members are dependent on the others, the family can neither reject members nor recruit new ones, and members are involved with each other emotionally. He further notes that all these factors affect the efficiency of the group:

The family as small group

The family carries on a great variety of activities, and its activities are characterized by diffuseness rather than specificity. It does not specialize in one or a small number of activities as do most other functioning groups, such as a children's play group, or a planning committee. In the mother-child relationship, for instance, the mother reacts to all the child's behavior and even anticipates his or her needs—her concern is all-inclusive. She is cook, waitress, nurse, protector, and giver and receiver of affection. The relationships in the family are characterized by emotional or affective behavior, and the relationships themselves, rather than impersonal goals, determine what is done.

Members of the leadership coalition (mother and father) do not think of the family in terms of specific functions—as a consumption unit or a child training unit, for instance. The family is different from other groups in that there is variety in its activities as well as in the roles that its members play.

The family is also at a disadvantage in comparison with other groups because its success or failure is largely tied in with the activities of only one of its members, the major breadwinner. . . . In sum, the family, when compared with other groups, is intrinsically "a puny work group and an awkward decision-making group."

A nonfamily group

For the purposes of comparison, consider a homogeneous task-oriented group which is trying to solve a problem. Six people are building a house: an architect, a constructor, a plumber, an electrician, a carpenter, and a laborer. Each has been engaged because of particular skills or attributes and is to be paid for his or her contribution. All must work cooperatively with the constructor, who is the manager or coordinator. The group members will work together until the house is completed, after which they may agree to collaborate on another project. They may, however, choose to take separate jobs since they have no commitment to one another, or if one does a poor job, the others may decide to stay together and replace that individual.

A family group

Consider a family of two parents and three children—a boy of 19, a girl of 16, and a girl of 10—who are planning a family vacation. The father has 3 weeks off in late June and early July; the mother works on weekends in a supermarket and can get only two weekends off. The boy is at college and is looking for a summer job. The older girl has a job as a lifeguard starting July 1, while the younger one belongs to a swimming team that practices every day. The father wants to rent a cottage, but the mother would prefer to go camping; the son doesn't want to spend a holiday with the family, and neither daughter wants to go out of town. Since the father never wanted the mother to take a job, he insists that the family members take their vacation together.

The family endures

This group is not homogeneous and is engaged in a continuing process of some 20 years' duration. The immediate goal of planning a vacation is perceived differently by all members. There are various degrees of authority as seen by each individual, and the relative autonomy of the individual members is in a state of flux. Despite the conflict, there are bonds of affection, a sense of responsibility, and a sense of belonging that continuously draw the family together. No one can abdicate completely from the family, although the teenagers, who are approaching the phase of relative autonomy that exists between leaving one's family of procreation and establishing one's own family, could be said to be capable of temporary and partial abdication.

When it functions as a small group that is trying to complete a task, the family is often inefficient and ineffective. Its strength as a group lies in creating a milieu in which its members can develop as individuals, become socialized, and establish bonds which will offer them emotional support.

The family performs five basic functions: socialization, care, provision of affection, reproduction, and provision of status. *Socialization* involves the development of social skills, including the development of interpersonal relationships. It includes learning how to deal with other people both in the same age group and in other generations. Socialization may start in utero, but it first becomes obvious when the mother and baby make early social contact, including eye contact. *Care* involves the provision of shelter, warmth, food, and protection. *Affection* involves love, warmth, worry, and caring. *Reproduction* involves sexual relationships with or without contraception. *Status* involves socioeconomic, educational, and occupational factors but also includes the simple legitimacy provided by the legal marriage of the parents.

Weaknesses and strengths

Five family functions

ROLE OF EACH FAMILY MEMBER

Traditional expectations exist for all family members: mother, father, and child. However, in present-day society these expectations are changing. It is nevertheless worthwhile to review the traditional roles in order to appreciate how differences from the usual or the expected may affect the younger generation and understand the expectations of the more traditional older generation.

The schema first presented by Epstein et al.[2,3] is valuable for the understanding of family function, and the subsequent discussion is based for the most part on that model.

The traditional role of wife and mother was until recently considered as largely expressive or affective; it included mothering, homemaking, sexual activity, and modeling "female" behavior to children.

The husband and father role was traditionally considered more instrumental, involving breadwinning and responsibility for major decisions (including money decisions), ultimate authority, sexual activity, some degree of child care, and the modeling of "male" behavior.

The child's role has often been looked on as a passive one but is increasingly being seen as active. The child receives the general attention of parents and siblings, learns and practices many new

Changing family roles

Mother

Father

Child

skills, and is a major source of education for parents by virtue of passing along things learned at school.

Role change related to social class

Changes in role expectations, such as more sharing of tasks previously designated as either the mother's or the father's, have recently been seen in western culture. Families in which the father is the breadwinner and the mother stays home with the children now constitute a small minority of American families. Social class seems to have a significant impact on the degree to which the roles have merged, with lower socioeconomic classes holding more to the older, traditional expectations.[4]

Expectations of each other

In assessing family functions, it is useful to explore the expectations of family members about their own and each other's proper duties. For example, if premarital counseling succeeds only in clarifying for the prospective partners their expectations of each other, it may prevent many marital problems.

COMMUNICATION IN THE FAMILY

The basics

The basics of every act of communication include a sender (S), a message (M), and a receiver (R). When communication takes place, S→M→R, problems can occur in any part of the system. For example, the sender may not deliver the message clearly, the message may be ambiguous, or the receiver may appear to hear without really listening.

Three levels of communication

As a special kind of small group, the family can be assessed according to its communication patterns. Epstein et al.[2] outlined three levels of communication within a family.

1   The first level describes *what* is being communicated. The "what" may be either feelings or information. If it is related to feelings, it is called *affective communication*. If it is related to accomplishing the usual tasks of living by passing on information or doing mechanical tasks, it is called *instrumental communication*.

2   The second level of communication concerns whether the delivery of the message is *clear*, obvious, and undisguised or *masked*, ambiguous, and confused.

3   The third level of communication concerns the receiver of the message. *Direct communication* points clearly to the intended receiver. *Displaced communication* may point at someone other than the person for whom it is intended.

Examples of all three types of communication follow.

Instrumental: Pass the salt.
Affectional: I love you.
Clear: I can't stand you.

Masked:	I don't like your dress [meaning I don't like you].
Direct:	You make me feel good [to one person].
Displaced:	You make me sick [to a group, although intended for one person].
Masked and displaced:	Men are chauvinists [by a girl to her boyfriend].

When a family fails to function, affective communication suffers first. When instrumental communication also breaks down, the family is probably in severe trouble; masked and displaced communications are more likely to occur as families become more disturbed in their functioning.

Family dysfunction

It has been suggested that disrupted families first show failure in affective communication. It is therefore important to note whether a family *can express emotions* when appropriate, to an appropriate degree, as a group as well as individually, and with appropriate degrees of personal involvement. Basic emotions may be expressed as positive, or *welfare,* emotions. e.g., happiness, tenderness, love, or sympathy, or as *emergency* emotions, e.g., rage, anger, fear, or depression. If emotions are not being expressed, one must determine whether instrumental functions have also broken down. Table 2–1 contains some questions that are useful in assessing family function.

Assessing affective and instrumental communication

ORGANIZING FAMILY INFORMATION

If knowledge of the structure and function of families is relevant, its usefulness depends on its immediate availability. Family-oriented records[5] and genograms[6] can provide an instant review of genetic, medical, and psychosocial information about the family of a patient presenting for medical advice. The bulkiness of paper records (one receptionist protested carrying 40 lbs of family-grouped records for an afternoon session) will soon be remedied by computerized systems. Innovative supplements to coordinated (family) information such as Smilkstein's family APGAR add to the basic data we can record.[7]

Records reflect family care

SUMMARY

Although the family can sometimes be a disruptive influence in the management of a sick member, generally it is a useful though often

Table 2-1　Checklist to Assess Family Function

1　How many are there in the family?
2　Who lives at home?
3　In what phase of the family life cycle is the family?
4　What problems does this raise for them?
5　What major problems has the family had in the past? (Inquire about death, separation, major physical or mental illness, financial crisis, etc.)
6　Does the family feel these problems were dealt with satisfactorily?
7　Is there any history of alcoholism, drug abuse, or delinquency in the family?
8　How are the major decisions made in the family and by whom?
9　a　What does each parent expect of each child, both on a day-to-day basis and for the future?
　　b　What do the children expect of each parent?
　　c　Are these expectations realistic?
10　What does each member of this family have to do to get attention?
11　How much tolerance for individual differences is there in the family?
12　What are the goals, interests, and values (including religious values) of the family?
13　Do all the family members work together toward these goals?
14　What is the educational level and financial status of the parents?
15　Are the in-laws and relatives helpful? Do they create problems for the family?
16　Do the family members have many friends in the neighborhood? To what groups or clubs do family members belong?
17　What sorts of community resources (health care services, community service agencies, police, etc.) has the family used? Would the family members use them again?
18　Has this family not used community resources at times when it would have been appropriate?

underutilized resource for the doctor, nurse, physiotherapist, or other health professional. If we understand how a family functions, we can use it more effectively. If we educate families to help ill members and if we expect more of them, we will almost without exception make our jobs easier and provide better patient care as well.

REFERENCES

1 F. M. Martinson, *Family in Society,* Dodd, Mead Company, New York, 1970.
2 N. B. Epstein, J. J. Sigal, and V. Rakoff, *Family Categories Schema,* The Family Research Group of the Department of Psychiatry, Jewish General Hospital, in collaboration with McGill Human Development Study, Montreal, Canada.
3 B. Epstein, D. S. Bishop, and S. Levin, "The McMaster Model of Family Functioning," *Journal of Marriage and Family Counseling,* pp. 19–31, October 1978.

4 J. Newson and E. Newson, *Patterns of Infant Care in the Urban Community,* Penguin, New York, 1971.
5 D. M. Shapiro, "A Family Data Base for the Family Oriented Medical Record," *Journal of Family Practice,* **13**(6):881–887, 1981.
6 H. T. Milhorn, "The Genogram: A Structured Approach to the Family History," *Journal of the Mississippi State Medical Association,* **22**(10):250–252, 1981.
7 G. Smilkstein, "The Family APGAR: A Proposal for a Family Function Test and Its Use by Physicians," *Journal of Family Practice,* **6:**1231, 1978.

Chapter 3

The Family as the Unit of Care

B. K. Hennen, M.D.

*The family is the cause of many health-related problems. It is also a re-
source for solving them and for preventing illness. A doctor who fails to take
advantage of available family resources is not practicing family medicine
effectively. Similarly, a doctor who fails to recognize when family resources
are deficient or nonexistent may neglect to ensure that alternative resources are found.*

**The family
survives**

The family is our basic social unit. Though family stability is constantly challenged by changing social forces, it is nevertheless true
that a large majority (80 percent in Canada[1] and 75 percent in the
United States [2]) of individuals live in family units, and most people
(92 percent in the United States[3]) hope the family will continue as
the basic unit. High divorce rates are countered by high rates of
remarriage among the divorced, suggesting that, even for those
whose marriages have failed, the state of marriage (and its insepa-
rable familial implications) is considered desirable.[4]

**What is family
care?**

There is ongoing debate about the relationship between families and family medicine and about what is meant when the family
is considered the unit of care. Family care can mean taking care of
all individuals in the family one by one "when it makes sense and

when I (the physician) can."[5] It can mean influencing family members to change factors affecting an individual's health. It can mean dealing with the family as an object of management ("the family as patient").[6]

Some family doctors believe that the relationships they have with families in their practice are similar to the relationships present within those families. Carmichael[7] reports that his role with the family can be well described by four characteristics: affinity, continuity, intimacy, and reciprocity. He emphasizes the importance of human relationships without focusing on "the family as the unit of care." He and others question the usefulness of medical practitioners arranging their education and practices to provide family-oriented services.

Carmichael's analysis of 40 families from his practice confirmed for him the fact that patients are largely unaware of family care and do not consciously seek out a physician to care for all family members. Family physician training programs offer an inadequate background in family studies, and few behavioral scientists in such programs have been trained to work clinically with families.[5] The practical drawbacks of family practice include a lack of space for comfortable family interviews in most offices, finding time in busy schedules to sit down with families, arranging payment for such services, and organizing efficient family-based records.[5,8]

Our view is summarized by Ransom: "The family is still our most pervasive and enduring context of human relatedness. . . . There is no way to intervene in an individual's life and not affect his or her 'family.'"[6]

As the basic social unit, the family constellation may be a major source of health problems. Since one must generally deal with the cause, the family often becomes the focus for the management of health problems that derive from its own dysfunction. The family is also a prime resource for solving health problems in general, even when their cause lies outside the family.

Questioning family care

Drawbacks

Problem and solution

THE FAMILY AS THE SOURCE OF HEALTH PROBLEMS

The death or illness of any family member creates stress that affects all members.[9] Stress also results when families are separated, for example, by job requirements or as a result of divorce. Any disruption of family functioning takes a toll of all family members.

Sources of stress

An illness in the family has emotional consequences, such as anxiety, depression, and behavior problems.

Illness causes anxiety

My office practice was suddenly and noisily interrupted one afternoon when a man charged through the waiting room and past my nurse, demanding to see me because his wife was "dying in the hospital." He was in a panic; he had just left his wife because he couldn't get anyone at the hospital to help her. She was in the hospital for knee surgery, and as far as I knew, having seen her a few hours before, she was progressing well. I phoned the hospital and learned that she had had an episode of hyperventilation; she was being seen by the intern at that moment and was feeling much better but was worried about what her husband had done after he had disappeared from her room.

The husband, a 5-year European Canadian who still had some difficulty with English and more difficulty with Canadian culture, had a great fear of doctors as a result of previous experiences. He had been passively opposed to his wife's operation in the first place and was also finding it difficult to cope with the children at home. When his wife suddenly began to hyperventilate during his visit, it was more than he could handle. His reaction was an understandable, if dramatic, expression of a husband's anxiety.

Acting out

A serious or prolonged illness in a family can be expected to cause situational depression in one or more members. This is particularly likely if the sick member is a child, if the illness makes heavy demands on the family's physical and emotional resources, or if the illness is known or perceived to be fatal. Children are particularly liable to act out when siblings or parents are sick.

A father of three children suffered multiple complications of abdominal surgery for an inflammatory condition and was hospitalized for a prolonged period. The adolescent son threw a large and noisy all-night party, causing considerable upset to siblings, neighbors, and particularly his mother. The absence of the father, the frequent absences of the mother, and the threat of the father's death all contributed to this unusual behavior on the son's part.

Stress illnesses

Psychosomatic illnesses, such as acid-pepsin disease or smooth muscle spasm diseases (colic, enuresis, asthma, and spastic colitis), also are frequently exacerbated in situations of family disruption.

Family transmits disease

The family itself can be a unit for the transmission of illness because of physical closeness, lifestyle, and inherited factors. Infectious disease, poor nutrition, and diabetes are examples of diseases that are easily transmitted within the family.

In short, the family can be the source of all types of illnesses, psychological, psychosomatic, or somatic.

THE FAMILY AS A RESOURCE FOR SOLVING HEALTH PROBLEMS

The family as resource

The family is often called upon to manage health problems which arise from its own dysfunction. The dysfunction may be caused by a specific illness of a family member and the inability of the sick person, the family, or the health care providers to deal with it. An example may serve to clarify.

An old friend whom I hadn't seen for a long time moved to where I was practicing and came to see me. She had cancer but didn't know it. She had had surgery about 9 months before she came to me; she was operated on for gall bladder disease, but when they opened her abdomen, they found she didn't have gall bladder disease but diffuse abdominal cancer. The doctors advised her husband and their two adult children that it was best for her not to know. For 9 months the two children and dad played games—cat and mouse games. They knew their mother had cancer and they knew she only had so much time, but their mother didn't know. What could they do when she said, "Why am I not feeling better? I had my operation." "Oh, you will feel better in a few days." They looked at each other knowingly across the room. The daughter would slip out to cry, and someone else would go in to help the mother. This continued for 9 months. Family communication was disrupted, since all conversation in the mother's presence was guarded, and family dysfunction ensued. The greatest potential resource—the family—was immobilized and unable to help its sickest member.

The husband decided to take his wife on a trip to Florida, to give her a holiday. Once there, the husband was under all kinds of pressure, and after a short time suddenly had a coronary. He had a cardiac arrest in the hospital and had to spend 3 weeks there. The bills were high, and there was insufficient insurance to cover them. Meanwhile, the mother, instead of having a nice holiday on the beach, spent most of her time going from motel to hospital. The couple finally got back to Canada, and that was when they came to me.

My attitude has been, except for rare occasions, that people should know what their problem is. I admitted the woman to hospital. By this time she had lost about 40 lb and was still asking why she was not feeling better. We did a few tests and confirmed the diagnosis with her previous doctors. I sat down with her and said, "Remember that operation you had 9 months ago? Were you told specifically what they found?" She said, "No, I really wasn't." I said, "Well, they found you had cancer." She looked at me and she smiled as if suddenly many things were clear and said, "Has Thomas known all this time?" (Thomas was her husband.) I said, "Yes, he has known all this time." She smiled and said, "I wonder what else he has been keeping from me?" This was the first time he had ever, to her knowledge, kept a secret of importance from her. She was surprised that she had not recognized the significant fib.

That's how she accepted it. From then on everybody was able to talk openly about her illness. She understood why she felt as she did, and her family was able to help. She went to visit her brother, who lived out West, for a last visit. When her medication made her hair fall out, she bought wigs. She was able to deal with her illness by discussing it with her family in an honest and positive way and by making plans with them to complete her unfinished business. She died within the next 6 months, but the last few months were productive because her family was able to help her come to terms with her illness. She, in turn, could help them.

Physician recognizes family potential

In this example, cancer in one family member and the attempts to keep the diagnosis from the patient disrupted the family's usually honest way of operating. The solution to the solvable problem (the cancer was not curable) was to restore to the family unit its basic style of functioning, i.e., frank and open discussion. To presume at the time of initial diagnosis that the family as a whole and the patient in particular were incapable of accepting the disease was to fail to recognize the family unit's potential for solving its own problems. The family physician, as an outside influence, should have been the person to place the illness in a context that would have allowed the family to use its strengths.

Preventive family medicine

The family is also a major resource in prevention. The family physician can give reinforcement and advice about the family's activities in health maintenance and preventive care. Pless points out that selected family physicians studied in Canada, Great Britain, and the United States had remarkably limited knowledge about the families of the patients they were treating. When "there is little doubt that the family does serve as a crucial resource unit in health care," Pless urges more research to show the importance to doctors of knowing more about the family.[8] Epstein et al.[10] suggest useful categories for considering the family's function in prevention, which are listed in Table 3-1.

THE FAMILY PHYSICIAN

Family physician's advantages

The doctor who looks after *all* members of the family has many advantages over the personal physician of any kind who only looks after individuals. This is not to deny that any capable physician, when considering a plan of assessment and management, will make inquiries about and take into consideration the family from which the patient comes and to which he or she must return. The family physician, however, not only inquires about the family and has it continually in mind but also possesses detailed personal knowledge about the health of the other family members and of the family structure as a whole.[11,12] The family physician who cares for the whole family has more frequent contacts with the family than any other care giver.

Opportunities to communicate

Consider, for the moment, that in Canada each individual visits the physician about five times per year on the average.[13] Given that the average Canadian family consists of 3.6 members, the family

Table 3-1 Areas for Family Participation in Prevention

Primary prevention

1 Lifestyle diseases: diet, addictive behavior, leisure activity, basic living habits
2 Health maintenance: immunization, screening activities
3 Family life education: sexuality, marriage, prenatal care, problems of aged members

Secondary prevention

1 Monitoring of well-being by physician and patient
2 Encouraging sick members to seek appropriate help
3 Compliance monitoring regarding specific management

Tertiary prevention

1 Balanced support between compliance monitoring and the appropriate independent activity of members with chronic illness
2 Adjustment of all members to changes necessitated by chronic illness in one member
3 Coping with crises created by a serious illness such as a congenital anomaly or by a dying family member

Source: Modified from Epstein et al.[10]

physician has many more opportunities per year to communicate, if only indirectly, with each family member than would be the case if the family members had their own individual doctors.

For example, the family physician may meet a new couple shortly before or after marriage. Ideally, perhaps, the doctor would see them in a premarital counseling situation. Generally, however, the woman is seen for contraceptive counseling prior to or shortly after marriage. In many families, pregnancy occurs within 2 years. This means that the woman is seen 10 or 12 times in the prenatal period, during which time considerable knowledge is gained not only about her as an individual but also about her relationships with her husband and their expectations as parents. (Some practitioners encourage husbands to participate in prenatal visits.) Then, for the first year of the baby's life, there are frequent visits during which much can be learned about the baby, the mother and mother-child relationship, the father and the family interaction at home, the interaction of parents-in-law, the siblings, etc. As the doctor learns, the partners also learn about themselves and about each other, especially if the doctor's interviews are appropriate and facilitate open discussion between them.

In the case of a young couple with a 1-year-old child, some 40 scheduled contacts with the doctor are possible, assuming the family has no illness. These 40 opportunities allow the doctor to (1) get to know the family's resources, weaknesses, and potential prob-

Opportunities to learn and teach

Frequent family contacts

lems, (2) offer preventive counsel and practical health education, and (3) establish a working relationship. They give the family doctor an advantage over physicians who separate their practice on the basis of age, sex, or problem.

> We recently observed a pediatrician seeing a child who presented with behavior problems and hyperactivity. The pediatrician, an expert in the field, got every available bit of information from the mother (a single parent) and the child about the child's behavior, then contacted community resources and the educational system to determine how the child was perceived. The doctor gave the mother excellent advice on how she should relate to the school system. An excellent management plan? Not once during the interview did the pediatrician indicate to the mother that he understood that it might be difficult for her to handle the child and her own feelings about the child. As a result of the consultation, the child may have become better behaved and more controlled, particularly at school, perhaps with the help of medication, but an opportunity to get at a major source of the problem—the mother's inadequacies, both perceived and real—was missed.

Caring for those without families

Although we have emphasized the family as a unit of care, we do not wish to imply that this should prevent a family doctor from looking after individuals who are single, those who live alone, or those who have other members of their family attending other physicians.

Look for alternatives to family

In fact, approximately one-third of patients who attend family practitioners do *not* have other family members who attend that same practice.[10,11] Some persons have no immediate family alive, others have no family members living in the same area, and still others have family members who attend other doctors. Most family practitioners accept such individual patients.

A lack of family is nevertheless worthy of note, because the family is probably the most important resource available to both patients and professionals. When that resource is absent or fails to respond, the task of those professionals is usually more difficult.

Lack of family makes cure more complex

Even if only two thirds of our patients come to us as members of whole families, are we not better able to understand the other third by recognizing the implications of the fact that they are missing members of their families for whatever reasons? We will probably be more aware that an old widower who has no one to nurse him will require more community resources than one who has a sibling or a child living nearby. Are we not more likely to consider that a young woman at university who becomes acutely ill may be missing her parents, who have until now nursed her through illnesses? Will we not be more likely to pick up the phone to call a colleague who looks after other members of the family to find out whether our patient's sore throat is a strep, or if someone else in the family is depressed, or to ask our colleague to consider seeing both members of a couple together because of the nature of the problem presented? These things are more likely to happen if we continue to focus on the family as a unit of care.

> An amusing example concerns a World War I army veteran who, at the tender age of 78, went to a government clinic for his regular visit. On the way out, he asked the doctor, "By the way, Doc, can I have a bottle of cough medicine for my wife?" "Sorry, Bill, we only look after you. You will have to buy your wife's cough medicine." "But Doc, *I* can't sleep because *her* cough keeps me awake." Wisely, the government physician handed over a bottle of medicine. The family *is* the unit of care.

CONFIDENTIALITY

A family focus does not preclude the confidentiality of the doctor-patient relationship with any one member of the family. If we look on the family as a unit of care, our patients will come to know that that is our perspective. We must facilitate communication within the family, however, in such a way that those matters which are considered confidential remain so. We must not be party to the cloak and dagger games that sometimes tear apart otherwise healthy families.

Maintain confidentiality

WHAT THE FAMILY PHYSICIAN NEEDS TO KNOW ABOUT FAMILIES

Epstein et al.[10] have outlined what they feel are the minimal elements of knowledge and skill which a physician needs in order to deal with families. These include the following:

Minimal knowledge for family physicians

1 An understanding of family structure and function
2 An awareness of how families communicate
3 Skills in observing how families operate
4 The ability to relate to the family as well as to the individual
5 Willingness to reinforce the central function of the family, that is, the provision of a milieu for the social, psychological, and physical development of its members.

In later chapters, we shall continue to consider these elements, stressing what we find most useful in practice.

REFERENCES

1 "Households by Types for Canada and Provinces, 1971," *1971 Census of Canada,* vol II, pt. 1 (Bulletin 2.1–12), Ministry of Supply and Services, Ottawa, 1973.
2 U.S. Bureau of the Census, *Statistical Abstract of the United States: 1978,* 99th ed., Government Printing Office, Washington, D.C., 1978.
3 *The Tricentennial Report: Letters from America,* Atlantic Richfield Company, 1977, p. 78.
4 G. H. Spanier, "The Changing Profile of the American Family," *Journal of Family Practice,* **13**(1):63, 1981.
5 W. T. Merkel, "The Family and Family Medicine: Should This Marriage Be Saved?" *Journal of Family Practice,* **17**(5):857–862, 1983.
6 D. C. Ransom, "On Why It Is Useful to Say That 'The Family Is a Unit of Care' in Family Medicine: Comment on Carmichael's Essay," *Family Systems Medicine,* **1**(1):19, 1983.
7 L. P. Carmichael, "Forty Families—A Search for the Family in Family Medicine," *Family Systems Medicine,* **1**(1):12–15, 1983.
8 I. B. Pless, "The Family as a Resource Unit in Health Care: Changing Patterns," *Social Science and Medicine,* **19**(4):385–389, 1984.
9 E. G. Olsen, "The Impact of Serious Illness on the Family System," *Postgraduate Medicine,* **47** (February 1970).
10 N. B. Epstein, S. Levin, and D. S. Bishop, "The Family as a Social Unit," *Canadian Family Physician,* **22**:1411–1414, 1976.
11 P. G. May and R. Kaelbling, "The Family Doctor as a Current Source of Continual Comprehensive Medical Care," *Ohio State Medical Journal,* **67**:1007–1013, 1971.
12 M. Hill, R. G. McAuley, W. B. Spaulding, and M. Wilson, "Validity of the Term 'Family Doctor': A Limited Study in Hamilton, Ontario," *Canadian Medical Association Journal,* **98**:734–738, 1968.
13 S. Judek, *Canada.* Royal Commission of Health Services Medical Manpower in Canada, Ottawa, 1964.

Chapter 4

The Family Life Cycle and Anticipatory Guidance

B. K. Hennen, M.D.

The normal stages of family development are fraught with stresses. By anticipating such stresses and placing them in perspective, the physician may be able to help patients cope with them before they become dysfunctional.

A useful concept in family medicine is that of the family life cycle. Just as individuals go through a developmental process:

Fetus → newborn → infant → toddler → preschooler → schooler → teenager → young adult → middle age → elderly

Individual life cycle

so do families. The stages of family development can be divided in different ways. One way is as follows:

Courting → marriage → childbearing → child rearing → child launching → empty nest → retirement → death

Family life cycle

This division names each of the stages according to a dominant function. *Courting* is a stage that is of importance as a potential time for preparatory education. *Death* is a stage that emphasizes the necessity of considering the survivors in terms of their loss of the complete family.

Duvall[1] depicts eight stages: married couples (without children), childbearing families (oldest child newborn to 30 months), families with preschool children (oldest child 2½ to 6 years), families with schoolchildren (oldest child 6 to 13 years), families with teenagers (oldest child 13 to 20 years), families as launching centers (first child gone to last child's leaving home), middle-aged parents (empty nest to retirement), and aging family members (retirement to death of both spouses). This classification separates child rearing into three stages and does not include courting and death. The stages are named in terms of structure rather than function.

Time phases in the cycle

Glick has used U.S. census data to document the average length of each stage in the life cycle of the family.[2] Figure 4-1 amalgamates these data into an average developmental profile for an American family. The concept, with its ability to help us anticipate what usually can be expected, is more important than the accuracy or currency of the figures. Changes in the figures over decades, however, may serve to identify trends in families.

To summarize the information presented, the following points about the average North American family are worth noting.

1   Couples are married about 2 years before the first child is born.
2   The average family size is 3.6 (that is, 1.6 children per couple in Canada in 1975).
3   The last child is born about 6 years after the marriage.
4   The first child leaves home within 16 to 18 years after the marriage.
5   The last child leaves home within 18 to 20 years after the marriage.
6   An adult relative moves in within 18 to 24 years after the marriage in about half the homes in the United States.
7   The basic couple is without children at home for the last 14 to 15 years of the marriage.

Individual and family life cycles

The normal course of a family's development takes its members through a cycle of events which, within a particular society, has some degree of predictability. Most families go through this cycle, which may include courtship, marriage, the birth of each child, the schooling of each child, the final leaving of home by each child, the retirement of either or both wage earners, and ultimately the death of one of the original partners. At the same time, each person within the family is going through an individual cycle of events that is also somewhat predictable.

The family doctor who "knows the family" can quickly place

Figure 4-1 Family life cycle.

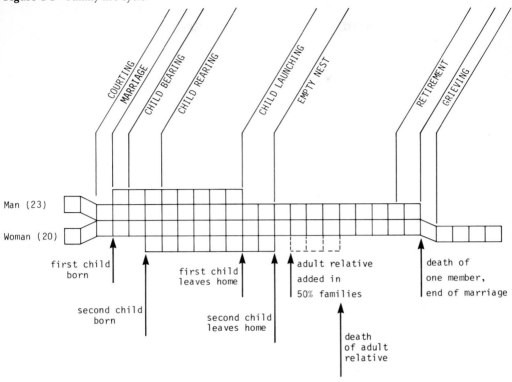

the patients in terms of individual and family developmental stages. In addition, the physician may be aware of some of the external life events affecting the family and, through a few searching queries, may identify others.

In the area of study of external life events, we are indebted to Holmes and Rahe[3] who have developed a system that gives a numerical score to particular life changes as they occur. The score depends on the impact of the changes on the individual. The theory is that when the impact of an event or sum of events passes a certain threshold, stress that is sufficient to impair function may result. In one study stressful life change was found to be an independent predictor of physical illness, whereas developmental stress was not.[4]

The most stressful life-change event according to Holmes is the death of one's spouse, which he scores as 100. Even happy or positive events can be stressful, such as marriage, which is scored as 50,

Holmes's life-change events

Table 4-1 Anticipatory Guidance Checklist

Individual development stage	Family development stage	External life events*
Fetus	Courting	+ + + Death of family member or friend
Newborn	+ + Marriage	
Infant	+ + Childbearing	+ + + Trouble with the law
Toddler	+ + Child rearing	+ + + Divorce
Preschooler	+ + Child launching	+ + + Marital separation
School-ager	+ + Empty nest	+ + Illness
Teenager	+ + Retirement	+ + Job problem or change
Young adult	+ + + Death	+ + Debt
Middle age		+ + Sex difficulties
Elderly		+ + New relative in house
		+ + Change in frequency of arguments
		+ + In-law problems
		+ + Outstanding achievement
		+ Change of residence
		+ Change in social, church, or recreational activities
		+ Change in sleeping or eating habits
		+ Holidays

*See Holmes et al.[3]
Note: + + + = severe stress, + + = moderate stress, + mild stress.

or vacation, which is scored as 13. In our table, in which a life-change event scored by Holmes is included, we have rated scores of above 60 as + + +, scores from 20 to 60 as + +, and scores from 0 to 19 as + (Table 4-1).

At the very least, by alerting patients to events that are known to have some likelihood of occurring, the physician may make them aware of problems they may not have anticipated. The offer to help in solving these problems is implied by the interest shown. A simple comment by the family doctor or the investment of a few moments during a visit initiated by a specific problem may pay significant dividends. A warning is, however, in order. The doctor must use discretion in timing such interventions. The presenting problem should be dealt with first. A woman who is worried about the significance of rectal bleeding will not appreciate an inquiry about her last son having gone off to school until she is reassured that she doesn't have cancer; a man with the fever and chills of influenza will not feel like talking about his new job.

By considering the place of the individual in his or her development and in family development and by checking out significant external life events (Table 4-1), the family doctor can anticipate normal problems. When appropriate, the physician can tell the patient what he or she perceives and perhaps offer preventive guidance.

Anticipating problems can become part of every office visit. This requires little expenditure of time and offers considerable potential for preventive counseling. For example, a family doctor, who has the license to prescribe contraceptives, generally knows when sexual activity begins for a couple and when or whether marriage is planned. The physician is then in a position to alert the couple (or at least one member of the couple) not only about the use and side effects of the medication but also about the likelihood of common relationship problems.

Preventive potential

> Two young people about to marry may never have jointly discussed their expectations of each other. I recall two couples who postponed marriage plans subsequent to a premarital counseling session. In one case, the young man had not planned on his wife's working independently outside the home to the extent that the woman had intended. In the other case, the woman's admission that she didn't really want to change her church made both partners reconsider the importance of religion to them in their forthcoming marriage.

The concept of anticipatory guidance has been established in child care practices,[5] a common example being that mothers are warned to lock up poisonous materials and medicines before their babies become toddlers. However, the concept can be applied to a family even though the presenting person may not be the one who is directly or solely at risk.[6]

Anticipatory guidance not new

> Seeing the wife of a recently promoted executive husband, the physician might ask, "Have you (has he) considered how his traveling might separate him more from you and the children?"

Anticipatory guidance can be seen as an attempt to prevent a problem before it is possible to detect its presence, as opposed to screening and early detection, which depend on the existence of evidence of the "illness."

Definition

The example in Table 4-2 shows how the anticipatory stage precedes the screening stage.

Often the physician gets no apparent reward from anticipating problems for patients. It is sometimes difficult to prove even to

Table 4-2   Stages of Problem Recognition

Anticipatory stage	Screening stage	Symptomatic stage
Things are right for problem to happen, given individual and family development stages.	Problem is happening but is not yet apparent.	Problem is evident.
Man in late forties ponders a late career change; wife is having hot flashes and feels she's lost her figure; oldest child is due to enter university away from home.	Man feels unfulfilled but can't risk job change; happens upon attractive and sympathetic receptionist at work; wife drinks alone in afternoon watching soap operas; child is doing well at university.	Man has affair; wife takes overdose.

one's own satisfaction that teaching patients to anticipate health risks makes any difference in outcomes. Nevertheless, I would like to offer a few examples of one-line openers that can be considered anticipatory in nature.

Examples of anticipatory guidance

For the late prenatal visits of a woman carrying her second baby: "How do you think the baby will be received by his older sister?"

For the mother of a child starting school: "How do you feel about Susie going off to school?"

For an adolescent: "Do you find your parents understand how you feel?"

For a middle-aged mother whose youngest child is about to leave home: "What plans do you and your husband have to fill the space left by Mary moving out to work?"

For a new widow: "Why don't we make an appointment for you to drop in next week?"

For a 64-year-old man: "Do you and your wife have any plans for retirement?" The doctor might explore the retirement plans, the adequacy of a pension, and the degree to which the husband's and wife's plans are in agreement. It may turn out that the wife has hopes for travel and a new home that are not in keeping with her husband's or that are beyond their financial means. With a year to go before retirement, there is time to arrange counseling and initiate a dialogue that may prevent an unhappy outcome.

These are simple examples of how the family physician can anticipate problems and explore areas of concern with the patient before deciding whether the potential problem deserves intervention.

In most cases, the family physician deals with one individual in the office. By assessing that individual not only in the context of personal development but also in the context of family structure, function, and state of development, the physician can anticipate potential problems.

REFERENCES

1 E. M. Duvall, *Family Development,* 4th ed., Lippincott, Philadelphia, 1967.
2 P. Glick, "The Life Cycle of the Family," *Marriage and Family Living,* **17:**3–9, 1955.
3 T. H. Holmes and R. H. Rahe, "The Social Readjustment Scale," *Journal of Psychosomatic Research,* **11:**213–218, 1967.
4 A. D. Blotcky and B. I. Tittler, "Psychosocial Predictors of Physical Illness: Toward a Holistic Model of Health," *Preventive Medicine,* **11:**602–611, 1982.
5 *American Academy of Pediatrics, Standards of Child Health Care,* 2d ed., American Academy of Pediatrics, Evanston, Ill., 1972.
6 K. F. Pridham, M. F. Hansen, and M. Conrad, "Anticipatory Care as Problem Solving in Family Medicine and Nursing," *Journal of Family Practice,* **4:**1077–1081, 1977.

Chapter 5

Illness Behavior

B. K. Hennen, M.D.

To understand how a patient decides that he or she has a problem that warrants the doctor's attentions is to set the stage for the most appropriate management, often before a specific diagnosis is made. Why did the patient come with that problem today? should be asked of themselves by all physicians in regard to each and every patient.

Self-care is common

Although many professional health services are available, people in Western society continue to look after many of their illnesses by themselves, within their own families, and without consulting a doctor. White showed that in the United States in 1961, one-third of the illnesses occurring during 1 month were presented to a doctor.[1] The Canadian Royal Commission on Health showed that on any given day in Canada 15 of every 140 persons who saw themselves as being ill took their problems to a doctor.[2] It seems that the majority of people who see themselves as ill look after their own health problems.

The challenge

One of the challenges of primary care is to see that persons who would benefit from medical services get those services while people who have sicknesses that they can look after by themselves learn how to do so appropriately.

Table 5-1 Stages in the Career of the Patient

1 Some *discontinuity* is perceived in usual function.
↓
2 The discontinuity is perceived as *illness*.
↓
3 Some form of *self-care* is attempted.
↓
4 Family serves as the first-line *external resource*.
↓
5 Other *external nonprofessional resources* are tried.
↓
6 *Professional, nonmedical resources* are consulted.
↓
7 *Physician* is consulted.*
↓
8 *Diagnostic assessment.*
↓
9 *Management plan.*
↓
10 *Cure or chronic illness or death.*

*The crucial decision to go to the doctor is based on factors which McWhinney[5] has categorized.

Before we can meet this challenge, we must understand better what steps people go through when identifying and managing an illness and what factors they consider when deciding that they should take their problems to the doctor.

Understanding why patients see doctors

The career of the patient (the steps through which the person developing an illness becomes a "patient") has been analyzed sociologically.[3,4] The rate at which a person progresses from stage to stage depends on the nature of the illness, the type of person, the familial and community context, the availability of resources, etc. Generally there are 10 stages, as shown in Table 5-1.

Stages in becoming ill

Most health problems experienced by the individual (about 80 percent) are resolved before they get to the seventh stage, which usually occurs in the doctor's office or the hospital emergency room.

Twenty percent of illnesses get to a doctor

What makes people decide to seek the doctor's advice has been discussed by McWhinney in his classic paper "Beyond Diagnosis,"[5] in which he describes seven categories of patient behavior. These can be combined into two main groups: problems and nonproblems. The problems may present directly or indirectly. *Direct problems* are those which the patient offers without apology or camouflage. *Indirect problems* are those which the patient covers up in some way to make them more acceptable to the doctor or those which are discovered when the patient has come for another reason. McWhinney's seven categories are as follows.

Why people go to the doctor

1 *Limit of tolerance:* The symptoms are causing pain, discomfort, or disability that has become intolerable (a problem presented directly).

2 *Limit of anxiety:* The patient visits the physician not because the symptoms are causing distress but because of their implications (a problem presented directly).

3 *Signal behavior:* The presenting illness or symptom is used as a ticket of admission to the doctor so that some underlying problem can be presented (a problem presented indirectly).

4 *Administrative:* The sole purpose of the visit is administrative, for example, to obtain a certificate of illness for an employer (a nonproblem).

5 *Opportunity:* The patient mentions a symptom solely because the opportunity has arisen; for example, a mother bringing her baby for a well-baby check mentions a symptom of her own (problem presented directly).

6 *No illness:* Visits are for preventive purposes, such as antenatal or well-baby care (a nonproblem).

7 *Lanthanic:* The doctor discovers a condition of which the patient is unaware (a problem presented indirectly).

Determine why the patient came

If we consider both the stages in a person's illness and the reasons why that person has chosen to visit the doctor, we will have a better understanding of the patient and the apparent severity of the illness (as the patient sees it). We will also have a better base on which to plan management.

An example

An example of how such information may be helpful can be seen in the case of a 38-year-old housewife and mother presenting with chest pain. Two doctors, A and B, approach the problem differently.

Doctor A: How can I help you?

Patient: I have a pain in my chest.

Doctor A: What kind of pain?

Patient: Oh, I don't know, a sharp pain.

Doctor A: Sharp like a knife?

Patient: Yes.

Doctor A: When do you get it?

Patient: When I reach up to the kitchen cabinet.

Doctor A: How long have you had it?

Patient: Two or three weeks.

Doctor A: How long does it last?

Patient: Just a few moments.

Doctor A: Does it hurt to breathe?

Patient: No.

Doctor A: Any cough?

Patient: No.

Doctor A: Fever?

Patient: No.

Doctor A: Let me examine you. Just take your top off. [Takes temperature.] Show me where. [Inspects part of body indicated. Palpation produced reaction indicating slight tenderness, but percussion and auscultation are clear.] It's nothing serious. We call it costochondritis. It's an inflammation of the cartilage between the breastbone and the ribs. Take two aspirins four times a day and avoid reaching over your head for a week. If it doesn't go away in a week or two, come back to see us. Okay?

Patient: Yes, thank you, Doctor.

Doctor B: How can I help you?

Patient: I have a pain in my chest.

Doctor B: Can you tell me something about the pain?

Patient: Well, it's a jabbing pain, rather sharp. I notice it when I reach up to the kitchen cabinet. It's annoying.

Doctor B: Anything else?

Patient: It lasts only a moment or two. What else can I tell you?

Doctor B: Is it interfering much with your usual activities?

Patient: Not really.

Doctor B: And you have had it for how long?

Patient: Maybe three weeks.

Doctor B: What made you finally decide to come in today?

Patient: Well, my neighbor came in yesterday, and her husband had a coronary a few weeks ago and died and—

Doctor B: That must have made you worry.

Patient: It sure did. Do you think I could have had a heart attack?

Doctor B: Well, your pain certainly doesn't sound like it, but let's examine your heart. Just slip off your top. Do you think you'd have come to see me if your neighbor hadn't dropped in?

Patient: Probably not. The pain seemed to be going away anyway.

In the first instance, although it may have been satisfying to give the patient a label that wasn't "heart," the doctor never really defined the patient's whole problem.

As the interview with Doctor B shows, the key questions to be answered include the following:

Three key
questions

1 What made the patient decide to contact her doctor?
2 What does the patient think is wrong?
3 What does the patient expect of the doctor?

Indirect
presentations
can be
decreased

It has been shown that physicians can decrease the frequency of complex presentations of indirect signals by encouraging frank discussion of psychosocial problems or problems of daily life. Such presentations of indirect signals accounted for as much as 13.9 percent of presentations in a study conducted in our group teaching practice.[6] Doctors who listen to everyday problems make it easier for patients to come quickly and directly to them without having to request unnecessary assessment of very minor symptoms. In the example we have presented, one hopes that when that patient next presents to Doctor B, she will say at once, "When my neighbor had a coronary last week, I thought I'd better get this chest pain I've been having checked out."

REFERENCES

1 K. L. White, F. Williams, and B. Greenberg, "Ecology of Medical Care," *New England Journal of Medicine,* **265:**885–892, 1961.

2 R. Kohn, *The Health of the Canadian People,* Queen's Printer, Ottawa, 1965.

3 I. K. Zola, "Pathways to the Doctor—From Person to Patient," *Social Science of Medicine,* **7:**677–689, 1973.

4 D. Mechanic, *Medical Sociology: A Selective View,* Free Press, New York, 1968.

5 I. R. McWhinney, "Beyond Diagnosis: An Approach to the Integration of Behavioral Science and Clinical Medicine," *New England Journal of Medicine,* **287:**284–287, 1972.

6 M. A. Stewart, I. R. McWhinney, and C. W. Buck, "How Illness Presents: A Study of Patient Behavior," *Journal of Family Practice,* **2:**411–414, 1975.

Chapter 6

The Family and Stress

B. K. Hennen, M.D.

No matter how well the family functions, there will be times in its evolution when it will be called on to deal with threats to its integrity, development, or even survival. These stresses are dealt with in different ways by different families and indeed by different members within the same family.

Individuals who face stress may call upon many resources, some of which are to be found within themselves. For most persons, the second line of resource is provided by the family. Coping with stress depends on being able to counter stress factors with adequate resources; personal, familial, or external. External resources include community services, health professionals, neighbors, and so on. Figure 6-1 illustrates the balance between stresses and resources.

Everyone deals with stress constantly. When the amount of stress experienced exceeds the individual's ability to cope with it, normal function breaks down. The ensuing dysfunction may present in a social, psychological, or physical form, but ill health is a likely consequence. The physician must be aware of the patient's and family's stresses and coping abilities.

Stress and illness

Figure 6-1 Balance relationship of stress and coping mechanisms.

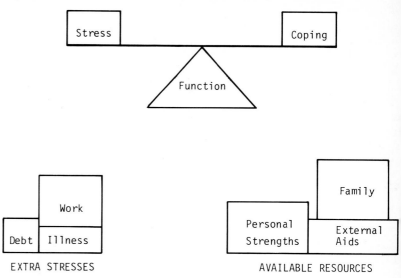

EXTRA STRESSES   AVAILABLE RESOURCES

A 20-year-old woman from another part of the country was attending a local community college. She presented with a peripheral neuropathy, which was considered nutritional because she had been on a faddist vegetarian diet for several months. For the previous 2 weeks, since she was out of money, one can of soup per day had been her sole intake. Local welfare regulations made it difficult to provide emergency funding, but a long-distance call to a sister provided sufficient money to supply a better diet and vitamin supplements, thereby effecting recovery. Longer-range finances come from student loans.

Providing
resources

The girl's resources were insufficient to cope with the stress of illness and poverty. Resources other than her own helped initially to define her problem, establish a medical diagnosis, and begin treatment. The family provided short-term financial aid; the government provided long-term financial aid. This is an example of professional and instrumental resources being provided.

A new mother who is in the hospital is visited regularly by her husband, who assures her that the apartment is not filling up with dirty dishes, that the final touches are completed on the baby's room, and that the bills are paid. Her own mother arrives at the home the day before she and the baby are discharged from hospital, just in time to do the dishes and prepare the apartment. The community health nurse drops in after a few days, just in time to adjudicate the debate between mother and grandmother as to whether the baby should be fed on demand or by schedule. Later the new father's mother offers to baby-sit so that the young parents can go out alone for an evening.

In this example, the resources were sufficient to cope with the stress of having a first child. The extended family offered caring and supportive resources, the nurse provided professional counseling, and the father provided personal support to his wife and received some instrumental help (cleaning up) from his mother-in-law.

If the sister's help had been removed in the first example and that of the two grandmothers in the second, alternative resources would have had to be sought. When alternatives cannot be found, the likelihood of dysfunction increases. When their coping resources are depleted or threatened, families will present in crisis.

Adequate resources

No resources

CRISIS

A crisis can take place when the stresses gradually (over varying periods of time) build up to a point beyond which the individual or family can muster adequate resources. This kind of situation has been referred to as *exhaustive crisis*.

An *acute crisis* occurs when a sudden stress overbalances the immediately available resources, even though further resources might be forthcoming in sufficient time.

Within the family, crises can be classed into four groups:

Exhaustive and acute crises

Four groups of family crises

1 Shifts in status
2 Abandonment
3 Addition
4 Demoralization

Modifying Hill's classification of family crises,[1] Smilkstein has described these four groups.[2] Crises that involve shifts in status include sudden impoverishment, prolonged unemployment, sudden wealth or fame, and political declassing. Crises of abandonment include the death of a child or spouse, a runaway child, and divorce. Crises of addition include unwanted pregnancies, new children by birth or adoption, gain of a stepparent or stepsibling, and the expansion of a household when members of the extended family or friends move in. Crises of demoralization include adultery, alcoholism, drug abuse, and delinquency.

During my teaching practice in 1974, a study by Wilson[3] identified 47 (11.6 percent) of 405 families in the practice as high users of our professional services. (A high-using family made twice the use of our services as the expected average of all practice families, with corrections made for age and sex.) Compared with a control group, the high-using families had the same number of medical problems but had more behavioral problems and twice as many social and economic problems. Altogether the high-using families

Families which use more services have more socioeconomic problems

had 229 problems compared with 153 problems in the control group. Marital problems, alcoholism, and illegitimate pregnancies were predominant in the high-using group.

Balancing stress with resources

Such families are sometimes named "problem families" or "sick families." A more apt name might be "chronically stressed families" or "families of limited resources." If we can identify the stresses and the resources, we can balance function more appropriately by relieving the stress, strengthening the resources, or both.

> A young, unwed, pregnant woman might be pleasantly surprised by the support that would come from her family if she could be encouraged to reach out to them.

> A teenage grandson may be pleased to move in temporarily with his grandparents in order to help his grandmother nurse her husband with pneumonia.

List resources on the record

A good case can be made for recording family problems and risk in more detail than is usually considered necessary. Some practitioners now keep family as well as individual problem lists.[4] A more positive approach would be to also keep *resource lists* for each family. These might be categorized according to Smilkstein's social (S), cultural (C), economic (E), educational (Ed), and medical (M) groups.[2]

> Mr. Watson, who is recently retired and has had a paralytic stroke, lives at home with his wife. Examples of problems and resource lists for Mr. Watson and his family are shown in Table 6-1.

Supplement family resources

If individual and family resources are not sufficient to deal with stress, the physician may suggest that they be supplemented by community resources. Meals-on-Wheels, professional home-makers, Red Cross sickroom supplies, home-visiting physiotherapists, clergy, and stroke clubs are examples of resources that may help the family cope at a reasonable level.

To be a good resource, the family must function adequately. By asking specific questions about function (see Table 2-1), the doctor will quickly find out what family resources are available.

Be specific in identifying strengths

Family physicians themselves are one external professional resource available to families, and as such they have long been facilitating the use of other resources: community health nurses, community services, and medical consultants. The family doctor is often the first professional contact for families in a crises. In the past, physicians depended intuitively on family resources. But if they identified their patients' resources more specifically and made

Table 6-1 Examples of Problem and Resource Lists

Individual problem list	Family problem list	Family resource list
1 Moderate essential hypertension	1 Alcoholic son	1 Mrs. Watson, practical nurse (Ed)
2 Retired	2 Dependent daughter-in-law and grand-children	2 Mr. Watson, resilient sense of humor (S)
3 CVA with residual hemiparesis on right (dominant) side		3 Grandchildren available for errands and chores (S)
		4 Adequate retirement income (E)
		5 Mortgage-free home (E)

others aware of them, the resources could be used to better effect by all those who provide health care to the families involved.

Knowing what resources patients and their families can muster to cope with stress provides the physician with one more element of information, which can be integrated into continuity of care.

REFERENCES

1 R. Hill, "Generic Features of Families under Stress," **39:**139–150, 1958.
2 G. Smilkstein, "The Family in Trouble—How to Tell," *Journal of Family Practice,* **2:**19–24, 1975.
3 J. L. Wilson, "Family Utilization of a Medical Center," *Journal of Family Practice,* **3:**991–996, 1977.
4 N. T. Grace, E. M. Neal, C. E. Wellock, and D. D. Pile, "The Family Oriented Medical Record," *Journal of Family Practice,* **4:**91–98, 1977.

Chapter 7

The Chronically Disabled Child and the Family

B. K. Hennen, M.D.
M. Seitz, Ph.D.
B. Seitz, M.A.

Families that have children with disabilities often need help and support in dealing with the difficulties of diagnosis, management, and treatment. Each chronically disabled child has special characteristics and individual needs, as does each family. The family may be looked at as a potential resource for the child with a chronic disability. An excellent book by Chenn et al.[1] emphasizes the importance of communication with families who have disabled children.

THE ROLE OF PARENTS

Family is a major resource

For a child with any type of chronic handicap, a well-functioning family is generally the most important resource outside of himself or herself. The strong family unit is usually able to meet the challenges presented by a handicapped child. The adaptability, acceptance, and resourcefulness demonstrated by such families never cease to impress professionals who are trained in the field.[2]

Emotional Reactions

Parents suffer many reactions

The parents of a child with a chronic disorder are subject to, and are the subject of, mixed reactions. The feelings parents express in many different ways include confusion, anger, guilt, rejection, denial, and even anticipatory mourning when death or a major physical loss is anticipated. Their resentment may stem from loss of time or money or from the social embarrassment of having brought a defective infant into the world. High-risk situations exist when parents have had interpersonal problems prior to the identification of the child's problem or when the preexisting child-parent relationships have been strained.

Ambivalence

One of the most common expressions of the confusion felt by parents of children with chronic disorders is the tremendous ambivalence they show about the care of the child and the expectations they have of the health care system and, in particular, of the doctor. On the one hand, they recognize the child's need for special attention and demand that the doctor or nurse take particular interest in the child's disability. On the other hand, their inherent need to consider the child normal obliges the physician to try to treat the child as normal; "these people are, in fact, both normal and abnormal."[3] The physician who is not aware of this ambivalence may misinterpret it as rejection or as an expression of anger which he or she cannot explain.

Social Problems

Many social impairments are suffered by the parents of handicapped children. To begin with, they have difficulty getting babysitters. Even grandparents, aunts, and uncles generally cannot cope with the actual or potential problems. Consequently, parents may develop a pattern of entertaining at home, requiring their friends to visit them and reciprocating less frequently.[4] In addition, only the most accepting friends or family members will be able to provide a relaxed and "childproofed" environment in which the handicapped child and his or her family can be comfortable.

Baby-sitting

Entertaining

Visiting

For youngsters who require wheelchairs, crutches, or prosthetic devices and for those who are blind or deaf, transportation both inside and outside the home is a major problem. Special considerations have to be taken in planning family moves to ascertain whether the new community has the necessary medical, educational, and social resources. Often the child's special needs are the prime determinant in the parents' decision to move to a different community.

Transportation

Moving

Financial Consequences

The financial consequences of having a chronically disabled youngster can be devastating even when health insurance is readily available. Proud and independent parents sometimes suffer considerable financial loss because they believe that seeking out available community resources is tantamount to asking for a handout.

Extra costs

Other parents are simply ignorant of existing financial and community resources and thereby miss out on the help that is available. A wheelchair ramp, a nebulizer or mist tent, a special school, taxis, special camping arrangements, and travel to special clinics are examples of additional financial burdens that families may have to bear.

Protection versus Independence

Overprotectiveness

The difficult balance between providing protection and guidance for the child and encouraging the child to be independent has to be constantly reviewed. The physician is often either the most appropriate person or the only person able to counsel the family members, redirect their thinking, and seek out any new evaluations required. For example, for parents with a paraplegic child to contemplate the youngster's ever doing something as simple as going to the store, there has to be participation, preparation, and support. The isolation the family offers may protect handicapped children from the ugly world, but when such youngsters finally feel ready to go out on their own, they may be unable to cope with the outside world. Moreover, the constant stress of dealing with the child's feelings and the fatigue resulting from the extra physical work can result in illness in the parents. In one case, the parents of a child with meningomyelocele both suffered severely (the mother from migraine, the father from neurodermatitis) until their daughter was 13 or 14 years old, when she started to show them that she had the potential to live independently and probably would not be their problem forever.

Fatigue

Favoritism

A parent may overindulge and center attention on a handicapped child to the exclusion of all other family members, including the spouse. Parental guilt often leads to overcompensation and results in attempts to make up for the imposed problems. Guilt often extends to siblings, who are made to feel responsible in part for the problems the disabled sibling suffers.

Guilt

Initiative and Aggressiveness

Creativity

As in any family, the ability of the parents of a disabled child to improvise and to be creative is a great asset. For example, one family with a paraplegic child was able to take her camping in spite of the fact that her wheelchair would not fit into the trailer. They acquired an old stenographic chair on rollers that fitted comfortably into the main part of the trailer and allowed the youngster to be quite mobile.

Aggressiveness

A degree of aggressiveness on the part of the parents may also be an asset, especially in communities in which the resources are either inadequate or poorly organized. In a small community, an aggressive parent may be able to put pressure on a school board which is reluctant to accept specifically handicapped children into the classroom or may persuade the school board to hire special education experts. Such parents have an advantage over those who passively accept the status quo. In one case, the parents were more successful in dealing with the problems of their own disabled children after having tackled similar problems at the community level.

Shopping for Doctors

Parents who have not accepted the truth about a child or those who have not received accurate information about a youngster's disability or its management and are not satisfied with their doctor often go from doctor to doctor. They may be looking for a more acceptable diagnosis, a better management plan, or a specific treatment or cure. This process can be extremely costly. Doctors who have become aware that a family has left them may still have a responsibility to point out either to the family or to the subsequent physician that this constant shopping can constitute a problem in itself.

Shopping can be expensive

Condemning shopping does not, however, suggest that parents who are dissatisfied with a physician should not make a change. If the parents feel that the doctor has not adequately accepted their child and the problem, the doctor will be of limited use to them, and a change will be in order.

Changing doctors may be necessary

Some dissatisfied parents may not seek other opinions. This may occur because of their loyalty to the doctor on the basis of previous services, because they have no real alternative in a small community, or because of traditional acceptance of the doctor's authority, among other reasons.

In view of the special needs—for education, travel, recreation, or treatment—of most affected children and their families, the greatest challenge for all concerned is to meet the demands of day-to-day living: the caring and sharing, the eating and sleeping, the washing and dressing, the talking and listening.

Ordinary living is difficult

THE SIBLINGS

Siblings of handicapped children often become yardsticks for measuring the child's development. The authors have seen several instances in which the parents did not accept the fact that a child was disabled or significantly affected until a younger sibling passed the affected child in particular developmental milestones.

Parents deny

Siblings of the affected child are apt to show jealousy because of the attention the affected sibling gets and may constantly question the love of their parents, acutely aware of the fact that the parents have less time for them. If siblings do manifest jealousy or

Jealousy

resentment, the family as a whole, not just the affected child, may have a pervasive problem. The basis of the difficulty may not be the disabled member, even though he or she becomes the scapegoat. The fault may lie in the family constellation and its lack of general problem-solving and coping abilities. Siblings who feel neglected or left out may show their feelings through demanding and aggressive behavior that is often directed at the affected child or at one or both of the parents. In the prepubertal years, siblings sometimes feel guilt and depression for reasons that are not obvious. They may feel responsible for the condition of the affected sibling and may sometimes find themselves wishing that the affected child would go away.

The disabled child may help   In such cases, the physician should keep in mind the norms of sibling relationships, which may still apply when one child has a chronic disability. A child confined to a wheelchair may still be able to fulfill his or her role as the older sibling in terms of providing advice, support, and a steadying influence for younger brothers and sisters.

PERSONAL RESOURCES OF THE AFFECTED CHILD

The affected individual's personal resources, personality, and basic attitudes, along with the way in which he or she interrelates with the other resources available, will ultimately be the determinant of success or failure in coping with the disorder. For a child with an acquired disorder, a premorbid deficient personality and established poor attitudes will have a negative effect on the response to the condition.

Premorbid personality   The behavior of a child with an acquired disorder may be predicted from the child's basic personality and development prior to the illness or event leading to the disability. A child who has always had difficulty separating from the parents (for example, staying with baby-sitters or going off to school) is more likely to have difficulty adjusting to hospitalization for an acquired disorder. A child who has demonstrated a phobic response to anxiety in the past may show inordinate fears of even minor procedures such as blood taking or even some aspects of a physical examination. A child who was very active before a disability may have great difficulty if immobilization is required. A child who resented or feared authority before the injury or illness may have great difficulty relating to doctors and nurses. A shy and withdrawn child may demonstrate unusual or excessive self-consciousness in the examination room.

Generally, what would be perceived by most people as negative characteristics in personality and attitude may be greatly exaggerated when compounded by a disability acquired during childhood.

In the case of an acquired disability, it is important to understand clearly the family situation at the time the disability occurred. A child already excessively jealous of a new sibling will be more likely to associate the disabling illness with the sibling.

A child with an acquired disorder can be expected to grieve over the loss of function or loss of body part in much the same manner as one experiences the loss of a loved one; reactions may include denial, questioning, anger, depression, and ultimate acceptance. Even children born with a disorder may go through these stages once they realize the degree to which they are different from most other children. As in the grieving process, however, not all children will go through all the stages, nor will the stages be experienced in any particular order.

Grief and loss

The personality, attitudes, and ultimate behavior of a child who has had a disability since birth will be an integral part of the disorder, affected by the way in which the family and society have reacted to it.

Each youngster's personality is unique. Also, the problem is unique, the family is unique, and the community is unique. A child who has acquired a disfiguring burn obviously has different problems than a child who has a hearing loss without physical deformity. A child raised in an atmosphere of approval will respond differently than one hidden in isolation and shame by parents. A child raised in a community that accepts such disabilities as "God's will" or an act of fate may expect less community support than a child raised in an aggressive and resourceful community that is frequently changing to adjust to new ideas.

The community setting

A disabled child still goes through most normal developmental changes. Drawings often reflect vividly how growing children see themselves. The use of a simple "draw-a-person" exercise can be very revealing.[5]

Youngsters age 10 to 15 seem to be particularly vulnerable. This is a time of self-awareness, awareness of interpersonal relationships and relationships with the opposite sex, and awareness of one's own body image. It can be a time of extreme frustration for an affected child who realizes how different he or she is from peers and what different potentials each may have.

Age 10 to 15 especially difficult

Sometimes the disordered youngster will demonstrate exaggerated responses to normal stresses. A child with cerebral palsy who develops to normal size, learns self-care, and has warm interpersonal relationships with family members may, at the expected times for normal children, become unusually frustrated with the social problem of language and the inability to make others understand. A frustrated child who can't keep up may regress to childlike behaviors or may associate with younger children. A child who is overindulged because of a handicap may become increasingly de-

Many behavioral responses

pendent. The parents may in turn respond to guilt feelings with overindulgence, creating an interdependence of parent and child that is detrimental to both. Older children, recognizing their dependence, may seek to break out on their own at inappropriate times and times of unreadiness. A child frustrated by repeated failure to manage the problem may end up feeling that nothing will work and may refuse to try new modes of therapy.

A moderate degree of self-assertion and opposition to authority (especially toward treatment methods) will be found in most youngsters struggling with a handicap, as is seen in normal children. It is not unusual, however, for a child with a minimal handicap to have greater difficulty coping with it than a youngster who has a readily apparent, obvious disability. This is probably the case because the expectations for the obviously disabled are more reasonable and less demanding.

Contacts with the health care system

The problems facing the individual with a chronic disorder include struggles against constantly being perceived as one who is always "sick" and has to be helped. It is probably impossible to get used to being stared at, and it is tiresome to have to constantly explain one's inability to participate in normal activities. The necessary contacts with many different professionals and the resulting complex ties with the health care system constitute a special problem for a chronically disordered youngster. Few people with chronic disorders can be expected to be completely satisfied with the care they receive, and both they and the professionals who are trying to help them must from time to time assess their progress objectively.

Generally speaking, children who cope successfully with a chronic disorder are more likely to possess the following characteristics.

1 They view the disability as a dynamic problem, not a static one; that is, they accept the fact that the disability is subject to change.

2 They ultimately learn to deal with being different from others but not necessarily "sick."

3 They work cooperatively with health professionals as co-therapists or co-planners of their management.

4 They make the most of their abilities and the best of their disabilities.

5 They are capable of sharing experiences with others who are similarly handicapped and in return are able to make use of the experiences of others.

6 They can regard frustration as positive evidence of active struggling against the problem.

7 They show a readily apparent and admirable enthusiasm for coping with life ("psychic energy").

8 They generally have a good sense of humor.

If the child is able to assess his or her limitations, strengths, and resources accurately and can emotionally accept the disorder, he or she is likely to develop a realistic approach to life and cope optimally with the disability.

PROFESSIONAL ATTITUDES

One doctor observed unnatural and aggressive behavior in a 15-year-old boy he had delivered. When the doctor learned that a psychiatrist was considering the possibility of an organic component in the etiology of the behavior, he was struck by confusion and guilt and sought out the old delivery records to see whether in fact the delivery had been as unremarkable as he remembered. Doctors, too, are subject to feelings of guilt toward patients for whose problems they feel they may have been responsible or whose problems they cannot solve.

Doctors also suffer guilt

The physician who forgets to consider the normal developmental progression of a chronically disordered youngster is as negligent as one who fails to recognize the disorder in the first place. I recall asking a resident physician whether the blind young woman she had just seen was on the birth control pill. Shocked at her sudden awareness of what she had done, she said, "I didn't ask her. I assumed because she was blind that she wasn't having sex."

Don't neglect the normal aspects

Professionals must clearly understand their own attitudes about patients and the problems they present. Only thus can the doctor be in a reasonable position to deal honestly and usefully with patients. Nowhere is this more obvious than in dealing with chronically handicapped patients (Table 7-1).

Know your feelings

We can promote better attitudes in the general public by striving for greater acceptance of handicapped children and their increased participation in normal activities. We can get ourselves and other members of our community to stop avoiding children in wheelchairs, with crutches, with abnormal spastic gaits, with canes,

Set an example

Table 7-1   Checklist for the Professional Who Deals with a Child with a Chronic Handicap

1   Am I clear how I feel about this youngster?
2   How does the child perceive the problem?
3   Are the parents' attitudes and expectations realistic?
4   Have we made full use of the child's strengths?
5   Have we dealt as well as possible with the handicaps?
6   Have the family's resources been well used?
7   Has attention been paid to the needs of all family members?
8   Are the appropriate community resources being used?
9   Is there a clear plan of management for the child and family over both the short term and the long term?

with peculiar speech defects, children who use sign language, and children who have visible hearing aids. We can use our professional influence to support better community and educational facilities for these children. This will make it easier for the handicapped to develop at their own speed and eventually to participate in society to the limits of their abilities. As one chronically handicapped girl said, "All people are handicapped. In some of us it doesn't show."

REFERENCES

1 P. C. Chenn, J. Winn, and R. H. Walters, *Two-Way Talking with Parents of Special Children: A Process of Positive Communication,* C. V. Mosby, St. Louis, 1978.
2 F. Bishop, "The Effects of Chronic Childhood Illness on the Family," *Australian Family Physician,* **3:**76–78, 1974.
3 M. A. Murphy, "The Family with a Handicapped Child: Review of the Literature," *Developmental and Behavioral Pediatrics,* **3**(2):73–82, 1982.
4 "Life with a Brain Damaged Child," *The New York Times,* March 23, 1973.
5 F. L. Goodenough and D. B. Harris, *Goodenough-Harris Drawing Test,* Harcourt Brace Jovanovich, New York, 1963.

Chapter 8

Child Abuse and the Family

G. MacDougall, M.S.W.

With the introduction of the term battered child syndrome *by Kempe[1] in the early 1960s, a new era of public and professional awareness of the physical abuse of children began. The 1970s brought a recognition of the widespread practice of "wife battering," and in the 1980s there has been an increasing awareness of the existence of child sexual abuse and the incidence of incest.*

It can be said that the prevalence of family violence is a reflection of a society which has become more violent and more tolerant of violent acts within the community and in the media. Amid the changing values and mobility of contemporary society, the family has undergone significant structural change during the past 80 years. The extended family with its many "built-in" supports has become the smaller nuclear family which has adapted to the demands of a highly mobile and technological society. The nuclear family, cut off from its traditional supports, is more isolated both socially and emotionally. The result is a family unit made more vulnerable by the stresses generated by contemporary life.

INTRODUCTION

A systems approach to the family recognizes not only that each family is a collection of individual relationships but also that the unit as a whole has characteristics which transcend the individual

Family dysfunction

relationships. Viewed within this context, any change in an individual, whether through illness, injury, or an external factor such as unemployment, is reflected throughout the family system. What in one view can be seen as an individual problem is more appropriately seen as a family problem. Within this framework, the abused child or the perpetrator of violence is not an "isolated problem." The existence of such individuals reflects the fact that the family system has become severely dysfunctional. The abuse situation, then, is more accurately assessed and treated within the family system where possible.

Situations involving child abuse of any type are difficult to identify, assess, and treat. These situations are both personally and professionally demanding, and for that reason family physicians and other health professionals have found it difficult to voice their concerns to parents and to refer families to appropriate child welfare agencies for assessment and treatment. Abuse situations require a multidisciplinary approach and can present complex management problems. However, child abuse is a serious situation, and the danger to the life and well-being of children is very real. As Paradis points out, abuse "has been shown to recur in approximately fifty percent of cases when intervention is not instituted and, in thirty-five percent of these, a child will be severely injured or killed."[2]

Life-threatening

Value judgment

One of the difficulties in assessing the presence of child abuse is the distinction between physical punishment and physical abuse. Personal standards and values may play a role in such a situation. For example, a physician who uses a physical punishment such as spanking in his or her own family may not be as concerned when a parent indicates that he or she used physical discipline as a physician who does not use such methods within the family. The rule of thumb is that any injury that requires medical treatment has gone beyond the limits of appropriate discipline and should be considered a potential abuse situation.

DEFINITION

The issue of the definition of child abuse is important. There are many definitions of child abuse, but the following descriptions are consistent with the literature. Child abuse is generally broken down into three types.

Physical abuse

1 *Physical abuse*: "acts of commission or omission on the part of the parent or custodian of a child which results in injury to a child. This includes, but is not necessarily restricted to, physical beating, parental deprivation, a cutting, burning, or physical assault, and failure to provide reasonable protection for the child from physical harm."[3]

2 *Emotional abuse*: "conveys the idea of 'mental injury' resulting from psychologically aggressive action. This includes overt rejection and repeated belittling of a child, open 'disowning' of the child, unreasonable demands for competence and repeated threatening or frightening responses to the child's failure to meet such demands, including close confinement which may cause serious emotional injury, combined with a cold withholding of comfort from an upset or distraught child. . . . When a child's future psychological development is at risk because of a caretaker's actions or failure to act, that is child abuse."[4]

3 *Sexual abuse*: "sexual conduct on the part of a parent or custodian towards a child which can range from rape, intercourse, oral-genital contact, masturbation, fondling and nudity."[3]

Emotional abuse

Sexual abuse

EXTENT

The extent of child abuse in North American society is just beginning to be understood. Child abuse has been underreported because of the nature of the problem and because of confusion arising from the use of differing definitions and diagnostic criteria to determine the presence of physical, emotional, or sexual abuse. Thus, the extent of the problem is generally acknowledged to be greater than has been reported. In areas where public awareness campaigns have been staged, there has been an increase in the number of abuse situations reported to child welfare authorities.

Underreported prevalence

It is estimated that 2 million children in the United States are abused each year, among whom 2000 to 5000 die. For children 1 to 5 years of age, death from violence is second to death from accidental causes.[5]

In 1980, Canadian estimates indicated that 3 in every 1000 children under the age of 16 known to provincial government child welfare agencies were suspected of having been victims of sexual abuse. In 1977, child sexual abuse was listed separately, and 300 children were identified. In 1980, 1593 cases of sexual abuse were reported, for an increase of 431 percent in reported cases over 3 years. This can probably be attributed to increased professional and public awareness, improved reporting mechanisms, and the establishment of services for sexually abused children.[6]

With increasing numbers of cases of physical and sexual abuse of children, the role of the primary-care physician has become an important one. It is to the family physician that the parents may bring a child with injuries that appear to be of a suspicious nature.

Table 8-1   Child Abuse Alert Checklist

Parent

1   Expresses fear of or shows evidence of losing control.
2   Shows detachment from the child.
3   Gives indication of abuse of alcohol or drugs.
4   States that child is "always injuring self."
5   Complains that there is no one to "bail him or her out" when "uptight" with child.
6   Is reluctant to answer questions, is defensive, and becomes angry with questions.
7   Indicates that he or she was raised in a "motherless," harsh way.
8   Shows unrealistic expectations of the baby or child, indicating lack of knowledge of normal development.
9   Shows a marked lack of concern for child's welfare and little or no remorse.
10 Treats siblings differently, with obvious preferences and dislike for one child.
11 Appears to be under considerable stress but does not seek help. Seems sad.

Child

1   Has an injury or marks which are unexplained or inadequately explained.
2   Has received no apparent medical attention for an injury.
3   Shows evidence of repeated injury.
4   Is unusually fearful of adults, perhaps of one sex more than the other.
5   If a baby, shows a "frozen watchfulness" with adults; shows a failure to thrive.
6   Shows unusual apprehension when an adult approaches while the child is crying.
7   Is frequently overtired and/or inappropriately dressed for the weather.
8   Is unusually aggressive, disruptive, or nervous.
9   Arrives early at school, leaves late, and indicates that the parent(s) won't care about absence.
10 Has difficulty in sitting, has genital-area discomfort, shows resistance to being touched at all by an adult.
11 Craves attention and affection but is easily hurt and mistrustful.

INDICATIONS

In all types of child abuse, there are indicators which may help the physician detect abuse situations[4] (see Table 8-1).

Hidden clues

A list such as the one provided in Table 8-1 serves to underscore the possible meaning of certain responses in a parent or child. Part of the difficulty for the primary care physician lies in the fact that such problems present in a fragmented way as they are developing so that the total meaning of the problem is not always apparent. Attention to these signs and an open-mindedness to the possibility of some form of abuse, even in families well known to the physician, may enable an early intervention before the situation becomes extremely dangerous to a child.

Physical abuse indicators such as the presence of old injuries, a child who has frequent injuries, and parents who are evasive in their explanation of the cause of injuries and/or who give inappropriate explanations may be important signs of child abuse. A parent who has unrealistic expectations of his or her child may be giving very harsh punishment for failure to measure up. An example of this is the parent who spanks a 13-month-old child for not being toilet-trained.

Unexplained trauma

Emotional Neglect

Emotional neglect is more difficult to detect. The family physician who provides continuous care may be in a position to observe a child who is not developing well. Knowledge of the physical and emotional stages of development will facilitate understanding and detection of a child who is being neglected emotionally. Behavioral changes inconsistent with normal development, such as moodiness, hostility, withdrawal, and antisocial behavior, may be indicative of a child who is suffering from emotional neglect.

Behavior change

Sexual Abuse

When a child indicates that he or she has been sexually abused by a family member or another individual, it is important to follow up on the statement. Children do not lie about sexual abuse and are often under pressure not to disclose such events. Sexually provocative behavior in a young child, a drop-off in school attendance, running away in an adolescent girl, and other altered behavioral patterns may be signs of sexual abuse or incest. The possibility of abuse should be raised in a sensitive fashion, and reports should be made to the appropriate child welfare agency.

ROLE OF THE FAMILY PHYSICIAN

The family physician, with his or her approach to the family as the unit of care, is in a position to assess not only the injury but the child and the parents as well. Identification of the family at risk through knowledge of any past history of violence, incest, and emotional neglect as well as an understanding of the impact of current stresses such as unemployment, alcohol abuse, marital breakdown, divorce, or acquisition of a new stepparent may lead to intervention before the problems increase in number and severity. For example, the intervention of a community health nurse or social worker may strengthen the parents' skills in child management and lead to the use of support services such as day care, with subsequent improved health and child care in the family. Through the

Family assessment

use of these techniques, further deterioration of family functioning may be prevented.

Community agency supports

The use of community resources such as child welfare services, community health nurses, day care, parent education groups, lay support, and counselors can prevent family breakdown. The family physician has a role to play in providing service for families who are in difficulty. The family physician is often the first professional individual or family contact, and this accessibility may lead to early intervention.

In situations where there is concern about child abuse, most physicians prefer to discuss their concerns with the parent(s). It is important to discuss the need to further assess the injuries, possibly through hospital admission. It is also necessary to know the legal requirements for referral of suspected abuse to a child welfare agency for follow-up and treatment of the family. The task is a difficult one for physicians and other professionals; they may find it difficult to acknowledge the fact that young children can be severely abused by the parent or care giver. Physicians also fear that

Approach to family

discussion of their concerns will lead to a severance of the relationship with the family. However, if parents are approached in a positive, nonjudgmental, and supportive fashion, this should not occur. The parent or care giver may well be relieved that the physician has intervened in a pattern of abuse which the family has been unable to break. The family members can then continue the relationship with the physician and by so doing have the support of a trusted family physician as they attempt to deal with the family problems.

When talking to parents or care givers about suspected abuse, it is important to allow them time to express their frustrations and concerns. Supportive statements and open-ended questions may help them describe the problems as they have experienced them. The family physician can offer specific help and support for these children and parents. The goal is to protect the child from further abuse and, for the physician, to initiate the process of assessment and treatment.

Legal Issues

In all cases of suspected abuse, the law in almost every jurisdiction in North America requires anyone who suspects child abuse to report it to the child abuse registry or the local Child Welfare Agency. Failure to do so may result in prosecution. Following notification, the child welfare specialists or the hospital-based child abuse team will begin an assessment process which, in cooperation with medical and sometimes police personnel, will identify the specific problems and the degree of risk to the child and then prepare treatment plans for the family. The goal is to keep the family members together or to reunite them after a placement period for the child. In circumstances where this is not possible, permanent placement of the child may be the only resort.

Hospitalization

In cases of suspected abuse, the family physician may wish to admit the child to the hospital for full medical, psychological, and social evaluation. If the parent(s) are uncooperative, the local Child Welfare Agency can intervene and ensure that the child will receive the required assessment and treatment. In all circumstances, the physician must report all cases of suspected abuse, as the safety of the child is the primary concern.

Child safety

Child Abuse Register

Many provinces and states in North America maintain a child abuse register to provide a vehicle for better reporting of all suspected cases of abuse. Improved reporting provides a basis for better service and more accurate knowledge of the extent of the problem. Information is recorded in the register only after careful evaluation of each situation confirms actual abuse. Individuals whose names are entered in the register are informed of this step and may appeal if they wish. The information in the register is used to help child welfare personnel identify children and families at high risk for abuse.

SUMMARY

The family physician has a key role in the detection of all forms of child abuse: physical, emotional, and sexual. The assessment and treatment of abusive families requires a multidisciplinary approach. However, family physicians can intervene in situations of family distress and work to prevent further problems from developing. The ability to provide families access to community services and resources is very important. In any form of abuse and in cases of suspected abuse, the children are being victimized and cannot "get out" on their own. In many cases, the family physician will be the only person who can intervene in the cycle and initiate steps to protect the child from emotional and physical harm.

Multidisciplinary approach

REFERENCES

1 C. H. Kempe et al., "The Battered Child Syndrome," *Journal of the American Medical Association,* **181**:17, 1962.

2 G. Paradis, "Psychological Problems in Adults: Violence in the Family," in J. C. Seely (ed.), *Working with the Family in Primary Care*, Praeger, New York, 1984, p. 419.

3 A. Taylor (ed.), *Child Abuse Manual*, The Registered Nurses Association of Nova Scotia, 6035 Coburg Road, Halifax, Nova Scotia, 1984.

4 Ontario Association of Professional Social Workers, *Child Abuse: A Handbook for Social Workers in Ontario*, O.A.P.S.W., 185 Bloor Street East, Toronto, Ontario, 1983.

5 M. C. McNeese and J. R. Hebelu, "The Abused Child," *Clinical Symposia*, **31**:4, 1979.

6 R. Badgley et al., *Sexual Offenses against Children: Report of the Committee on Sexual Offences against Children and Youths*, Canadian Government Publishing Centre, Supply and Services Canada, vol 1, 1984.

Chapter 9

Understanding Families

D. Curtis, M.S.W.

Orientation to the family as the unit of care has been discussed in an earlier chapter. This chapter looks at the family with a problem and, using the McMaster model of family dysfunction, provides some practical pointers for family physicians to understand family interactions and their effects on the presentation and management of illness.

Being a family member is a nearly universal experience. Understanding how families function is our common pursuit. Why is it, then, that knowledge of family function is one of the most elusive, difficult tasks that family physicians encounter?

This is in part due to our training as gatherers of detailed factual information and the putting together of this information in a very logical fashion. True understanding of how a family functions seems to lie beyond the facts. It is also necessary to understand the "process" of what goes on in the family, or how the individuals interact together over time. As opposed to the "left brain" logical putting together of data, conceptualization of family function is often thought of as nonlinear, or right-brained, in nature.

To get the facts and keep an eye on the process of what goes on is literally to do two things at once. One method of overcoming this problem is to have two interviewers at a family session, each performing only one of these tasks.

Another problem in understanding families is that they are all too familiar to us. If the brain is thought of as an information-receiving organ, one of its major functions is to screen out information and select what is important. The best example of this would be to point out that you probably do not notice the clothes you are wearing or the chair on which you are sitting. Similarly, if you registered everything that went on within your own family, you would be overwhelmed with information. You habitually tune out most of it, and tuning it back in is not an easy task.

Diagnostic structure

One way of overcoming this unique problem of being both familiar and unfamiliar is to learn a simple, somewhat familiar structure with which to view the family. In the remainder of this chapter, a simple diagrammatic model will be provided that can easily be recalled to assist a doctor in understanding family functioning. The model is in the shape of our main area of interest, the human body.

THE McMASTER MODEL

Functional model

This figure is in fact a simple outline of the McMaster model of family functioning. This model puts forward the idea that every family must perform certain basic tasks: putting food on the table, providing shelter, and nurturing the various family members.

To accomplish this, the family should function relatively well in the following dimensions. They must be able to *problem solve*; one could even regard the family as a problem-solving unit. To problem solve effectively one must *communicate*, get people to do what they should by means of *role* assignment, be emotionally *involved* and care about each other, have the ability to *respond emotionally* to each other, and properly *control* the behavior of the others. If all this is done well and correctly, individual family members will be nurtured both physically and emotionally.

ASSESSING THE FAMILY

Assessing the family involves asking the family members about these various dimensions in order to see how they accomplish their tasks. Part of this takes place while you observe the family members and how they interact, and the other part takes place while you gather facts by asking them about problem solving, etc.

For illustrative purposes, let us assume that you are going to interview the Smith family, consisting of the father (age 33), the mother (age 30), and two children, John (age 6) and Mary (age 2). Just a week ago you saw Mrs. Smith and John together with the complaint that "John isn't doing very well in school." It turned out

Figure 9-1   McMaster Model. Adapted from "The McMaster Model of Family Functioning," Epstein, Bishop and Levin, *Journal of Marriage and Family Counseling*, October, 1978. I.E.C. August 1984.

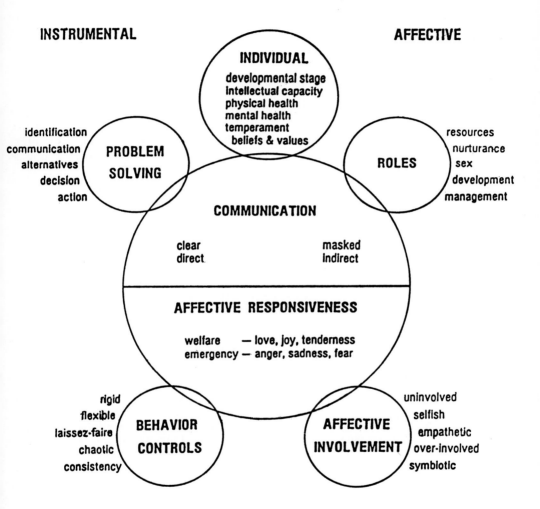

SCHEMATIC REPRESENTATION OF THE
McMASTER MODEL OF FAMILY FUNCTIONING

INSTRUMENTAL   AFFECTIVE

INDIVIDUAL
developmental stage
intellectual capacity
physical health
mental health
temperament
beliefs & values

identification
communication
alternatives
decision
action

**PROBLEM
SOLVING**

ROLES

resources
nurturance
sex
development
management

COMMUNICATION

clear
direct

masked
indirect

AFFECTIVE RESPONSIVENESS

welfare   — love, joy, tenderness
emergency — anger, sadness, fear

rigid
flexible
laissez-faire
chaotic
consistency

**BEHAVIOR
CONTROLS**

**AFFECTIVE
INVOLVEMENT**

uninvolved
selfish
empathetic
over-involved
symbiotic

that the school had requested that Mrs. Smith see her family doctor because John was not doing well academically in grade 1 and had a behavior problem. He had been throwing temper tantrums and on occasion had hit other children. They thought that "something must be wrong."

On that occasion you checked out John, the *individual*, represented on the diagram by the head. Now you quietly discuss things with Mrs. Smith.

Background
data

John's physical exam proved to be normal. He had passed his developmental milestones within the expected parameters and appeared to have an average intellectual capacity. Mrs. Smith informed you that the school psychologist was going to see him concerning this in the near future. Temperamentally speaking, it turns out that John has always been an extremely active youngster, very assertive and quick with his temper. Mrs. Smith, who had a relative who was sensitive to certain foods, asked whether you thought he should be seen concerning that possibility.

SETTING UP THE FIRST FAMILY INTERVIEW

Family process

Families tend to develop certain patterns and habits that they find very difficult to stop. A vital part of any assessment is to recognize these little bits of process, as they are often quite subtle. The interviewer should interfere with this process as little as possible, at least initially, and be a good observer.

The interview begins before they arrive with the arranging of chairs in a semicircle, with your chair obviously placed. This allows the family to pick a seating pattern, usually out of habit, and can give you an idea as to the allegiances within the family.

Initial clues

The interview actually begins in the waiting room as you observe who is doing what, who is sitting with whom, and who is talking with whom. This also gives you some early idea about what people do in this family so that you can ask some questions and cross-check your early impressions at a later point.

Observation proved useful in this case as the waiting room was a buzz of activity with the mother trying to corral two active children. The father, who proved to be very pleasant and amiable and greeted you with a huge smile, had been sitting over to the side reading a *Road and Track* magazine. Some of the statistical data you had gathered at the first interview started to fit at this point. Mr. Smith is a salesman, frequently away from home, and Mrs. Smith had hinted that a lot of the burden of raising the children seemed to fall on her. She is a full-time housewife, without any extended family support, living in a moderate-income apartment in the downtown area. Once in the interview room, the children sit to either side of the mother, while the father takes his chair and separates from the three of them a little, getting a bit closer to you. He then strikes up an animated conversation.

THE INTERVIEW

After appropriately introducing yourself, learning everyone's name, and suggesting to the parents that they assume the management of the children and "just carry on as if you were home," you might begin with the following:

"Before we get going, I would like to make sure we are all here for the same reason. I think I know why you are here, but I just want to make sure that everyone else is here for the reasons I think they are here. You never know; occasionally I find we are here for five different reasons, and I don't discover this until the middle of the interview. So, I would like to ask you why are you here as a family talking to me today. Could I then ask any one of you who wishes to begin."

Explaining the rules

At this point most interviewers will scan the family to indicate that anyone can answer, pick a neutral spot to look at, and wait. If all goes well, the waiting will not be too uncomfortable and eventually someone will speak up. It is important to see who takes the lead, as that person may well be the spokesperson for the family. In some families that are especially uncomfortable, the scapegoat will be pushed forward for the proverbial sacrifice, to ask the first question. If the silence is agonizing, you might remark rather neutrally, keeping in mind not to interfere too much at this point, "Hmm, it seems to be difficult to answer this question." Having received a reply, and possibly clarified it, one might then turn to the other members of the family and ask them, "Well, what do you think of that?" picking a neutral spot and waiting again to see who replies.

Encouraging dialogue

Some interviewers then start to gather statistical data at this point (if they haven't done it before) and watch the interaction while they are obtaining the data. Besides names, one would want to know ages, occupations, grade in school, living place, years of marriage, amount of time lived in any one place, ethnic origin, support groups such as extended family, etc.

During this relatively brief segment you observed that it was the mother who answered your question about why they were here today. She stated that John has a problem. When you were asking what others thought, John replied that he had been a bad boy. Interestingly, the father who previously had been quite talkative, didn't say much at this time.

PROBLEM SOLVING

The strong right arm of any family is its ability to solve problems. A rather simple method of assessing this problem-solving ability while at the same time gathering data is to give the family members a problem about themselves.

"Since we agree we are all here because of John's behavior in school, I would like to pose this problem for you. Why do you think John is having a problem with his behavior in school? I want to mention that

Provide examples

Table 9-1   Seven Stages to the Process

1   Identification of the problem
2   Communication of the problem to the appropriate resource(s)
3   Development of action alternatives
4   Decision on one alternative
5   Action
6   Monitoring what action is taken
7   Evaluation of success

there may be one or many reasons, and I would like to find out what you think about this while at the same time getting an idea as to how you in fact solve problems and look at them."

There are seven basic stages in problem solving (Table 9-1), and it is useful to know how far along a family can go without stalling. They may not be able to articulate these stages but most likely just do it out of habit. However, you should be able to assess the stage they are at.

You were aware that the members of the Smith family are not skilled in terms of solving problems of an emotional nature. John's behavior had in fact been identified by the school, not by the family. While it was apparent to you that John had a behavior problem from observing him in the waiting room, it was not something the parents were prepared to identify as a problem. Nonetheless, the mother led off by vaguely stating that she felt he was nervous in school and was being bullied by the other children. When asked to comment on that, the father said that John could "take care of himself" and went on to say that he really wasn't all that sure there was a problem and that John was just "a normal kid." You got the impression that the mother was being quite protective of him and that the father didn't want to admit there was a problem.

Resisting the temptation to go on and ask them about their seeming differences of opinion concerning the child, you ask if there are any further problems they would like to identify and add to the list you are making. The mother wonders if the teachers are skilled in controlling John. You point out that she is having a lot of trouble controlling him herself and that she had mentioned this in the previous interview. The father chimes in at this point in vigorous agreement, indicating that "with a few good whacks" he would certainly teach him, but his wife won't let him do that.

Significantly, the family doesn't identify John's very immature behavior (in the form of temper tantrums), his extreme activity which the school has complained about, and his aggressiveness toward his little sister. While gathering the statistical data, you learned that there are no financial problems, and this couple seems to be able to handle problem solving of a physical nature, but it obviously has a lot of difficulty in the emotional area. They haven't been able to make it to stage 1. The rest of the interview should reveal to you why they are so poor at problem solving with emotional issues.

COMMUNICATION

Diagrammatically speaking, communication is considered to be the heart of the matter. What is *said* to whom is often just observed by the interviewer rather than questioned and inquired about. It is defined as how the family exchanges information.

A simple method of assessing communication is to decide whether the message is clear and is directed to the proper person.

Clarity of messages

> *Clear and direct:* "Doctor, you make me angry because you think I am away too much." The father is clearly telling you that he is angry at you and exactly why he is angry.
> *Clear and indirect:* "People make me angry when they question me about John." The message is clearly that the mother is angry, and about what, but you are not sure if it is you she is angry at.
> *Masked and direct*: "Doctor, you really tick me off." You know the father is angry at you, but you are not sure of the reason.
> *Masked and indirect*: "Doctors give me a pain in the neck." The mother is obviously upset, but about what and whom is not clear.

Being clear and direct is the most desirable form of communication, while being masked and indirect is the least desirable form. The father appears to be able to communicate much more effectively than the mother, especially when it comes to the expression of negative emotions.

ROLES

This has been assigned to the left hand, and the "emotional" side, of the diagram. Who does what to whom is defined as "repetitive patterns of behavior by which individuals fulfill family functions."

Certain necessary family functions must be carried out by a healthy family. Roles are usually assigned to these functions (Table 9-2).

> A well-functioning family will have clearly allocated roles and account-ability built in. In this family, it turns out that the father's role as the provider and the mother's role as the homemaker are fairly well defined. John was able to say that if he had a problem he would go to his mother, but it turned out that it was not clear to either adult whom they should talk to about emotional issues. Mrs. Smith thought she might go to her next-door neighbor first. Neither of them has identified John's problem at school, though that seemed to be Mrs. Smith's

Identifying responsibilities

Table 9-2   Family Functions

Necessary family functions	Questions family might be asked to assess
Physical	
Provision of resources	Who earns the money? Who does the housework?
Emotional	
Nurturance and support	May ask each member, "If you have a problem, whom do you go to?"
Sexual gratification of marital partners	May privately inquire of adults concerning their ability to satisfy each other sexually.
Physical and emotional	
Life-skills development	"When John had trouble in school, who helped him out?"
Systems management and maintenance	Who is the leader, and who makes the decisions?

Table 9-3   Emotions in the Family

Types of emotions	Questions you might ask individual members
Positive: love, tenderness, happiness, and joy	How do you let others know you are happy? Are you affectionate?
Negative: anger	If you are upset, angry, or just ticked off, how do you let others know?
Sadness	If you are down, sad, or feeling blue, how do you let others know about this emotion?

role, and it wasn't clear who was the leader in terms of emotional issues.

AFFECTIVE RESPONSIVENESS

This is designated on the diagram as a "gut issue." The ability to use one's emotions is defined as "the ability to respond to a range of stimuli with the appropriate quality and quantity of feelings." (See Table 9-3.)

> The well-functioning family member will be able to use all emotions in an appropriate amount and quality. It turned out the Smiths have particular difficulty in terms of negative emotions. The father admitted to having no problems with anger, but on further questioning it

Table 9-4 Family Relationships

Relationship	Questions you might ask
Couple	What do you do as a couple separate and away from the kids?
Family	What do you do as a family, all together?
Father	What do you do as father and son?

turned out that he expresses his anger all the time over the littlest things, and on occasion he has exploded almost dangerously. On two occasions he hit Mrs. Smith, and she is quite fearful of him. She had been abused by her own father in her family of birth. Mrs. Smith further states that because of her difficulties in her family of origin, she tends to keep her anger to herself and is quite underassertive. Both parents, as it turns out, have problems with anger, with the father being overassertive and the mother being the opposite. John appears to have patterned himself after his father in terms of both temperament and the expression of anger. They have particular difficulty agreeing how to handle John's assertiveness. Positive emotions are at a low ebb in this family at this point, with very little affection except between mother and children. Sadness is something that is not dealt with at all, except by "doing" something.

AFFECTIVE INVOLVEMENT

This has been assigned to the left foot, and the "emotional" side, of the diagram. This involvement with each other is more clearly defined as "the degree to which the family shows interest in, and values the activities and interests of, other family members."

Family integration

Family involvement extends all the way from the uninvolved (boardinghouse) family to the symbiotic (you can't tell where one member begins and the other ends) family. In between, you will find involvement with a tremendous amount of self-interest, appropriate empathetic involvement, and overinvolvement (Table 9-4).

Some clinicians consider the question, What do you do as a couple? to be the important question one can ask a family. This is based on the observation that couples who really care about each other and enjoy each other will make sure that they have time together and that they are the most important unit in the family. As it turned out, the Smiths at this point do practically nothing together, though they did initially in their marriage. The mother turned out to be overly involved with the children, while the father did practically nothing with them. It was a rare event for the family to get together as a total unit and go on outings.

Table 9-5   Family Control

Behavior control	Questions you might ask
Adults controlling children	
Dangerous	What do you do when John puts his finger in the electrical outlet?
Psychobiological (food and drink, sleep, sex, elimination, and aggression)	What if John does not eat? What about bedtime?
Social	What if John has a temper tantrum in the store?
Adults controlling adults	
Dangerous	What did you do about your husband drinking and driving?
Psychobiological	So, what do you do if he bugs you a lot to make love? [asked privately]
Social	And what did you do when your husband wouldn't leave the party?
Children controlling adults	
Psychobiological	You might inquire what John does that makes his parents let him stay up late at night.
Social	You might wish to find out what behavior John exhibits that ends up making his parents buy him whatever he wants.

BEHAVIOR CONTROLS

Patterns of behavior

This is diagrammatically represented (for the sake of memory) as the strong right foot. The general methods individuals use to control each other are defined as "the pattern the family adopts for the handling of behavior."

Behavior control is usually considered to involve adults controlling children, but it also involves children controlling adults and adults controlling each other. Families tend to adopt a certain style which it is useful to identify, ranging from *laissez-faire* to *chaotic* through the more desirable *flexible and consistent* to *rigid* (Table 9-5).

Diagnostic/ management planning

The Smiths have a lot of trouble with behavior control. Because of their difficulties with anger, they don't seem to be able to get together to control John's behavior properly. In addition, Mrs. Smith doesn't control her husband's behavior very well, as indicated by some of the data that came out of the interview. You tell them, based on your assessment, that they have problems in the area of problem solving of emotional issues, more specifically, anger. Because of these difficulties, they are having trouble not only between themselves but with their son. You recommend that they be seen in family therapy and that two specific issues be dealt with: first, that child management techniques be taught, and second, that they resolve their difficulties in terms of expression of anger. In the meantime, the psychological testing will be carried out, and the Smiths are going to consult a specialist concerning their son's hyperactivity.

SUMMARY

This chapter briefly summarizes one model (the McMaster model) to describe family discordance and therapeutic intervention as a method by which family physicians can understand and assist families in trouble.

This chapter has been adapted from the "McMaster Model of Family Functioning," written by Epstein, Bishop, and Levin and published in the *Journal of Marriage and Family Counseling,* October 1978.

The schematic representation of the McMaster Model of Family Functioning was designed by Dr. Ivan Carter, Assistant Professor of Psychiatry, Dalhousie University, Halifax, Nova Scotia, as an "aide-mémoire" for medical students. It is adapted from the McMaster Model but not identical to it. In particular, it adds an individual "head" which is not described in the McMaster Model (although it is a component of the Model's predecessor, the Family Categories Schema) and each of the "limbs" has only five "digits" which necessitated some rearranging of the original material.

Part Two

Common Problems

Chapter 10

Common Health Problems and Principles

B. K. Hennen, M.D.
D. B. Shires, M.D.

The family physician sees a different range of problems, presented differently, than the specialist or hospital physician. Not only must the family physician deal with clinical and social aspects for which highly technical hospital care has limited solutions, he or she must also try to provide continuous care, involve the family, deal with the many dimensions of illness, and manage illness in its early undifferentiated stages.

The following chapters will outline 20 problems often seen in primary care. Each chapter and problem illustrates one or more principles of family medicine as well as giving information on diagnosis, management and therapeutic plans, and special features or problems.

In 1973, the Canadian College of Family Physicians' committee on objectives identified the most common presenting symptoms in ambulatory family practice in Canada.[1] More recently, a study by Marsland et al. looked closely at the presenting diagnoses of patients in over 100 practices in Virginia over a 2-year period.[2] However, the study identified diagnoses as opposed to presenting problems, and there is of course a great difference. For example, a patient presenting with chest pain could end up having many of the most common diagnoses listed in the Virginia study. Chest pain can be the presenting symptom for hypertension, contusion, bron-

Most common symptoms

Most common diagnoses

Table 10-1   Important Common Problems

Highest ranked on emphasis index*	Most common physician-identified problem†
Obesity	Respiratory infection
Diabetes	Dermatitis
Iron deficiency	Anxiety and/or depression
Depression	Hypertension
Acute otitis media	Arthritis
Hypertension	Pain (spinal)
Asthma	Minor trauma
Acute laryngitis and/or tracheitis	Urinary infection
Pneumonia	Diabetes
Cholecystitis and/or lithiasis	Menstrual irregularity
Cystitis	Otitis
Appendicitis	Acid-pepsin disease
Acute bronchitis and/or emphysema	Marital social problem
Anxiety neurosis	Pregnancy
Insomnia	Cardiac disease

*See *Canadian Family Medicine*.[1]
†Collated from our own practice experience.

chitis, muscle strain, obesity, depression, anxiety, abdominal pathology, congestive heart failure, pneumonia, osteoarthritis, influenza, rheumatoid arthritis, pulmonary infarct, and coronary heart disease.

Problems to be emphasized

The Canadian College of Family Physicians' committee on objectives attempted to identify those diagnoses which deserve the greatest emphasis because of their combined frequency, severity, and treatability. Finally, through analysis of problem-oriented patient charts from our own family medicine center, the authors have collected the most common physician-identified problems in our practice (Table 10-1).

Authors' own practice

From our subjective consideration of the data, we have selected 20 common problems whose management exemplifies the principles of family medicine listed in Table 10-2.

Family medicine principles

The principles of family medicine were described in this book's first edition. Other authors have described them in a different format.[3,4] In 1982, in Newcastle, Australia, four of us reconsidered the principles and found that there were about two dozen of them.[5] They depend on the nature of illness as it presents to the family doctor, the nature of the person with the illness and that person's family, the relationships established between the patient and the family doctor and between the family and the family doctor, the community setting in which the patient and doctor meet and the expectations of both in that setting, and finally, the tactics in which the family doctor must be skilled in order to do the job.

The specific problems discussed in the subsequent chapters demonstrate these principles. Each problem is intended to emphasize one or two principles, although most of the problems could be used to demonstrate many of the principles.

Table 10-2 Principles of Family Medicine: Example Problems

	Principle	Problem description
	Nature of the illness	
1	Disease is frequently seen at an earlier stage than the stage at which it presents to other physicians.	Abdominal pain
2	Illness is frequently undifferentiated when it presents.	Fatigue
3	Family physicians deal with a great deal of uncertainty in both assessment and management.	Dental problems
4	The family doctor must frequently manage both chronic and multisystem disease.	Diabetes
5	The family doctor sees a high prevalence of chronic, emotional, and transient illness.	Wheezing
6	Understanding illness behavior is crucial to teaching and understanding patients.	Chest pain
7	Illness is seen in the context of family life.	Diarrhea
	Nature of the person or family	
8	Illness may present with signals or tickets.	Depression
9	Psychosocial factors are an integral part of each problem.	Child abuse
10	Sometimes patients display symptoms that are most common to one illness when they actually have a different illness.	Confusion in the elderly
	Relationship with doctor	
11	Much of the family physician's work depends on his or her personal relationship with the patient.	Death and dying
12	Time is a diagnostic and management tool. Continuity of care is of major importance.	Lower back pain
13	The onus of lifestyle change is on family physicians, who must encourage patients to take responsibility for their health.	High-risk pregnancy

Table 10-2   Continued

Principle	Problem description
Community setting	
14 The family physician is the doctor of first contact.	Hypertension
15 It is necessary to make a decision on all new patients. The family doctor can't say, "I'm sorry, I can't help you."	Sexual dysfunction
16 Family doctors require an acute awareness of community epidemiology (e.g., knowledge about mining, industries, lifestyle, and epidemics in the community).	Sexually transmitted disease
17 Awareness of community resources is essential for management.	Cancer
18 Referrals are frequent and involve a wide variety of professional consultants.	Learning disabilities
Family practice skills	
19 Management is often related more to prognosis than to diagnosis.	Sore throat
20 A regional assessment is often sufficient.	Headache
21 Relief of distress is a prime concern.	Earache
22 Records must be succinct but should be useful.	High-risk pregnancy
23 A minor complaint may present an opportunity to approach a more serious health problem.	Sore throat
24 Pattern recognition is an important skill.	Diabetes

REFERENCES

1 *Canadian Family Medicine: Educational Objectives for Certification in Family Medicine,* The College of Family Physicians of Canada, Toronto, 1973.

2 D. W. Marsland, M. Wood, and F. Mayo, *Content of Family Practice: A Statewide Study in Virgina with Its Clinical, Educational, and Research Implications,* J. Geyman (ed.), Appleton-Century-Crofts, New York, 1976.

3 I. R. McWhinney, *An Introduction to Family Medicine,* Oxford University Press, N.Y. 1981.

4 T. J. Phillips, "The Intellectual Roots of Family Practice," *Pharos,* Winter 1981, pp. 26–31.

5 B. K. E. Hennen, *General Practice in the Newcastle Undergraduate Curriculum,* Newcastle, Australia, The University of Newcastle, NSW Faculty of Medicine, 1981–82.

Chapter 11

Diarrhea in a Child

D. B. Shires, M.D.

PRINCIPLE

In planning management, assessing the family's ability to cope is often as important as assessing the patient's ability. This is especially true when the patient is a child. When the assessment and management of a child's problem are conducted over the telephone, an accurate evaluation of the parents' reliability as historians, observers, and providers of care is vital. Infant diarrhea presents such a challenge.

DEFINITION

For practical purposes, *diarrhea* can be defined as the passage of frequent (more than twice the norm for the individual or over eight per 24 hours), loose, or watery stools, which are often greenish-yellow.

PREVALENCE

Children account for 20 percent of cases of diarrhea seen in family practice.[1,2] Diarrhea is among the 10 leading causes of death in children ages 1 to 4 in North America and Europe.[3] In the Third World, acute infectious diarrhea is the leading cause of mortality in children.

ETIOLOGY

Diarrhea in an infant, while usually the result of mild self-limiting illness, has the potential of rapidly becoming serious if warning signs are ignored. Most diarrheal illnesses in children are associated with abnormal transfer of fluids and electrolytes across the bowel wall, probably as a result of microorganism interference with the wall's normal function. ROTA viruses are a significant cause of diarrhea in both the United States and Canada, [4,5] particularly during the winter in the north. In summer infectious bacteria peak, while in temperate regions all organisms are seen year-round.[6]

Illness patterns

In early childhood, the etiology of common diarrhea is rarely determined in the laboratory, and most cases of diarrhea are self-limiting in response to conservative management. Diarrhea in a child or infant is basically a management problem, and awareness of illness patterns in the community is helpful in its management (Table 11-1).

There would seem to be a June-to-October peak in enteroviral infection in America, with a higher incidence in lower socioeconomic groups.[7]

Table 11-1   Etiology of Acute Diarrhea in Developed Countries

Shigella

Salmonella (toxin)

Staphylococcus (toxin)

Enteropathic *Escherichia coli*

Enteroviruses

Adenoviruses

Secondary to general infection

Food and nutrition excess or deficiency

Parasites (usually chronic)

Weaning diarrhea

Iatrogenic

Source: Adapted from Gordon et al.[7]

Diarrhea is frequently associated with concurrent infections such as otitis, pyelitis, and pneumonia. It may result from the treatment of these conditions rather than being directly related to the primary infection. Antibiotics inhibit normal bacterial flora and allow the overgrowth of pathogens, causing diarrhea.

Inappropriate feeding (for example, too much fat or excess carbohydrate) can cause diarrhea, as can too large a feeding. Less common causes include enzyme deficiencies, enteritis, colitis, gastrointestinal allergy, endocrine disorder, behavioral disorder, vitamin deficiency, chemical or food poisoning, and ultraviolet light treatment for neonatal jaundice.[4]

PREVENTION

Breast feeding may help prevent diarrhea since it produces stools of low pH, low *E. coli* content, and high *Lactobacillus* content. Human milk contains greater amounts of IgA, IgG, and IgM than cow's milk, thus affording more resistance against some infectious agents.[8]

For artificially-fed babies, basic hygiene in terms of clean bottles and nipples is important. In most Western countries, sterilization of bottles and nipples is not necessary if there is a good water supply but this should be done when an infection exists in the home.

Associated factors

Isolating the affected family member with any infectious illness, and with diarrhea in particular, may reduce the likelihood of transmitting the infection.[5] Avoiding unnecessary antibiotics in the treatment of other infections can also reduce the frequency of iatrogenic diarrhea.

Poverty, poor hygiene, contaminated water supply, malnutrition, and ignorance have been associated with diarrheal illness in worldwide studies.[9]

Parents should be provided with knowledge about common infant illnesses such as diarrhea before they occur and should be prepared to manage them. We should provide guidelines for parents in order to help them decide when to seek professional help.

DIAGNOSIS

Assessing the Parent's Ability to Report and Manage

Most parents contact the doctor for infant diarrhea when the apparent discomfort of the infant and the inconvenience of loose stools persist for more than a few hours. A few parents are aware of the potential risk of dehydration.

Table 11-2   Considerations in Assessing the Reliability of a Caller

New patient

Compliance history

Comprehension

Concerns inappropriate

Distance and transportation

First child or nonexperienced

Panicky parent

Conflicting family advice

Anticipatory
guidance

Most new parents, especially those of a firstborn, worry when the baby seems to be sick. Such parents may seek help fairly early. The physician may find it useful to see a first baby early in the course of a diarrheal illness, not only to reassure the new parents but also to teach them about the management of the illness. Competent, experienced parents are more likely to make contact later in the course of an illness, when their initial management has failed or seems not to be working quickly enough.

One's first priority is to assess the parents' ability to cope. The following questions may help in such an evaluation:

Assessing
coping
mechanisms

1   How well do I know the family?
2   What has been the parents' past performance in accurately representing symptoms and complying with treatment?
3   How well do the parents seem to understand the significance of the important symptoms?
4   What degree of anxiety do they show?
5   Do they seem to disagree about assessment or management techniques? Is a grandparent involved?
6   Is distance or transportation a problem? Would it be easier to see the patient now even though the problem seems to be minor? (See Table 11-2.)

A crucial step is to decide on the basis of the initial information whether the child needs to be seen right away or can be cared for by the parent, assuming that the parent's report is accurate.

Questions for
parents

In questioning a parent over the phone or directly, one needs to know the frequency, size (volume), and color of the stools; the presence or absence of blood or mucous or both; whether the infant is vomiting and how much; what the feeding pattern has been for the last 24 hours; and whether there are other symptoms that suggest a primary infection elsewhere.

Dehydration

It is important to assess the degree of dehydration by asking

Table 11-3 Signs of Acute Dehydration on Examination

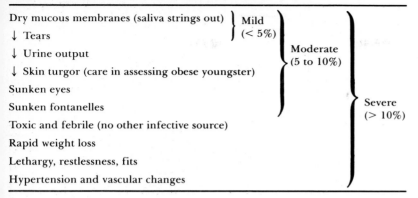

Dry mucous membranes (saliva strings out) } Mild (< 5%)

↓ Tears

↓ Urine output Moderate (5 to 10%)

↓ Skin turgor (care in assessing obese youngster)

Sunken eyes

Sunken fontanelles

Severe (> 10%)

Toxic and febrile (no other infective source)

Rapid weight loss

Lethargy, restlessness, fits

Hypertension and vascular changes

about the moisture of the mucous membranes, the frequency of voiding, the degree of lethargy or irritability the infant shows, the number of stools per hour, and the baby's temperature. If the child has fewer than one small-volume stool every 3 hours and the parents are coping well, management can begin without seeing the patient. More frequent stools, voluminous stools, stools for which the volume is not clearly described, and diarrhea associated with other worrisome symptoms are reasons for direct observation and examination of the patient by the physician. Signs of acute dehydration on examination are shown in Table 11-3.

MANAGEMENT

Infants usually respond to conservative treatment using clear oral fluids made up of glucose and electrolyte components. Antibiotics are rarely indicated in North America even for bacterial kinds of infection (an exception is made for *Shigella* with toxicity). Generally, a diet of clear fluids offered in the form of flat cola, apple juice, commercial water/electrolyte formulas, and gelatin desserts or Popsicles in small amounts is sufficient. No solids should be given for 24 hours. The WHO oral rehydration therapy (ORT) solution is ideal (Tables 11-4 and 11-5).

Fluid replacement

If vomiting accompanies the diarrhea, Parker advocates nothing by mouth for 6 hours, then 15 ml of flat cola every 10 minutes, doubling the volume each time until a volume of 180 ml an hour is reached and thereafter switching to clear fluids but avoiding citrus fruit drinks.[11]

In babies who are already on solid foods, on the second or third day one can reintroduce solids such as rice cereal, bananas, and apple sauce. Milk, beginning with 2 percent fat, may usually be

Gradual return to normal diet

1 DIARRHEA IN A CHILD

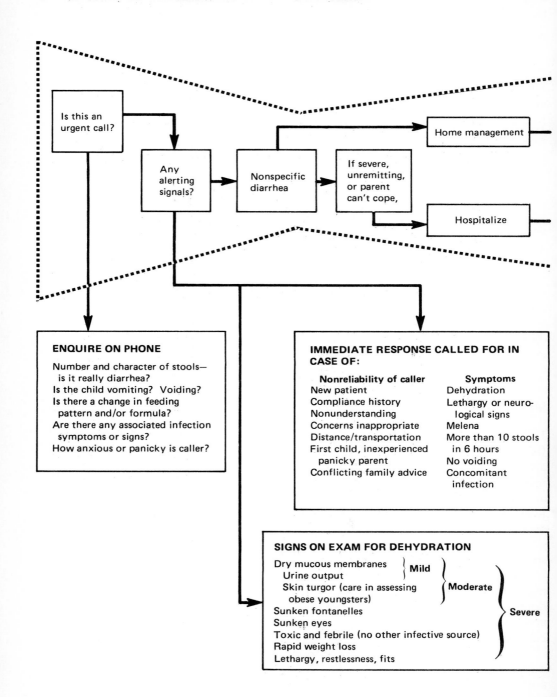

Is this an urgent call?	

Any alerting signals? → Nonspecific diarrhea → If severe, unremitting, or parent can't cope, → Hospitalize

Home management

ENQUIRE ON PHONE

Number and character of stools— is it really diarrhea?
Is the child vomiting? Voiding?
Is there a change in feeding pattern and/or formula?
Are there any associated infection symptoms or signs?
How anxious or panicky is caller?

IMMEDIATE RESPONSE CALLED FOR IN CASE OF:

Nonreliability of caller	**Symptoms**
New patient	Dehydration
Compliance history	Lethargy or neuro-
Nonunderstanding	logical signs
Concerns inappropriate	Melena
Distance/transportation	More than 10 stools
First child, inexperienced	in 6 hours
panicky parent	No voiding
Conflicting family advice	Concomitant
	infection

SIGNS ON EXAM FOR DEHYDRATION

Dry mucous membranes   } **Mild**
  Urine output
  Skin turgor (care in assessing   } **Moderate**
  obese youngsters)
Sunken fontanelles
Sunken eyes   } **Severe**
Toxic and febrile (no other infective source)
Rapid weight loss
Lethargy, restlessness, fits

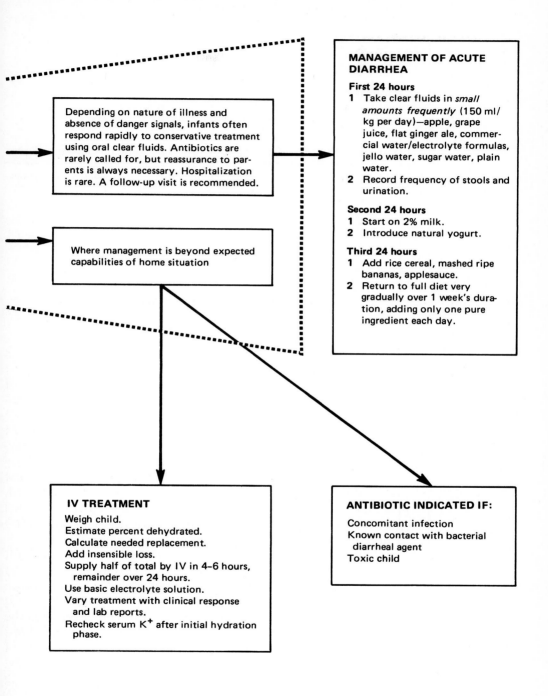

Depending on nature of illness and absence of danger signals, infants often respond rapidly to conservative treatment using oral clear fluids. Antibiotics are rarely called for, but reassurance to parents is always necessary. Hospitalization is rare. A follow-up visit is recommended.

Where management is beyond expected capabilities of home situation

MANAGEMENT OF ACUTE DIARRHEA

First 24 hours
1 Take clear fluids in *small amounts frequently* (150 ml/kg per day)—apple, grape juice, flat ginger ale, commercial water/electrolyte formulas, jello water, sugar water, plain water.
2 Record frequency of stools and urination.

Second 24 hours
1 Start on 2% milk.
2 Introduce natural yogurt.

Third 24 hours
1 Add rice cereal, mashed ripe bananas, applesauce.
2 Return to full diet very gradually over 1 week's duration, adding only one pure ingredient each day.

IV TREATMENT
Weigh child.
Estimate percent dehydrated.
Calculate needed replacement.
Add insensible loss.
Supply half of total by IV in 4–6 hours, remainder over 24 hours.
Use basic electrolyte solution.
Vary treatment with clinical response and lab reports.
Recheck serum K^+ after initial hydration phase.

ANTIBIOTIC INDICATED IF:

Concomitant infection
Known contact with bacterial diarrheal agent
Toxic child

Table 11-4 WHO Oral Rehydration Formula

	Grams/liter of water
Sodium chloride	3.5
Sodium bicarbonate	2.5
Potassium chloride	1.5
Glucose	20.0

Table 11-5 Electrolyte Composition of Some Rehydration Solutions

	Sodium, mmol/L	Potassium, mmol/L
WHO formula	90	20
Hydralyte	84	10
Lytren	30	25
Pedialyte	30	20
Apple juice	1.9	26.6
Coca-Cola	0.4	13

Source: Modified from Burey.[10]

introduced after 2 or 3 days. A return to a full diet within a week should be the goal.

Failure to show improvement as indicated by a continuation of vomiting or diarrhea or by other signs of worsening such as increased lethargy or irritability warrants seeing the child.

If the child fails to improve on such an oral regimen within 24 to 48 hours, hospitalization for monitored oral replacement therapy or parenteral fluid replacement should be considered. Any child deemed to be moderately or severely dehydrated when first assessed should be hospitalized. If severe dehydration is assessed, parenteral treatment should probably be started immediately. However, at least one study demonstrated the efficacy of the WHO oral rehydration therapy in moderately severe dehydration.[12]

Follow-up

If the initial management leads to recovery, a follow-up visit may be used to reassure the parents if they have been particularly anxious or uncertain and to teach them how to handle future episodes.

Parents want the diarrhea to stop. They should be told that the fluid/electrolyte balance is of more importance during the illness than nutrition. The management of diarrhea should be part of parent education at the first or second well-baby visit. The family-practice nurse or doctor can provide this education, explaining how to prevent diarrhea and how to manage it when it occurs. A competent and informed parent can care for most infant and child diarrhea.

REFERENCES

1 D. W. Marsland, M. Wood, and F. Mayo, *Content of Family Practice: A Statewide Study in Virginia with Its Clinical, Educational, and Research Implications,* J. Geyman (ed.), Appleton-Century-Crofts, New York, 1976.

2 D. Mundell et al., "Toxigenic Escherichia coli and Childhood Diarrhea," *Western Journal of Medicine,* **124**(5):357–360, 1976.

3 J. E. Rhode and R. S. Northrup, "Taking Science Where Diarrhea Is," *Ciba Symposium 42, Acute Diarrhea in Childhood,* Elsevier Excerpta Medica, North-Holland, Amsterdam, 1976.

4 A. Bakken, "Intestinal Lactase Deficiency as a Factor in the Diarrhea of Light-Treated Jaundiced Infants," *New England Journal of Medicine,* **295**(11):615, 1976.

5 A. Z. Kapikian, H. W. Kim, R. G. Wyatt, W. L. Cline, R. H. Parrott, R. M. Chanock, J. O. Arrobio, C. D. Brandt, W. J. Rodriguez, A. R. Kalica, and D. H. Vanlick, "Recent Advances in the Aetiology of Viral Gastroenteritis," *Ciba Symposium 42, Acute Diarrhea in Childhood,* Elsevier Excerpta Medica, North-Holland, Amsterdam, 1976.

6 "Diarrhea: When the Patient's Under Age 2," *Patient Care,* **19**:125–150, 1985.

7 J. E. Gordon, I. D. Chitkara and J. B. Wyon, "Weaning Diarrhea," *American Journal of Medicine Science,* **245**:345, 1963.

8 J. J. Bullen, "Iron-Binding Proteins and Other Factors in Milk Responsible for Resistance to Escherichia coli," *Ciba Symposium 42, Acute Diarrhea in Childhood,* Elsevier Excerpta Medica, North-Holland, Amsterdam, 1976.

9 J. T. Harries, "The Problem of Bacterial Diarrhea," *Ciba Symposium 42, Acute Diarrhea in Childhood,* Elsevier Excerpta Medica, North-Holland, Amsterdam, 1976.

10 S. Burey, "Oral Rehydration," *Nova Scotia Medical Bulletin,* April 1983, pp. 37–38.

11 K. Ross Parker, "Diarrhea and Vomiting in Infancy," *Canadian Family Physician,* **24**:1011–1013, 1976.

12 C. C. Carpenter, "Oral Rehydration: Is It as Good as Parenteral Therapy?" *New England Journal of Medicine,* **306**:1103–1104, 1982.

Chapter 12

Earache

D. B. Shires, M.D.

PRINCIPLE

Relieving distress is a prime concern for all physicians. As the first-contact health professional, the family physician has many opportunities to give reassurance to the anxious, compassion to the grieving, and relief to those in pain. The quicker the response, the quicker the relief. The child with an earache deserves quick attention.

DEFINITION

Otalgia

Pain in the ear (otalgia) is a common symptom in children. A child who is old enough to verbalize discomfort may still not be accurate about its exact description or locale. Itching or "popping" may be more apt descriptions of what the patient perceives. Pain originating from nearby structures may be inappropriately identified as being in the ear or may in fact be referred to the ear.

Pain in the ear in infants and young children may be revealed by irritability and/or crying. Pulling at the ears is not a reliable sign of earache in toddlers.

Table 12-1   Etiology of Earache

Of 100 patients presenting with earache:

    77 may be expected to have acute otitis media

    12 may be expected to have otitis externa

    6 may be expected to have a boil in the canal

    2–3 may be expected to have mumps

    1–2 may be expected to have a foreign body in the ear canal

    0–1 may be expected to have mastoiditis

Source: Based on review of the frequencies of these diagnoses reported by Hodgkin[2] and Marsland et al.[1] and the likelihood of each condition presenting with earache.

PREVALENCE

Approximately 1 of every 25 patients in family practice will present with an earache.[1,2]

ETIOLOGY

"Earache" may be due to acute suppurative otitis media but is an unreliable symptom of this condition.[3] It may also be a symptom of acute or chronic otitis externa, myringitis, a furuncle in the external ear canal, a foreign body in the canal, mastoiditis, trauma, or mumps parotitis. It may also represent referred pain from the teeth, tonsils, tongue, or temperomandibular joints.[4] (See Table 12-1 for details on etiology.)

APPROACH TO THE PATIENT

Once the symptom has been identified as pain and not as itching or a pop, one should find out about its duration and any previous occurrence and then try to determine the aggravating factors. Consider the following examples.

Aggravating factors

    1 Jaw movement (chewing or yawning) is more likely to stir up pain from otitis externa and temperomandibular dysfunction.

    2 Eating acidic food may aggravate mumps parotitis.

    3 Swimming or water in the ear from showering may trigger an episode of otitis externa.

    4 A recent cold may precede acute otitis media.

    5 Painful itching is most suggestive of chronic otitis externa.

Other details of the history of the disease may be extracted during the physical examination. A known habit or a recent history of putting foreign objects such as hairpins or match sticks into the ear may raise the possibility of traumatic injury to the canal or drum. Air travel or deep sea diving may cause barotrauma.

ASSOCIATED SYMPTOMS

Diagnostic discriminators

Some symptoms are highly specific, for example, dysphagia accompanying pharyngitis and tonsillitis, teeth grinding (bruxism) with temperomandibular dysfunction, and hearing loss from otitis. More often, the associated symptoms are nonspecific (e.g., nausea and vomiting) or unreliable. Fever occurs only in a minority of children over 6 years old who present with otitis media.[5]

EXAMINATION

How to examine a child

The young child is best examined held against the parent's chest while the parent's free arm embraces the child's trunk, including both arms.[6] During the external examination, the physician should look for pain on movement of the pinna or pressure on the tragus (found in acute otitis externa), swelling or tenderness over the mastoid (swelling in mastoiditis and tenderness in both mastoiditis and otitis media), swelling of the parotid gland (mumps), and adenopathy (most upper respiratory infections) as well as making general observations on how sick the youngster appears.

Dealing with wax

To examine the ear properly requires removal of cerumen that obstructs the view of the external canal and the tympanic membrane (drum). A metal applicator with cotton on the end, gentle suction, and gentle lavage with either hydrogen peroxide or tepid water are methods of removing wax. (If one holds the instrument between the thumb and index finger while resting the ulnar aspect of the same hand firmly against the side of the head, there is less danger from sudden jerks of the head.) Prior insertion of drops of olive oil or mineral oil is preferable to the use of a cerumenolytic agent to facilitate the procedure.

If the canal wax is packed hard in an uncooperative and distressed youngster who has a high probability of an inflamed middle ear, it is acceptable to institute specific antibiotic treatment as well as drops of oil in the ear and then have the patient return in 24 to 48 hours for another look.

Otitis externa

The external canal should be examined with the otoscope, probing gently on insertion for sites of local tenderness (often the early sign of a furuncle or "blind pimple") and assessing the integrity of the epithelium, noting especially redness and weeping exudate indicative of acute inflammation or the cobblestoned appearance of chronic irritation. In acute otitis externa, swelling of the canal may make observation of the drum initially impossible. The canal epithelium may be boggy and pale, nodes may be palpable both anterior and posterior to the ear, and the auricle itself may be inflamed and oozing or crusted.

Examination of the Drum

Observation of the drum in acute otitis media will show redness (two-thirds of the drum should be red to validate the diagnosis). Bulging of the drum, though a hallmark, was seen in only 54 percent of 500 patients diagnosed as having acute otitis media.[7] One out of five drums in acute otitis media has a perforation, and the physician must look carefully through such a perforation for evidence of granulation tissue or polyplike formation, which may represent cholesteatoma formation. Scarring of the drum suggests previous infection, while retraction suggests chronic serous otitis. Perforation without pus or drum distortion suggests trauma.

Acute otitis media

A flaming red drum with a bleb or vesicular swelling on it is typical of acute myringitis. A drum that is moderately injected without deformity may be part of a common cold or simply a result of prolonged crying. Pneumatic otoscopy may cause pain in an acutely inflamed ear.

Hearing loss may result from otitis media or otitis externa in which there is much edema or debris in the canal. Deafness also may result from a foreign body.

Deafness

MANAGEMENT

Acute Purulent Otitis Media

Management should relieve pain, promote drainage, specifically treat the likelihood of bacterial infection, and ensure a minimum of complications by means of adequate follow-up. Pain relief involves applying local warmth with a carefully monitored heating pad or hot water bottle, the warmth of a mother's breast, or topical drops of warm oil. Systemic analgesia with aspirin, acetaminophen, or codeine should be used as needed. Drainage occurs naturally by means of spontaneous perforation in about 20 percent of cases or can be effected through the eustachian tube by opening the tube with decongestant nose drops or systemic decongestants. The nose drops should not be used for more than 3 or 4 days. Oral decongestants in adequate doses without antihistamine are recommended. Many over-the-counter preparations contain antihistamines, which are indicated only if allergy is considered an etiologic factor.

General measures

The most common bacteria found in middle-ear aspirations are pneumococci and streptococci. *Hemophilus influenzae* has been found to be common in youngsters under 4 or 5 years of age and, more recently, in older children.[8] Infants may have *Escherichia coli.* Bacteria are found with varying frequencies (40 to 70 percent) in middle-ear aspirates. Fry[9] and Laxdal[10] advocate antibiotics for those who are severely ill, show no improvement in 48 hours, have had previous attacks, or are not readily accessible for medical follow-up; other patients should be treated symptomatically. All should be followed up with equal care.

Antibiotics   Antibiotic therapy should be instituted in the following way.

Children Under 10 Years of Age
Amoxicillin (50 mg/day per kilogram of body weight in three divided doses), for 10 days
or
if child allergic to penicillin
Erythromycin (30 mg/day per kilogram of body weight in four divided doses), for 10 days
plus
Sulfisoxasole (150 mg/day per kilogram of body weight in four divided doses), for 10 days
Penicillin-Resistant H. Influenza
Cefaclor (20 mg/day per kilogram of body weight in two divided doses), for 10 days
Children Over 10 Years and Adults
Penicillin in the usual dose
or
Trimethoprim-sulfamethoxazole in the usual dose

Our preference is for local heat, aspirin or codeine, phenylephrine (Neo-Synephrine) nose drops, and ampicillin (under age 10) for a week. When a child has been asymptomatic for 2 days, the nose drops can be stopped. A final follow-up at 3 to 4 weeks from the onset is warranted, at which time hearing is tested with a 512 tuning fork, a squeaky toy, and a whispered voice.

Myringotomy   A child who does not improve in 2 to 3 days should be seen again. If pain has persisted and is severe, myringotomy should be considered. The antibiotic may be changed after the doctor makes sure that the initially prescribed one was taken.

Complications   Complications of unresolved otitis media include: chronic serous otitis with hearing loss, mastoiditis, meningitis, and chronic cholesteatoma. All are serious and warrant every effort at prevention.

Otitis Externa

Once drum perforation has been ruled out, the canal must be cleaned by gentle lavage, using tepid water or hydrogen peroxide.

If the canal is acutely inflamed and swollen, insert a cotton wick soaked in 5% Burow's solution. This can be kept moist with solution drops for 2 to 3 days, when the canal usually becomes less painful and more open for cleaning.

Once the canal is open, ear drops can be inserted. The patient's head should be held laterally with the affected canal orifice up for at least 5 minutes. Acetic acid (2%) is particularly effective, as is topical gentamycin against *Pseudomonas,* the most likely bacterial pathogen. Neomycin is present in many topical preparations and is effective against the most likely pathogens. Neomycin therapy should be limited to 7 to 10 days; in rare cases, it causes local hypersensitization. Neomycin should be used with caution in patients with otitis externa complicated by chronic otitis media or by a perforated tympanic membrane because of possible absorption of the drug leading to ototoxicity. Local anesthetics used topically are more likely to cause sensitivity and should be avoided. If analgesia is required, local heat and systemic analgesia (aspirin or codeine) are preferable. Hydrocortisone in the drops helps settle inflammation and pain quickly. The canal should be initially cleaned out every 2 to 3 days if possible. — Local medications

Cultures need be taken only for patients who do not respond within 4 to 5 days and should precede the use of systemic antibiotics. — Culture

Persons subject to recurrences, especially swimmers and persons who bathe by showering, should keep their ears dry with a twisted piece of facial or toilet tissue in the canal. If necessary, prophylactic use of acetic acid (2%)–steroid drops is warranted.

Furuncle or Boil

If it is pointing, the furuncle can be incised. Otherwise, 5% Burow's solution, inserted on a cotton wick, and warmth may relieve discomfort. If fever is significant or if diffuse erythema suggests more widespread cellulitis, systemic antibiotics such as cloxacillin are indicated.

Mumps

Warmth, systemic analgesics, adequate hydration, and avoidance of acidic foods are important for mumps parotitis. Oral hygiene may have to be reinforced, and alternatives to toothbrushing, such as saline mouthwashes, should be suggested.

Foreign Bodies

Foreign bodies can usually be washed out or lifted out with thin thumb forceps. If some inflammation exists, drops of Burow's solution may make it possible to remove the object in 24 hours unless

2 EARACHE IN A CHILD

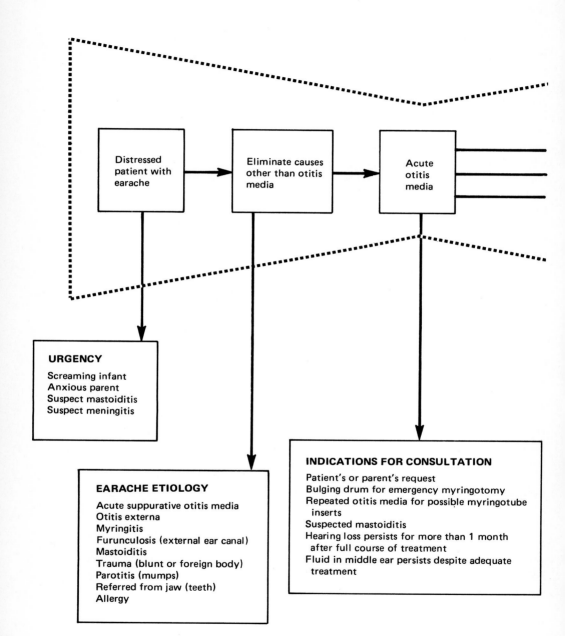

URGENCY

Screaming infant
Anxious parent
Suspect mastoiditis
Suspect meningitis

EARACHE ETIOLOGY

Acute suppurative otitis media
Otitis externa
Myringitis
Furunculosis (external ear canal)
Mastoiditis
Trauma (blunt or foreign body)
Parotitis (mumps)
Referred from jaw (teeth)
Allergy

INDICATIONS FOR CONSULTATION

Patient's or parent's request
Bulging drum for emergency myringotomy
Repeated otitis media for possible myringotube
  inserts
Suspected mastoiditis
Hearing loss persists for more than 1 month
  after full course of treatment
Fluid in middle ear persists despite adequate
  treatment

GENERAL

Rest
Analgesic—aspirin or codeine
Local heat (well-wrapped hot water bottle)
Avoid aggravating factors such as jaw movement,
  pulling on tragus, lying on side, etc.
Decongestant—systemic or short-term topically

SPECIFIC

Antihistamines only when allergy suspected
Topical drops of warm oil
Antibiotic
  Ampicillin (under 10 years old)
  Penicillin (over 10 years old)
  Sulfa-trimethoprim (alternative when indicated)

FOLLOW-UP AND PREVENTION

If no improvement, see again in 72 hours.
One week, then one month, after initial visit or
  diagnosis if improving.
Check hearing at 1 month follow-up visit.
Use chewing gum or decongestants early in future
  acute upper respiratory infections.
Refer early when indicated.

the object is likely to enlarge with wetness, as happens with a dried bean or pea. Occasionally general anesthesia is required. Oil drops will smother live insects and thus reduce distress caused by their movement.

Mastoiditis

Emergency consultation

Mastoiditis is an urgent complication of otitis media. Essentially the management should involve early consultation with an ear, nose, and throat surgeon. However, large doses of antibiotics, as described for acute otitis media, should be started at once, and investigation, including x-ray, should be conducted to establish the extent of the infection and assess the necessity for surgical intervention.

SUMMARY

Although a child with earache is most likely to have acute otitis media, other possibilities exist in approximately one out of four cases. A careful history of the pain and examination of the wax-free ear will usually lead to the correct diagnosis, but sometimes the child's inability to describe the quality and location of the pain and difficulties in cleaning the ear make diagnosis more difficult. Relieving the pain, promoting drainage, using appropriate antibiotics, and doing careful follow-up to prevent complications are the basis for treatment for any closed infection such as otitis media. A child with an earache is usually in acute distress and is at risk for chronic and serious complications. He or she deserves quick assessment and careful follow-up.

REFERENCES

1 D. W. Marsland, M. Wood, and F. Mayo, *Content of Family Practice: A Statewide Study in Virginia with Its Clinical, Educational, and Research Implications,* J. Geyman (ed.), Appleton-Century-Crofts, New York, 1976.
2 K. Hodgkin, *Towards Earlier Diagnosis in Primary Care,* 4th ed., Churchill Livingstone, Edinburgh, London, and New York, 1978.
3 L. Ingvarsson, "Acute Otalgia in Children—Findings and Diagnosis," *Acta Paediatrica Scandinavica,* **71**:705–710, 1982.
4 P. Blake, D. N. Thorburn, and I. A. Stewart, "Temperomandibular Joint Dysfunction in Children Presenting as Otalgia," *Clinical Otolaryngology,* **7**:237–244, 1982.
5 G. Smilkstein, "The Pediatric Lap Exam," *Journal of Family Practice,* **4**(4):745, 1977.
6 G. Strickler, M M. Rubenstein, J. B. McBean, L. D. Hedgecock, J. A. Hugstad, and T. Griffing, "Treatment of Acute Otitis Media in Children. IV: A Fourth Clinical Trial," *American Journal of Diseases,* **114**:123–130, 1967.
7 R. Schwartz, W. J. Rodriguez, N. K. Waheed, and S. Ross, "Acute Purulent Otitis Media in Children Older Than 5 Years: Incidence of Haemophilus as

a Causative Organism," *Journal of the American Medical Association,* **238**:1032–1033, 1977.

8 L. De Santo, and G. Strickler, "Acute Otitis Media in Children," *Postgraduate Medicine,* **45**(5):210–215, 1969.

9 J. Fry, "Antibiotics in Acute Tonsillitis and Otitis Media," *British Medical Journal,* **2**:833–866, 1958.

10 O. E. Laxdal, "My Child Has an Earache," *Canadian Family Physician,* **20**(9):65–66, 1974.

Chapter 13

Sore Throat

D. B. Shires, M.D.

PRINCIPLE

Many problems presented to the family physician are not susceptible to specific diagnosis. An acute illness, in particular, may be
sufficiently undifferentiated on the first visit to leave its etiology
obscure. Nonetheless, even a slight possibility of serious sequelae
in a particular disease may warrant treatment for that disease.

In such situations, management is often started without waiting for further evidence to confirm the diagnosis. The decision to
start treatment is based on what is called a *management diagnosis*. If
the patient recovers, we may never know whether the treatment
was responsible or whether the natural history of the illness made
it self-limiting. Such is the uncertainty of family practice.

DEFINITION

When a patient presents with a sore throat, he or she is usually
referring to dysphagia or pain on swallowing. In the case of a child,
we have found that unless the sore throat causes fairly severe discomfort on swallowing, it is less likely to cause the parent to bring

the child to the physician than its associated symptoms, e.g., fever, rash, cough, irritability, and lethargy.

PREVALENCE

Sore throat may be part of viral or bacterial pharyngitis, coryza, influenza, or mononucleosis. These combined illnesses account for 1 of every 12 visits in family practice. The highest incidence of sore throat occurs during the first 35 years of life.[1,2]

ETIOLOGY

One of three cases of pharyngitis is streptococcal. The accuracy with which beta-hemolytic streptococcal infection can be diagnosed is frequently disputed.[3] In one study, more experienced physicians demonstrated better clinical judgment than their younger colleagues, but both groups had error rates over 50 percent.[4] Clinical assessment without culture is not sufficiently accurate in children to warrant specific management decisions. Strep throat is less likely to occur in those under age 2 or over age 40. In adults (persons over 15 years of age), a clinical diagnosis of a viral infection can be made with reasonable accuracy. Hoarseness, for example, is rarely present in streptococcal pharyngitis.[5-7]

A viral diagnosis is more likely if there has been a prodrome of coryza-like symptoms, hoarseness, generalized muscle aches and pains, and known viral illness in the community. A diagnosis of streptococcal infection is more likely with scarlatiniform rash, strawberry tongue, or Pastia's lines in the skin creases or if there is a known streptococcal epidemic. In young children, crusting and excoriation of the nares is frequently bacterial in origin.

Viral infection

Strep throat

Diphtheria and gonorrhea are unusual but serious bacterial causes which should be considered in nonimmunized or at-risk persons. Mononucleosis is often accompanied by severe exudative pharyngitis and should always be considered a possibility.

Other causes

WHY PEOPLE PRESENT WITH SORE THROAT

Factors which prompt persons with sore throats to see a doctor include the following:

Presenting complaints

1 *Severity*: "It even hurts to swallow water."
2 *Duration*: "I thought it would pass, but it's been 5 days now."
3 *Potential or actual interference with work*: "I've got an important meeting in Chicago the day after tomorrow, and I thought you might be able to give me something to help me get through it."

4 *Encouragement by others for the visit*: "The secretary at the office told me I had better see my doctor."

5 *The potential seriousness*: "The school nurse said there has been scarlet fever around."

6 *Previous experience with doctors*: "Doctor Smith always gave me a shot of penicillin for this. Otherwise, I wouldn't have come and bothered you."

PRESENTING FEATURES

The likelihood of group A strep occurring in a child with a sore throat and no fever is small (3 percent or less).[7]

Fever

The degree of fever, the presence of exudate, and the presence of lymphadenopathy are not helpful in differentiating between viral and bacterial pharyngitis in children under age 15.[5]

Carriers

Social contacts are an important factor in the diagnosis. Healthy patients who had had contacts with persons with positively diagnosed streptococcal infections were found to have strep on culture in up to 25 percent of cases.[8]

MANAGEMENT

General measures

The administration of antibiotics to a patient with acute streptococcal pharyngitis shortens the duration of illness and improves symptoms, although it does not affect the natural history of the disease.[9] Antibiotic treatment does not appear to protect against the development of acute glomerulonephritis.[10] The strongest argument for the treatment of streptococcal pharyngitis has been the prevention of rheumatic fever.[11] Although uncommon, rheumatic fever still does occur; thus, streptococcal pharyngitis must be correctly managed.

Symptomatic Treatment

Symptomatic treatment should be offered to any patient with sore throat and may include fluids (cold or even iced, such as Popsicles), honey and lemon, hard candies to suck, acetaminophen for high fever or discomfort, and decongestant nose drops such as phenylephrine, oxymetazoline, and xylometazoline for 3 or 4 days for stuffy nose or sinus discomfort.

Penicillin

Specific treatment for presumed streptococcal infection is penicillin given as oral penicillin G 50 mg/day per kilogram of body weight in four divided doses for 10 days administered on an empty stomach or penicillin V 50 mg/day per kilogram of body weight in four divided doses for 10 days. In penicillin-sensitive individuals, give erythromycin 50 mg/day per kilogram of body weight in three

Table 13-1   Signs of Toxicity

High temperature (> 39°C)

Vomiting (more than twice)

Lethargy

Dysphagia even for fluids

"Sick" appearance

divided doses for 10 days. For children whose families have demonstrated poor compliance in the past or have been suspected of noncompliance in giving medication, intramuscular benzathine penicillin 600,000 units intramuscularly for children under 60 lb or 1.2 million units for older children or adults is recommended.[12]

Ampicillin has no place in the treatment of suspected streptococcal pharyngitis, particularly if there is a possibility of infectious mononucleosis. An interaction may occur between ampicillin and the autoimmune responses of infectious mononucleosis, resulting in a morbilliform rash. Confirmed or suspected streptococcal patients should be isolated for 24 hours after the start of appropriate penicillin therapy. Total compliance among ambulatory patients has been disappointingly low; if oral therapy is used, it should be accompanied by strongly reinforced explanations to patients and family, with close follow-up.

Some practitioners suggest follow-up cultures after treatment because of the relatively high rate of failure among patients in regard to compliance with therapy and to ensure that the treatment has been adequate.

Follow-up

Taking all this into account, we recommend a pragmatic regimen for dealing with sore throat.

PRAGMATIC REGIMEN

1   A toxic child with a sore throat should be given penicillin and symptomatic treatment without waiting for the results of a throat swab culture. If the child is not toxic and if culture service is readily available, do a throat swab and, while waiting for the results of a culture, initiate symptomatic treatment. If the culture is positive for strep, treat the patient with penicillin. If the culture is negative and the child is still not toxic, continue supportive therapy.[13] Signs of toxicity are described in Table 13-1.

Use of bacterial cultures

2   If culture service is not readily available, all children should receive symptomatic and supportive therapy, but only afebrile children who have not had prior antipyretic medication should be managed without antibiotics. This regimen will result in overuse of antibiotics, but it is warranted.[14]

3 SORE THROAT

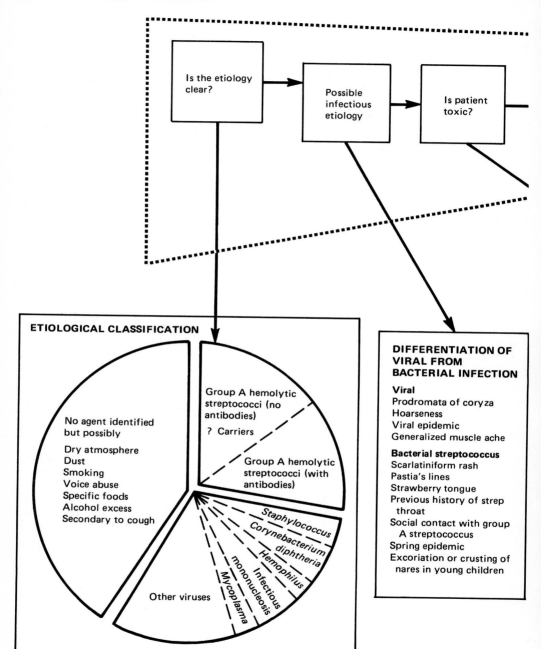

Is the etiology clear?

Possible infectious etiology

Is patient toxic?

ETIOLOGICAL CLASSIFICATION

No agent identified but possibly

Dry atmosphere
Dust
Smoking
Voice abuse
Specific foods
Alcohol excess
Secondary to cough

Group A hemolytic streptococci (no antibodies)

? Carriers

Group A hemolytic streptococci (with antibodies)

Staphylococcus
Corynebacterium diphtheria
Hemophilus
Infectious mononucleosis
Mycoplasma

Other viruses

DIFFERENTIATION OF VIRAL FROM BACTERIAL INFECTION

Viral
Prodromata of coryza
Hoarseness
Viral epidemic
Generalized muscle ache

Bacterial streptococcus
Scarlatiniform rash
Pastia's lines
Strawberry tongue
Previous history of strep throat
Social contact with group A streptococcus
Spring epidemic
Excoriation or crusting of nares in young children

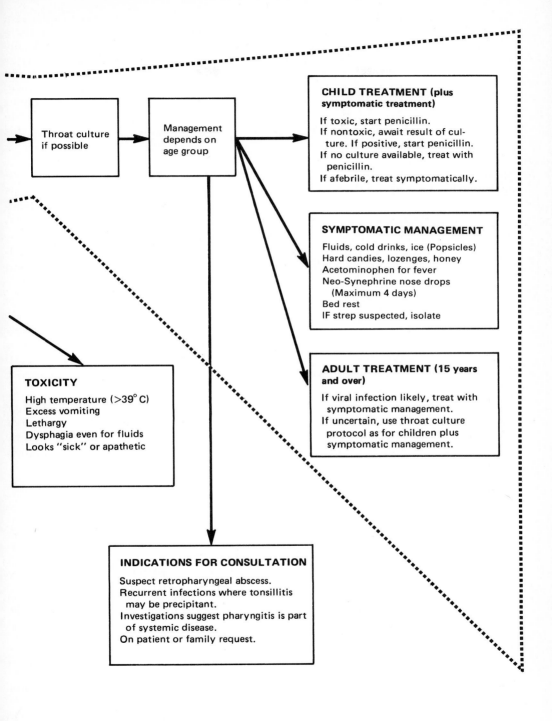

Throat culture if possible

Management depends on age group

CHILD TREATMENT (plus symptomatic treatment)

If toxic, start penicillin.
If nontoxic, await result of culture. If positive, start penicillin.
If no culture available, treat with penicillin.
If afebrile, treat symptomatically.

SYMPTOMATIC MANAGEMENT

Fluids, cold drinks, ice (Popsicles)
Hard candies, lozenges, honey
Acetaminophen for fever
Neo-Synephrine nose drops
  (Maximum 4 days)
Bed rest
IF strep suspected, isolate

ADULT TREATMENT (15 years and over)

If viral infection likely, treat with symptomatic management.
If uncertain, use throat culture protocol as for children plus symptomatic management.

TOXICITY

High temperature (>39° C)
Excess vomiting
Lethargy
Dysphagia even for fluids
Looks "sick" or apathetic

INDICATIONS FOR CONSULTATION

Suspect retropharyngeal abscess.
Recurrent infections where tonsillitis may be precipitant.
Investigations suggest pharyngitis is part of systemic disease.
On patient or family request.

Balancing risks of complications

3 For persons age 15 years and over, if symptoms such as a gradual prodrome with stuffy nose, coryza, generalized muscle aches and pains, and hoarseness are present, one can reasonably make a clinical diagnosis of viral infection. Adults have fewer risks than children for developing rheumatic fever from untreated streptococcal infection and greater risks of having adverse reactions to penicillin. Overall, it seems reasonable that if one cannot make a clinical diagnosis of viral infection, one should manage the adult in the same way as was recommended for children in this chapter.

Spotting an epidemic

Even when culture service is not readily available, a practitioner should send off cultures from three or four typical patients each week in order to determine the presence of a possible streptococcal epidemic in the community. When an epidemic seems evident (usually in the spring), overtreatment is usually justified.

Dry throat swabs taken at home by parents and mailed in adequately sealed envelopes can yield at least 80 percent accuracy and may be useful in isolated areas.[15]

Office cultures using blood agar plates and bacitracin sensitivity disks can be done for a few dollars.[16]

Finally, it is important to remember that many patients likely to have streptococcal infections never receive medical services. It is probably not an exaggeration to assume that there are some 10 persons at home with a sore throat for every 1 who presents to a doctor.

Treatment of the group A beta-hemolytic *Streptococcus* carrier state is a contentious issue. Beta-Lactamase-producing anaerobes may "shield" streptococci from the activity of penicillin, thereby contributing to their persistence. Thus, lindomycin and clindamycin are superior to penicillin in eradicating the "carrier state."[17]

REFERENCES

1 D. W. Marsland, M. Wood, F. Mayo, *Content of Family Practice: A Statewide Study in Virginia with Its Clinical, Educational, and Research Implications,* J. Geyman (ed.), Appleton-Century-Crofts, New York, 1976.

2 *Canadian Family Medicine,* sec. 6, "Presenting Symptoms and Problem Solving," The College of Family Physicians of Canada, 1974.

3 Faculty Survey, "Acute Sore Throat—Diagnosis and Treatment in General Practice," *Journal of the Royal College of General Practitioners,* **25**:126–132, 1975.

4 J. C. Shank and T. A. Powell, "A Five Year Experience with Throat Cultures," *Journal of Family Practice,* **18**(6):857–863, 1984.

5 A. Forsythe, "Selective Utilization of Clinical Diagnosis in the Treatment of Pharyngitis," *Journal of Family Practice,* **2**(3):173–177, 1975.

6 B. B. Breese and F. A. Disney, "The Accuracy of Diagnosis of B Hemolytic Streptococcal Infections on Clinical Grounds," *Pediatrics,* **44**:670–673, 1954.

7 L. H. Honikman, and B. F. Massell, "Guidelines for the Selective Use of

Throat Cultures in the Diagnosis of Streptococcal Respiratory Infection," *Pediatrics,* **48:**573–581, 1971.

8 K. Flicker, "Acute Pharyngitis—When to Treat," *Clinical Trends in Family Practice,* **5**(6):1–2, 1977.

9 C. B. Hall and B. B. Breese, "Does Penicillin Make Johnny's Strep Throat Better?" *Pediatric Infectious Disease,* **3**(1):7–9, 1984.

10 J. L. Taylor and G. R. Haire, "Antibiotics, Sore Throats and Acute Nephritis," *Journal of the Royal College of General Practitioners,* **33:**783–786, 1983.

11 R. Lave and J. R. Hodges, "Early Treatment of Streptococcal Pharyngitis," *Annals of Emergency Medicine,* June 1984, pp. 440–448.

12 M. Markowitz and L. Gordia, *Rheumatic Fever,* 2d ed., American Heart Association, Committee Report on Prevention of Rheumatic Fever, W.B. Saunders, Philadelphia, 1973.

13 S. M. Bell and D. Smith, "Quantitative Throat Swab Culture in the Diagnosis of Streptococcal Pharyngitis in Children," *Lancet,* **ii:**61–63, 1976.

14 E. A. Mortimer and B. Boxerbau, "Diagnosis and Treatment: Group A Streptococcal Infections," *Pediatrics,* **36:**930–932, 1965.

15 H. Jackson, J. Cooper, W. J. Mellinger, and A. R. Olson, "Streptococcal Pharyngitis in Rural Practice," *Journal of the American Medical Association,* **197:**385–388, 1966.

16 H. L. Moffet, et al., "Group A Streptococcal Infections in Children's Home. I: Evaluation of Practical Bacteriologic Methods," *Pediatrics,* **33:**5–10, 1964.

17 I. Brooke, "Treatment of Group A Streptococcal Pharyngtonsillitis," *Journal of the American Medical Association,* **247:**2496, 1982.

Chapter 14

Detection of Chronic Disabilities in Children: Communication Disorders

M. Seitz, Ph.D.
B. Seitz, M.A.
B. K. Hennen, M.D.

This chapter provides the physician with guidelines for identifying young patients at risk for chronic disabilities in general and more specifically for recognizing the early signals of communication disorders and initiating assessment and management appropriately.

Many children have chronic physical or mental disorders. Problems due to rubella, Down's syndrome, or a neural tube defect or other inherited genetic disorder can be anticipated or recognized prenatally. Others become known at birth or are caused by complications of birth that result from anoxia, conditions generally associated with a low Apgar score, and/or prematurity. Still other disorders become apparent only as the child matures beyond infancy; these include many hearing, language, and learning disorders as well as behavior problems. Finally, some disorders are acquired postnatally because of disease or accident. These acquired disorders may be acute, as in the case of a head injury or central nervous system infection, or slowly disabling, as in the case of diabetes or asthma.

Faced with such a variety of chronic disorders, how can the family physician best prepare for early identification and appropriate treatment? In this chapter, we propose a general approach that makes the most of available information and enables the physician to organize practice time more efficiently.

The first section presents a six-point plan for the early identification, assessment, and management of chronic disorders in children. The second section describes a group of chronic problems that are difficult to diagnose and treat: disorders of hearing and speech. These disorders are dealt with in some detail, and an attempt is made to demonstrate how the use of the suggested plan can facilitate their treatment. Chapter 10 suggested how to assess the resources of families with chronically disabled children and discussed the interactions between such families and the family physician.

EARLY IDENTIFICATION, ASSESSMENT, AND MANAGEMENT OF CHRONIC PHYSICAL OR MENTAL DISORDERS IN CHILDREN

Our plan contains six points designed to optimize the family physician's efforts in caring for children with chronic disorders (Table 14-1). Each point will be discussed in some detail to demonstrate how it can be beneficial to family management.

REVIEW OF THE PLAN

Prenatal and Birth History

A good case history and accurate case records are essential for long-term care. Thus, the first step in the identification of potential or real chronic disorders is to obtain an accurate prenatal and birth history. Any family history of potential hereditary or congenital problems should be specifically noted at this time.

    Factors that may affect the unborn child to the extent that he or she will be at risk for the development of a chronic disorder should also be carefully noted. The general course of the pregnancy and specific details of the labor and delivery process should become part of the child's health record so that potential problems can be carefully monitored later.

Accurate records

Include risk factors

At-Risk Factors

Table 14-2 lists conditions that in our opinion would put a child at risk for chronic disabilities. The list includes medical, genetic, and social conditions that have been found to cause or to be associated with chronic disabilities. It is by no means complete, but it indicates the broad range of problems that can adversely affect a young child's development and learning. It is wise to clearly mark the file of any child found to be at risk for one or more of the risk factors listed in this table so that the child can be observed more closely during early development for signs of chronic problems. A file marked in such a manner will alert the doctor to investigate more closely any deviance in development noted when the child is seen in the office. Inherited problems or syndromes such as Waardenburg's syndrome, Treacher Collins syndrome, and albinism are rarely seen in family practice but obviously do occur and must be considered.

Broad range of risks

Flag the record

Table 14-1   Early Identification, Accurate Assessment, and Management of Chronic Physical or Mental Disorders in Children

1   Obtain an accurate and thorough prenatal and birth history.
2   Put an at-risk indicator on the records of children who may be susceptible to developmental disorders or chronic disabilities.
3   Keep an accurate and up-to-date set of developmental norms for comparison purposes.
4   Emphasize the doctor-parent or doctor-child interview and the examination.
5   Use in-office screening procedures efficiently.
6   Develop an appropriate cadre of medical and nonmedical consulting resources.

Table 14-2   Causes and Conditions Associated with Children with Chronic Disorders

Prenatal conditions	Anoxia
	Rubella
	Other viral infections during pregnancy
	Ototoxic drugs
	Other drugs
	Fever
	Bleeding during pregnancy
	Potential genetic problems indicated by family history
	Any form of overindulgence by the mother, such as drugs and alcohol
Natal conditions	Birth trauma
	Hyperbilirubinemia
	Anoxia
	Apgar score lower than 5
	Birth weight less than 1500 g
	Prematurity
	Observable structural defects
Postnatal conditions	Viral diseases
	Meningitis
	Recurrent otitis media
	Ototoxic drugs
	Extreme noise
	Cerebral palsy
	High fever
	Convulsions
	Epilepsy
	Trauma, including burns
Social problems	Child abuse
	Inadequate parenting
	Isolation
	Large families with low income
	Excessive use of alcohol or drugs by one or both parents

Developmental Norms

The next task is to determine whether an at-risk infant is developing normally. All potential chronic problems must be viewed in
the context of what is normal. To facilitate judgments of normal
child development, physicians should have available in the office
some list of developmental norms, such as the Denver developmental tables.[1] These norms provide useful data about the physical, social, and behavioral landmarks of children by chronological
age. They provide physicians not only with an estimate of the patient's overall development but also with an indication of specific
areas of weakness, whether social, emotional, or physical.

Comparative
tables useful

The Interview and Examination

When assessing infants and young children, three main general
sources of information are available: (1) the child's birth and medical history, (2) age-specific developmental norms, and (3) the par-
ent-doctor or patient-doctor interview and examination. While
there are exceptions, the majority of parents are reliable observers
of their children's behavior. Their fears are often justified; they are
always real. However, parental observations may be affected by
fear, guilt, or anxiety about the child as well as about possible mistakes the parents may be making in raising the child.

Information
available

Parents are
good observers

The doctor must determine early whether parents' concern
about the child warrants immediate investigation as opposed to observation over time. This first decision is often the most critical
one; too often, it is made without sufficient investigation because
of time pressures in the practice setting.

Deciding when
to act

Office Screening Procedures

It is essential that potential problems be identified as early as possible and that an accurate assessment be made of disabilities which
are not always obvious. Physicians are not always aware of the extent to which early detection and management can result in successful and shortened treatment.

Early detection

Generally, the best screening tools are the patient's case history,
a record of updated developmental landmarks, and a careful and
accurate interview. However, screening tests are available to help
the physician make a more accurate diagnosis and referral if necessary. The Denver Developmental Screening Test (DDST) from
Mead-Johnson Laboratories[1] contains over 100 simple age-related
tests, and a child can be evaluated on approximately 20 of these
tests during one visit. The time required to administer the DDST
is about 15 to 20 minutes. The DDST evaluates not only gross motor skills but also fine motor skills and personal social areas.

A good
screening test

External Consulting Resources

The very nature of chronic developmental disorders often makes them hard to identify. Moreover, the diagnostic procedure, as well as the management, is often time-consuming and requires the help of outside consultants, both medical and nonmedical.

Medical and nonmedical consultants

Most doctors are aware of the availability of medical consultants. However, many of them overlook the nonmedical resource professionals who can help children with chronic disorders. Among these professionals are the following:

1   Clinical psychologist
2   Social worker
3   Community health nurse
4   Classroom teacher
5   Physical therapist
6   Speech–language pathologist
7   Audiologist
8   Educational psychologist
9   Special education teacher
10 Nutritionist
11 Prosthetic specialist
12 Guidance counselor
13 Occupational therapist
14 Teacher of the deaf
15 Dentist

Identifying available help

Such professionals can be found in local clinics, hospitals, schools, and workshops. The single best source of information about them is probably the social worker or the local office of community or public health. It is wise to keep a list of these local nonmedical resources for speedy referral and to remember that many of these professionals have heavy workloads so that scheduling an appointment for a patient may take a month or two.

COMMUNICATION DISORDERS IN CHILDREN: AN EXAMPLE OF A COMMON CHRONIC DISABILITY

Communication disorders were selected as an example to demonstrate the use of our plan. They have a relatively high incidence and often go unrecognized in the general population. It is estimated that hearing and speech problems that require professional treatment are present in 10 to 15 percent of the U.S. population.[2-4]

Disorders are common

These percentages break down in the following manner. Approximately 1 percent of the general population have profound hearing impairment, 5 percent have a hearing loss severe enough to need professional help, and another 7 percent have speech-related handicaps that require special treatment. Consequently, in any general patient population, the family physician can expect that about 10 percent of patients under 12 years of age will have a communication disorder requiring some form of diagnosis and treatment. Practices that have a high percentage of children and those which are situated in poorer socioeconomic areas may have even larger proportions of affected children, and their problems may be of greater severity.

Another reason for choosing communication disorders as an example is that slower than normal speech and language development is often one of the first identifiable symptoms of a broader underlying pathology. For example, a child who can hear but is slow in speaking and seems unable to understand simple requests may have some form of mental retardation, a child who speaks slowly and with effort may be exhibiting some form of dysarthria indicative of lower motor neuron disease, a child whose voice quality is hypernasal may have a submucous cleft or some form of soft palate dysfunction, and a child who is not responsive but is hyperactive and tends to act out may have a hearing loss or a neurological disorder. These are examples of cases in which awareness of speech and hearing development can help in the diagnosis of underlying medical problems.

Underlying pathology

Before discussing our plan in greater detail, we shall outline some basic information about speech and hearing disorders which will help family physicians in their assessment.

OVERVIEW OF DISORDERS

Hearing Disorders

Hearing disorders can be classified into three different types: (1) conductive loss caused by problems in the outer or middle ear, such as otitis media, (2) a sensorineural loss that affects frequency-specific areas of the cochlea, and (3) mixed hearing loss caused by malfunctioning of both the middle ear and the inner ear.

Hearing loss may affect one or both ears and may be continuous or intermittent. Regardless of the type or cause, early hearing loss, even of an intermittent type, can be detrimental to a child's language and learning abilities. If not diagnosed and treated early, hearing-impaired children may also develop behavioral or social problems.

Effects of undetected hearing loss

Speech Disorders

Speech disorders, which are not necessarily related to hearing impairment, can be divided into four basic types.

1 *Language and language-related disorders*: These disorders affect the way in which a child produces sentences or a child's language-generating capacity. Approximately 15 to 20 percent of the speech-disordered population will have language-related disorders.[3] These disorders are often of a more severe nature as they have a direct effect on the rate at which the child learns language. They may also be precursors of later learning difficulties such as dyslexia.

Words should be complete by age 3

2 *Articulation problems*: These disorders affect the child's articulation pattern, e.g., the way the child produces the sounds of speech, and thus interrupt or distort the formation of words. Articulation disorders constitute about 75 percent of all speech disorders.[3] As a normal child matures, he or she learns the sound system of the native language in the following manner. First, the child learns the vowels and those consonants which are produced by movement of the lips and the tongue and the lips. Some speech sounds, such as "s," "r," and "l," take longer to master than others. As the child learns to speak in syllables and words, there is an initial tendency to leave off word endings. It is important to note that this pattern of not completing words should not continue beyond age 3 years. In fact, a child who has multiple articulation problems, e.g., problems with two or more different speech sounds, after age 4 or 5 has a speech problem serious enough to warrant referral for a thorough speech and language evaluation.

Hoarseness

Nasal tone changes

3 *Voice disorders*: These disorders affect the vocal quality of the child's speech. Approximately 5 to 8 percent of speech-disordered children have voice-related disorders.[3] These range from vocal quality disorders such as the hoarse, harsh voice that sometimes accompanies or results from an upper respiratory infection to voices that are hypernasal (perhaps from soft palate insufficiency or a submucous cleft), hyponasal (resulting, for example, from enlarged tonsils or adenoids caused by chronic infection), or either too loud or too soft. Many of these vocal problems are associated with definite organic pathologies that require medical attention. Others are functional and, if not quickly self-correcting, will require special assessment and management. Most children with voice problems can benefit from voice therapy administered by a trained speech–language pathologist. Often therapy is needed to establish new and correct vocal habits and thus prevent chronic recurrence of the voice problem.

Stuttering

4 *Rate disorders*: These disorders are associated with the child's rate of speech and are more commonly known as stuttering or cluttering. They constitute about 5 to 8 percent of all speech problems. They may also be related to the organization of the flow of speech. Generally speaking, rate disorders are not amenable to medical treatment and are better treated by a speech–language pathologist or psychologist.

Other problems, such as cleft palate, cerebral palsy, anoxia, and rubella, also may be associated with hearing, speech, and language disorders, but these disorders will fit adequately into the classification given. For example, a child with cerebral palsy may have problems that include all four types of speech disorders discussed above.

Social and environmental factors also can contribute to communication problems in a young child. For example, alcoholism or drug addiction in one or both parents, isolation of a child from social contact, child abuse, and less obvious kinds of psychological or emotional disorders can profoundly affect a child's ability to learn language and/or desire to communicate.

Social causes

Early detection and management of chronic disorders can result in successful and often shorter treatment. Often the type of treatment needed is not medical but psychoeducational. This is the case for chronic disorders of hearing or speech, which are often better treated by qualified speech pathologists and audiologists than by physicians.

USING THE PLAN

We shall now show how our suggested plan (Table 14-1) can be used to provide efficient, early diagnosis and treatment of potential communication disorders in children.

Use of Birth History Information as an Indicator of Potential Problems

One of the first indicators of a potential chronic problem in a child may come from the birth history. If the birth record indicates that a child has one or more at-risk factors (see Table 14-2), the child may be significantly slower than normal children in developing language skills,[5] run a significantly higher risk of having a hearing disorder,[2] or experience significant learning delays later in life.[4]

Problems that can potentially affect speech and language include craniofacial anomalies such as cleft lip or cleft palate or both, Down's syndrome, metabolic abnormalities, and spina bifida. Prenatal use of ototoxic drugs by the mother or any history of diseases such as rubella, genital herpes, and other viral illnesses during pregnancy should also be noted since the fetus may have been affected by such conditions.

Use of Risk Factors to Identify Potentially Susceptible Children

The risk factors noted in Table 14-2 are not equal predictors of a child's susceptibility to developmental disorders. For example, the following subset of factors has been found to predict hearing disorders with greater accuracy: (1) family member with congenital sensorineural hearing loss (in first cousins or closer), (2) bilirubin levels greater than 20 mg per milliliter of serum, (3) congenital

Major risk factors

rubella, (4) defects of the ear, nose, or throat on routine physical examination, (5) birth weight less than 1500 g, and (6) chronic otitis media. [2,4,6,7]

Newborn hearing screening

In order for language and speech to develop normally, a child must have, among other things, adequate hearing, especially during the first 2 years of life. Recent research has indicated that one of the risk factors listed above was present in over 70 percent of children found to have severe hearing loss. In many hospitals in North America, newborn hearing screening programs have been established that use the first five of these six risk factors.[2,6] Although newborn screening programs are of great assistance in the early identification of profound hearing loss, many children are still missed. Unless family physicians become aware of the early signs of hearing loss, many affected children may well go undiagnosed and untreated for 2 years or more.

Many children develop chronic otitis media during the first 2 years of life; if not treated, this can cause later language and hearing delays.[4,8,9] Two recent studies [5,9] have demonstrated that children found to be at risk at birth are significantly slower in developing a broad range of language, cognitive, and motor skills. This in time affects their overall ability to perform both in and out of school.

Use of Normative Data for Early Assessment of Children

Child will not grow out of it

The physician who lacks knowledge of developmental norms will not understand the implications of parents' statements about their children, for example, "She doesn't seem to listen to me," "He doesn't talk as much as his brother," or "He is hard to understand." For the doctor to advise that the child will grow out of it or to say, "We'll check it again in 6 months," may mean that the opportunity for an accurate early assessment has been lost. It may also delay the start of a valuable early intervention.

Reference norms

When dealing with communication disorders, it is wise to refer to a set of norms that specifically define normal speech and hearing development in addition to using the general physical norms and landmarks. Norms that include data on speech and hearing can be found in Lillywhite,[10] Gesell and Amatruda,[11] Berry,[12] and Bzoch and League.[13] We have included as Table 14-3 a set of norms based on a chart prepared in the United States by the National Institute of Neurological Diseases and Stroke. The questions in the table are organized around general communication milestones and are designed to help the physician obtain answers from the parents that can be compared with the norms.

In-depth assessment

If the responses to such questions indicate problems, the next step is to begin an in-depth assessment, which may include screen-

Table 14-3 Landmarks to Use with the "Slow-To-Talk" Child

Average age	Questions	Average behavior
3 to 6 months	What does the child do when you talk to him or her?	The child awakens or quiets to the sound of the mother's voice.
	Does the child react to your voice when unable to see you?	The child typically turns the eyes and head toward the source of the sound.
7 to 10 months	When unable to see what is happening, what does the child do when he or she hears such things as familiar footsteps, the dog barking, the telephone ringing, candy paper rattling, or someone's voice?	The child turns the head and shoulders toward familiar sounds even when unable to see what is happening. Such sounds do not have to be loud to cause a response.
11 to 15 months	Can the child point to or find familiar objects or people when asked to? Examples: "Where is Jimmy?" "Find the ball."	The child shows an understanding of some words by appropriate behavior, for example, pointing to or looking at familiar objects or people on request.
	Does the child respond differently to different sounds?	The child jabbers in response to a human voice, is apt to cry when there is thunder, or may frown when scolded.
	Does the child enjoy listening to some sounds and imitating them?	Imitation indicates that the child can hear the sounds and match them with his or her own sound.
1½ years	Can the child point to parts of his or her body when asked to? Examples: "Show me your eyes," "Show me your nose."	Some children begin to identify parts of the body. The child should be able to show his or her nose or eyes.
	How many understandable words does the child use—words you are sure really mean something?	The child should be using a few single words. They are not complete or pronounced perfectly but are clearly meaningful.
2 years	Can the child follow simple verbal commands when you are careful not to give any help, such as looking at the object or pointing in the right direction? Example: "Johnny, get your hat and give it to Daddy."	The child should be able to follow simple commands without visual clues.
	Does the child enjoy being read to and points out pictures of familiar objects in a book when asked to? Example: "Show me the baby."	Most 2-year-old children enjoy being read to and shown simple pictures in a book or magazine and will point out pictures when asked to.
	Does the child use the names of familiar people and things such as "Mommy," "milk," "ball"?	The child should be using a variety of everyday words heard in the home and neighborhood.
	What does the child call himself or herself?	The child refers to himself or herself by name.

Table 14-3 Continued

Average age	Questions	Average behavior
2 years	Is the child beginning to show interest in the sound of radio or TV commercials?	Many 2-year-old children do show such interest, by word or action.
	Is the child putting a few words together to make little "sentences"?	These "sentences" are not usually complete or grammatically correct.
2½ years	Does the child know a few rhymes or songs and enjoy hearing them?	Many children can say or sing short rhymes or songs and enjoy listening to records or to parents singing.
	What does the child do when the ice cream vendor's bell rings out of sight or when a car door closes at a time when someone in the family usually comes home?	If a child has good hearing and these are events that bring pleasure, he or she usually reacts to the sound by running to look or telling someone what is heard.
3 years	Can the child show an understanding of the meaning of some words besides the names of things? Examples: "Make the car go," "Give me the ball."	The child should be able to understand and use simple verbs, pronouns, prepositions, and adjectives such as "go," "me," "in," and "big."
	Can the child find you when you call from another room?	The child should be able to locate the source of the sound.
	Does the child sometimes use complete sentences?	The child should be using complete sentences some of the time.
4 years	Can the child tell about events that have happened recently?	The child should be able to give a connected account of some recent experience.
	Can the child carry out two directions, one after the other? Example: "Bobby, find Susie and tell her dinner's ready."	The child should be able to carry out a sequence of two simple directions.
5 years	Do neighbors and others outside the family understand most of what the child says?	The child's speech should be intelligible, although some sounds may still be mispronounced.
	Can the child carry on a conversation with other children or familiar grown-ups?	Most children can carry on a conversation if the vocabulary is within their experience.
	Does the child begin a sentence with "I" instead of "me" and "he" or "she" instead of "him" and "her"?	Some pronouns should be used correctly.
	Is the child's grammar almost as good as that of the parents?	Most of the time the child should match the patterns of grammar used by the adults of the family and neighborhood.

Source: Modified from *Patient Care*, November 1, 1974. Based on *Learning to Talk*, National Institutes of Neurological Disease and Stroke, National Institutes of Health, Bethesda, Md. 20014.

ing tests that can be given in the office as well as more extensive use of developmental age norms. The individual physician's expertise and skill in the problem area under consideration should be the deciding factor in determining how far the investigation should go. If the doctor's knowledge is limited, he or she should ask for help at an early stage. If, however, the doctor possesses the particular interests and skills required, he or she may proceed further without consultation.

Use of Doctor-Parent and Doctor-Child Interviews during the Office Examination

No one is likely to argue with the statement that the examination and the concurrent doctor-parent interview constitute the most important part of any diagnostic and treatment process.

Many chronic problems in infants, particularly communication disorders, are difficult to assess accurately for the simple reason that very young children won't talk or communicate in the doctor's office. Perhaps the best approach is to try to put the parents at ease by paying close attention to their observations about the child and then asking a series of nonthreatening, nonblaming questions. A good opening question may be, How does your child make his or her needs known to you?

A gentle approach

Detailed examples of such questions can be found in an excellent article by Cantor et al.[14] Some of the questions Cantor suggests include the following. "Does your youngster stop crying when you start to talk?" (If not, suspect hearing or behavioral problems.) "Does your child cry at sudden loud noises?" (If not, suspect hearing loss.) "Does your child look at you when you speak?" (If not, suspect hearing loss or emotional disorders.) "Does your child seem to understand and yet produce little or no speech?" (If so, suspect developmental delay of some form.) "Does your child try to talk back when you talk to him?" (If not, suspect either hearing loss or developmental delay.) "Is the child uncomprehending and deficient in both oral and gestural language?" (If so, suspect retardation.) The doctor can easily ask questions like these in the office.

Useful questions

Use of In-Office Screening Procedures for Hearing and Speech Disorders

Screening for hearing loss in a young child may present a particularly difficult problem for the family physician. It is virtually impossible to determine by office screening procedures alone whether a child under 9 months of age has a hearing loss. In addition, physicians may place too much faith in currently used screening procedures, which are coarse at best. Informal screening

Office hearing tests have limitations

procedures such as the use of tuning forks, noisemakers, or variations in speech intensity may be sufficient for detecting fairly severe hearing losses in older children. However, a child with a moderate to severe conduction (middle-ear pathology) hearing loss that affects all frequencies more or less equally may not respond to these informal tests. A child with a high-frequency hearing loss may respond to the low tones of the human voice or to 256- and 512-Hz tuning forks but may be unable to hear 1024- or 2048-Hz tuning forks. Such a child may be able to hear the vowel sounds of speech but may miss many consonants, such as "s," "sh," "th," and "h."

An additional weakness of tuning fork tests given in the office is that the doctor cannot control either the intensity levels of the tuning forks or the ambient background noise. A tuning fork does not measure acuity; it indicates the site of the lesion. Office noise alone can often mask a suspected hearing loss entirely or make a moderate hearing loss appear to be more severe than it actually is. In general, if a hearing loss is suspected from behavioral data or informal screening tests, an early referral for audiological assessment should be made.

Better, earlier screening is coming

Physicians are not always aware of the extent to which new methods of early detection and management can result in successful and often shorter treatment.[15] In fact, new brainstem-evoked response audiometric (BERA) techniques [16,17] make it possible to obtain an accurate assessment of even a newborn's hearing. These procedures will soon be available in most large audiological clinics.

If behavioral social clues are present, refer

Even without BERA, audiologists can now obtain very accurate estimates of hearing thresholds in children as young as 6 months.[18] Therefore, there is little reason for delay in sending an infant for a hearing evaluation if hearing loss is suspected.

Often the type of treatment needed for hearing disorders is not medical but psychoeducational or audiological. When properly fitted hearing aids are supplied or programs of aural habilitation are begun at an early age, children with hearing loss can often go to a regular school to receive an education with their peers. With early treatment, such children need not become a burden to their families or to society in general.

Review of Screening Tests   Some screening tests are available to help the physician make a more accurate diagnosis and referral if necessary, among them the Denver Developmental Screening Test.

More specific screening tests

Even more specific tests may be employed for the diagnosis of suspected speech disorders. Two such tests are the Denver Articulation Screening Exam (DASE) (Mead-Johnson Laboratories)[19] and the Physician's Developmental Quick Screen for Speech Disorders (PDQ).[20]

These tests can be administered by the physician or by trained aides and can be very helpful in determining the existence of a developmental disorder that requires further investigation or referral. The DASE was specifically designed for use by physicians and others who work with children and who may not be familiar with speech development.[19] It is designed to differentiate between normal speech and significant speech delay as well as to help identify such related deviant conditions as hypernasality and hyponasality, lateral lisp, and the presence of tongue thrust.

The Developmental Quick Screen for Speech Disorders (PDQ)[20] was also designed for use by the physician. It covers five areas of speech: language, articulation, voice, speech rate or rhythm, and general structure and function of the speaking mechanism. The test contains 10 separate age-related forms for children 6 months to 6 years, each of which has its own constructions and age norms.

The College of Family Physicians of Canada recently completed a study, using its nationally distributed sentinel practices, to assess the value of a kit for the screening of hearing disorders in office practice.[21]

All these tests were designed with the medical practitioner in mind. By themselves they do not constitute definite diagnostic information. Rather, they provide a data base to help the physician determine the existence or severity of potential communication disorders. If the child is found to be within normal limits, further action may not be warranted. If, however, the child fails the screening test, the doctor should refer the child for a more complete speech and language or hearing diagnosis by a speech pathologist.

Nonmedical Referral Resources for Assessment and Treatment of Communication Disorders

The very nature of communication disorders frequently makes them hard to identify. Often the diagnostic procedure is time-consuming and requires the help of outside consultants, both medical and nonmedical. Nonmedical professionals who can help children with communication and learning disorders include the following:

Speech and hearing consultants

Speech and language pathologist
Audiologist
Oral rehabilitation specialist
Teacher of the deaf
Educational psychologist
Clinical psychologist
Special education teacher
Social worker

Table 14-4   Twenty Conditions That Signal Referral for Hearing, Speech, and Language Evaluation

1   The child is not producing intelligible speech by age 2.
2   Speech is largely unintelligible after age 3.
3   There are many missing initial consonants after age 3.
4   There are no sentences by age 3.
5   Sounds are more than a year late in appearing according to the expected developmental sequence.
6   There is an excessive amount of indiscriminate, irrelevant verbalizing after 18 months.
7   There is consistent and frequent omission of initial consonants at any age.
8   There are many substitutions of easy sounds for difficult ones after age 5.
9   The amount of vocalizing decreases rather than steadily increases at any period up to age 7.
10 The child uses mostly vowel sounds in his or her speech at any age after 1 year.
11 Word endings are consistently dropped after age 5.
12 Sentence structure is consistently faulty after age 5.
13 The child is disturbed by his or her speech at any age.
14 The child is noticeably nonfluent (stuttering after age 5).
15 The child is distorting, omitting, or substituting any sounds after age 7.
16 The voice is a monotone, extremely loud, largely inaudible, or of poor quality.
17 The pitch is not appropriate to the child's age and sex.
18 There is hypernasality or lack of nasal resonance.
19 There are unusual confusions, reversals, or telescoping in connected speech.
20 There is abnormal rhythm, rate, or inflection after age 5.

Deciding when to refer

These nonmedical professionals can offer help in the diagnosis of communication disorders as well as provide treatment programs for children. The younger the child is when referred for diagnosis and management of a communication disorder, the better the chance for normal growth and development of listening, speaking, and learning skills. The problem facing the physician is to decide when to refer for a consultation on a potential communication disorder. Lillywhite[22] has developed a list of 20 conditions (Table 14-4) that signal the need for a consultation.

REFERENCES

1   W. Frankenburg, J. Dodds, and A. Fandell, *1970 Denver Developmental Screening Test,* University of Colorado Medical Center. Available through Mead-Johnson Laboratories, Evansville, Ind.
2   M. P. Downs, "Early Identification of Hearing Loss: Where Are We? Where Do We Go from Here?" in G. T. Mencher (ed.), *Early Identification of Hearing Loss,* Karger, Basel, Switzerland, 1976, pp. 14–22.
3   W. H. Perkins, *Speech Pathology—An Applied Behavioral Science.* C. B. Murphy, St. Louis, 1977.

4 M. P. Downs, "The Expanding Imperatives of Early Identification," in F. Bess, *Childhood Deafness*, Grune & Stratton, New York, 1977.

5 J. Zarin-Ackerman, M. Lewis, and J. Driscoll, Jr., "Language Development in 2-Year-Old Normal and Risk Infants," *Pediatrics*, **59** (Neonatology Supplement): 982–986, 1977.

6 G. T. Mencher, J. T. Jacobson, M. R. Seitz, "Identifying Deafness in the Newborn," *Journal of Otolaryngology*, **7**:490–499, 1978.

7 S. E. Gerber and G. T. Mencher (eds.), *Early Diagnosis of Hearing Loss*, Grune & Stratton, New York, 1978.

8 V. A. Holm and L. H. Kunze, "Effect of Chronic Otitis Media on Language and Speech Development," *Pediatrics*, **43**:833–839, 1969.

9 B. J. McCulloch, S. L. Steck, and G. T. Mencher, "The University of Nebraska Neonatal Hearing Project—One Year Later," in G. T. Mencher (ed.), *Early Identification of Hearing Loss*, Karger, Basel, 1976, pp. 143–155.

10 H. Lillywhite, "Doctor's Manual of Speech Disorders," *Journal of the American Medical Association*, **167**:850–858, 1958.

11 A. L. Gesell and C. S. Amatruda, *Developmental Diagnosis: Normal and Abnormal Child Development*, Harper and Row, New York, 1965.

12 M. Berry, *Language Disorders of Children: The Bases and Diagnosis*, Prentice Hall, Englewood Cliffs, N.J., 1969.

13 K. R. Bzoch and R. League, *Receptive-Expressive Emergent Language Scale*, Tree of Life Press, Florida, 1970.

14 H. E. Cantor, R. L. Levee, L. J. Rutledge, W. S. Yancy and A. Zaner, "Why Isn't My Child Talking Right?" *Patient Care*, **8**:212–240, 1974.

15 J. A. Browder, R. B. Hood, and L. E. Lamb, "The Physician and the Child with Hearing Impairment: Guide to Early Recognition and Management," *Rocky Mountain Medical Journal*, **70**:42–46, 1973.

16 T. W. Picton and A. D. Smith, "The Practice of Evoked Potential Audiometry," *Otolaryngologic Clinics of North America*, **11**(2):263–282, 1978.

17 B. Mokotoff, C. Schulmann-Galambos, and R. Galambos, "Brain Stem Auditory Evoked Responses in Children," *Archives of Otolaryngology*, **103**:38–43, 1977.

18 "Life with a Brain Damaged Child," *The New York Times*, March 23, 1973.

19 A. F. Drumwright, *1971 Denver Articulation Screening Exam*, University of Colorado Medical Center. Available through Mead-Johnson Laboratories, Evansville, Ind.

20 S. Kuleg and K. Baker, *The Physician's Developmental Quick Screen for Speech Disorders (PDQ)*, University of Texas Medical Branch, Department of Pediatrics, Galveston, 1973.

21 Childhood Hearing Impairment, National Task Force on Childhood Hearing Impairment, College of Family Physicians of Canada, December, 1984.

22 H. Lillywhite, "Speech and Language Development and Disorders," in W. E. Nelson, V. C. Vaughan, and R. J. McKay (eds.), *Textbook of Pediatrics*, 10th ed., W. B. Saunders, Philadelphia, 1975, pp. 104–107.

Chapter 15

Dental Problems in Family Practice

A. E. MacLeod, D.D.S.

PRINCIPLE

Most physicians have relatively easy access to dental services. This is fortunate, since the training of family doctors in dental problems is, to say the least, deficient. This chapter does not give an exhaustive account of all the dental problems a family practitioner is likely to encounter but instead touches on the more common conditions and provides basic managerial advice.

The family practitioner should gain some practical instruction in common dental procedures before setting up practice. The chapter begins by describing the dental consequences of medical treatment, then discusses some common dental problems in office practice, and concludes with general comments on preventive dentistry and patient education.

MEDICAL TREATMENT AND DENTAL CONSEQUENCES

Drug Therapy

Before initiating treatment, most dentists ask patients whether they are taking medication. The purpose is to avoid possible interactions with drugs that dentists commonly use. If a physician knows that a patient on medication is planning a visit to a dentist, he or she should make sure that the dentist has been informed about the medications.

Anticoagulants can complicate routine oral surgery. Patients on *antihypertensive* agents who receive local anesthesia containing epinephrine risk cardiac stress. Similarly, the relatively rare use of *monoamine oxidase–inhibiting* drugs in managing depression can be seriously interfered with by epinephrine. Patients on *long-term sedation* do not normally present a problem; however, a dentist may contribute to the cumulative effect of their medication by unwittingly prescribing additional sedatives before treatment. This is particularly a problem in the elderly. With prior information, these interactions can be avoided.[1]

Drug interaction with dental medication

Tetracycline Pigmentation

The administration of tetracycline to children results in gray-black pigmentation of their permanent teeth. This pigmentation is irreversible (Figures 15-1 and 15-2). The most susceptible years for tetracycline pigmentation in a child's development are from birth to age 8 years, when the anterior permanent teeth are being formed. From 8 to 12 years, tetracycline also causes pigmentation. However, the affected teeth are toward the rear of the mouth and are much less noticeable. It is helpful, therefore, to select an alternative antibiotic when treating children in the age groups that have a high risk for pigmentation.

Dental side effects of drugs

Dental Problems in Pregnancy

Dentists today scoff at the legend that mothers lose a tooth for every child born. There is, however, some truth in the notion, since pregnancy is a time of risk for dental problems. Pregnant woman usually manifest a higher than normal rate of decay and periodontal (gum) inflammation (see the section "Swelling in the Mouth" in this chapter). The causes of these problems, which appear to be associated solely with pregnancy, are an increasing basal metabolic rate and endocrine function and a tendency to satisfy hunger between normal mealtimes with refined carbohydrate foodstuffs. Good oral hygiene is therefore of prime importance for pregnant women.

Dental risks to fetus

Pacemakers

Patients with pacemakers present an unusual problem in the dental office. The current inducted into the body of such patients by an

Pacemaker advice

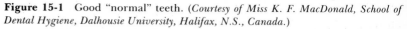

Figure 15-1 Good "normal" teeth. (*Courtesy of Miss K. F. MacDonald, School of Dental Hygiene, Dalhousie University, Halifax, N.S., Canada.*)

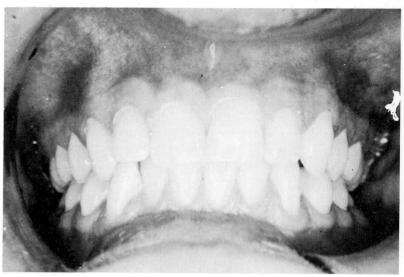

Figure 15-2 Teenager's teeth, pigmented by tetracycline. (*Courtesy of Dr. D. P. Cunningham, Dental Faculty, Dalhousie University, Halifax, N.S., Canada.*)

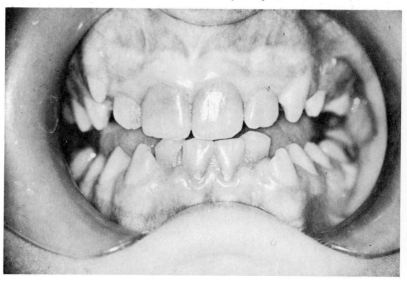

electrosurgical tissue-cutting instrument is potentially dangerous since it may shut down a pacemaker or interfere with its rhythm. Accordingly, when pacemaker patients are referred, dentists should be advised, and patients should be aware of the risk of treatment involving electrosurgery, ultrasonic scaling instruments, ultrasonic cleaners, and even the old-style (arcing) belt-driven handpiece drills.

Bacterial Endocarditis

Bacteremia is the link between dental treatment and bacterial endocarditis. Tooth extraction is the most obvious dental cause of infection, but simple scaling and cleaning of teeth (in which bleeding often occurs) can also lead to bacteremia. For patients at risk for bacterial endocarditis (especially those with structural or rheumatic heart problems or a prosthetic heart valve), a prophylactic antibiotic regimen is strongly recommended. The organisms most commonly implicated are alpha-hemolytic streptococci. The American Heart Association has made specific recommendations about the prevention and treatment of bacterial endocarditis.[2] These should be available from the librarian of your professional association or from a medical school library.

Antibiotic cover for dental procedures

Anxiety

Many patients perceive dental treatment as being stressful. When a physician has defined a patient as exceptionally anxious, he or she should apprise the dentist of this fact before the start of dental treatment so that anticipatory measures can be taken.

The principal strategies used to manage anxiety in the dental office are extra explanation, very gentle management, premedication, and a combination of all three.

It is possible for a patient to receive dental treatment under a general anesthetic (GA). This is best done when the GA is administered by an anesthesiologist using an endotracheal tube. Blocking off the trachea is essential in view of the debris thrown in the air by a high-speed drill and the proximity of the operating area to the entrance to the lungs.

General anesthesia

DENTAL PROBLEMS IN THE MEDICAL OFFICE

Toothache

Toothache can be divided into two broad types: toothache with external signs and toothache with only internal symptoms.

Figure 15-3   Cellulitis from dental abscess. (*Courtesy of Dr. D. P. Cunningham, Dental Faculty, Dalhousie University, Halifax, N.S., Canada.*)

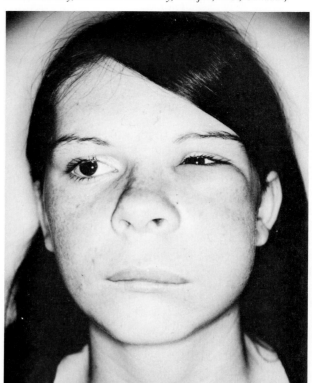

Dental abscess   **External Signs**   The contents of the nerve canal are inflamed by bacterial infection. The visual signs are swelling of tissues around the tooth, face, eye, or neck. The infected tooth is tender to percussion. The most common form of pain associated with swelling comes from an acute abcess. When a dental abscess develops, the infected contents of the pulp chamber in the tooth invade the surrounding bone and soft tissue, causing pressure pain (Figure 15-3). The choices for treatment are extraction, drainage of the abscess, and antibiotics. Today dentists frequently manage acutely abscessed teeth by first draining the pus through a channel cut into the crown of the tooth. Later they sterilize the root canal, pack it with filling material, and fill or crown the tooth with rigid materials. If a dentist is not readily available, pain and infection can be managed by means of analgesics and antibiotics. Definitive treatment by a dentist should be arranged before discontinuation of the antibiotic.

Internal Symptoms The nerve is irritated by decay or exposure, etc. The patient complains of tenderness or sensitivity to hot or cold stimuli. Treatment is achieved by means of analgesics such as acetaminophen with codeine (Tylenol 3). Definitive treatment by the dentist will sedate the nerve and seal off the tooth from painful stimuli.

Toothache

There are two deceptive types of toothache, as follows.

1 *Trigeminal neuralgia*: The patient describes excruciating facial pain associated with the tooth. Fast dental evaluation should be arranged in order to confirm or rule out a dental component before intensive medical treatment.

2 *Temporomandibular (TM) joint pain*: This is a remarkably common condition, most frequently described in women age 25 to 50 years. It often presents as pain on opening the mouth. A possible cause is irregular locking of the teeth, forcing TM joints into unnatural closure and muscle spasm. Dental treatment will smooth out the occlusion. This syndrome, however, appears to be primarily associated with psychological stress that is clinically demonstrated by trauma caused by grinding of the teeth while sleeping. Relief can be provided by fabricating a mouth guard. However, if the primary cause of pathological clenching and grinding of the teeth is psychological, a psychological remedy will be necessary.

Nocturnal teeth grinding

Postextraction Hemorrhage

Dentists are responsible for any postoperative complications (e.g., hemorrhage) which follow their treatment. The basic steps in managing the postextraction hemorrhage that is associated with about 1 percent of tooth extractions are as follows.

Dental bleeding

1 Advise no rinsing for 24 hours in order to prevent dislodging of the initial clot and restarting of the hemorrhage.

2 Have the patient apply pressure directly onto the socket by means of tissues rolled into a pad (opposing jaw applies pressure) for 15 minutes at a time.

3 If the first two measures fail, have the patient use a wet tea bag in the same manner. A tea bag has an ideal physical shape for this task. Also, the tannic acid in tea acts as a clotting agent.

4 In the unlikely event that these measures fail to arrest the hemorrhage, infiltrate tissue around the socket with local anesthetic, remove the contents of the socket, pack the socket with resorbable sponges (Gelfoam if available), and suture across the socket, using a minimum of two sutures. Repeat step 3.

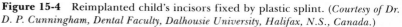

Figure 15-4 Reimplanted child's incisors fixed by plastic splint. (*Courtesy of Dr. D. P. Cunningham, Dental Faculty, Dalhousie University, Halifax, N.S., Canada.*)

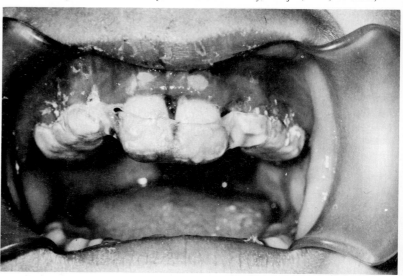

5 In the unlikely event that step 4 fails, refer the patient to a dentist or emergency room for radiographic evaluation and treatment of the cause, e.g., sequestrum, fracture, or blood dyscrasia.

Examination of the Mouth after Trauma

Dental injury

Trauma to the mouth is usually associated with extreme injury to the face. In view of the proximity of the mouth to the airway, it is wise to complete an examination of the mouth before managing external injuries. The following guidelines should be used.

1 Look for bleeding sockets and account for all dislodged teeth and dentures or parts of teeth and dentures. If the number found does not match the number of sockets and dentures, take steps to rule out their presence in the airway. Tooth fragments in the stomach can be ignored.

2 Close all intraoral wounds.

Fracture of mandible

3 Check for fractures of the maxilla and mandible. Fractures involving mobility of the parts are easy to recognize; simple fractures not involving mobility can be difficult to recognize visually. One method of determining the presence of a fracture is to oppose the teeth of both jaws (i.e., close the jaws). If there are sufficient teeth and no fracture is present, the opposing teeth will not mesh together because of distortion from muscle tension.

Figure 15-5 Same teeth, splint removed 3 weeks later. (*Courtesy of Dr. D. P. Cunningham, Dental Faculty, Dalhousie University, Halifax, N.S., Canada.*)

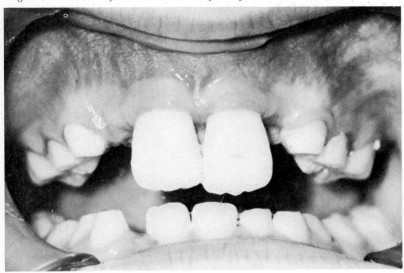

4   Once a fracture has been detected, arrange for its reduction and fixation.

5   Ask a dentist to advise on the care of the mouth once the first four principal management steps have been completed.

Teeth Knocked Out of the Mouth

It is practical to reinsert teeth knocked out by a blow to the face in children up to 10 years of age. Only permanent teeth should be considered; the younger the child, the better the chances of success.

The extruded tooth should be placed in a wet tissue or held by the child under his or her tongue. The child should be seen by a dentist immediately, i.e., within 1 hour. The sooner the child has the tooth reimplanted, the better. If 6 hours has passed since the accident, it is pointless to attempt reimplantation.

The dentist will fix the tooth in its socket by wiring it to the adjacent tooth or securing it with a quick-setting plastic splint. Depending on the age of the child, the nerve may be removed and the canal sealed off before reimplantation. Reimplanted teeth do not last indefinitely. Their roots slowly reabsorb throughout a maximum life of 7 to 10 years. By this time the child's jaw will be close to maturity, and a permanent replacement for the damaged tooth can be planned (Figures 15-4 and 15-5).

Reimplanted teeth

Figure 15-6   Bilateral torus of mandible: a "normal" bony swelling of mouth. (*Courtesy of American Dental Association.*)

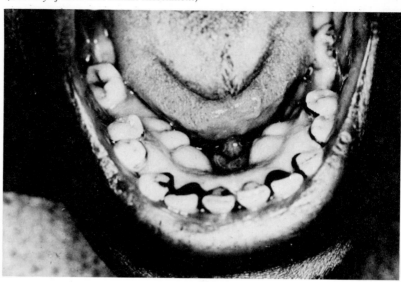

Swelling in the Mouth

Gum swelling

The oral tissues are subject to the same range of pathological change as any other part of the body. However, the following "normal" swellings are common.

Osteoma torus

1 *Hard, bony swelling*: Benign osteoma torus (exostosis) shows as central swelling in the hard palate and as bilateral bumps in the mandible just lingual to bicuspid teeth. These osteomas are very common; treatment is not required unless a denture is planned (Figure 15-6).

Vitamin deficiency

2 *Swelling and bleeding of gum tissue*: This is very common and is usually caused by a lack of oral hygiene. In rare cases, the condition may be associated with a deficiency of B-complex vitamins. The first remedy is stepped-up brushing and flossing by the patient, and the second is scaling by the dental hygienist.

Pregnancy

3 *"Pregnancy" tumors*: These are due to soft tissue swelling, which presents as benign epithelial growths around teeth. Such tumors are apparently caused by temporary endocrine disturbance and disappear after parturition (Figure 15-7). No special dental treatment is required other than careful oral hygiene by the patient and/or dental hygienist.

Drug swellings

4 *Dilantin hyperplasia*: Widespread epithelial thickening around the teeth is directly related to the use of diphenylhydantoin (Dilantin) in treating epilepsy (Figure 15-8). No special dental treatment is required apart from careful oral hygiene by the patient and/or dental hygienist.

Figure 15-7 Common appearance of pregnancy tumors. (*Courtesy of American Dental Association.*)

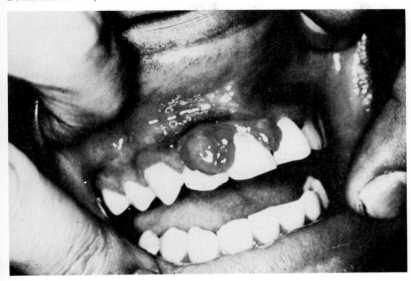

Figure 15-8 Hyperplastic gingival tissue associated with long-term ingestion of dilantin. (*Courtesy of American Dental Association.*)

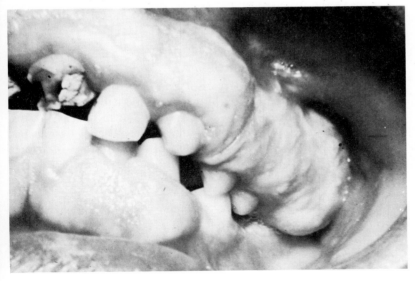

Figure 15-9 Leukoplakia involving palatal aspect of maxilla. (*Courtesy of Dr. R. W. Priddy, Faculty of Dentistry, University of British Columbia, B.C., Canada.*)

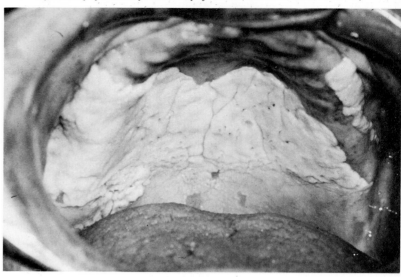

Impacted
molars

 5 *Impacted third molars*: Inflammation associated with impacted mandibular wisdom teeth frequently presents as swelling and pain in the area of the ear or the side of the face. Refer the patient to an oral surgeon.

Geriatric Patients

Leukoplakia

 Oral Cancer   Elderly persons are more prone to oral cancer than younger ones. When carrying out a physical examination of anyone over 50 years of age, it is a good idea to check the lips, tongue, floor of the mouth, and palate for epithelial neoplasms. Leukoplakia—dry, white keratinization of epithelium—often precedes neoplastic degeneration; if spotted in time, it can be successfully treated (Figure 15-9).

Cheilosis

 Wearers of Full Dentures   Older persons who have worn full dentures for a long time tend to lose the vertical height of the bony ridges under their dentures; this results in impaired masticatory function and, frequently, tympanic pain. Visually, the problem can be identified by creases at each corner of the mouth with escaping saliva causing chronic inflammation of skin tissue (angular cheilosis). Such individuals should be referred to a dentist for denture replacement to restore normal facial appearance and relieve any tympanic pain (Figure 15-10).

Figure 15-10 Angular cheilosis—associated with loss of natural chewing teeth or worn down dentures. (*Courtesy of Dr. B. B. Harsanyi, Dental Faculty, Dalhousie University, Halifax, N.S., Canada.*)

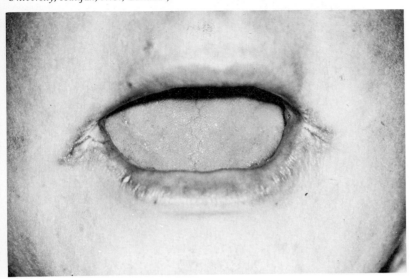

Pediatric Problems

Neonatal Teeth   A baby's first set of teeth (deciduous or primary teeth) start to appear around the age of 6 months. Mothers are understandably puzzled when a baby is born with teeth already in place. There are two types of neonatal teeth.

Type 1   The teeth involved are commonly the two lower deciduous incisors. These are true teeth that happen to have erupted 6 months ahead of schedule. Mistiming in the activity of the thyroid gland has been suggested as a likely cause. The occurence rate of this phenomenon is about 1 per 3000 births. If at all practical, these teeth should be retained, not removed. At a later date in the child's development, they will be required for mastication; even more important, they are needed for the formation of a normal dental arch and subsequent avoidance of orthodontic treatment when the permanent teeth erupt.

A problem may arise if the incisal edges of prematurely erupted teeth are very sharp. Such teeth can irritate the baby's tongue or lips. If the baby is being nursed, the mother's nipple can be lacerated. In such cases, a dentist should be requested to smooth down the sharp edges by means of careful disking. If prematurely erupted teeth are so shaky that the baby can dislodge them, it is wise to remove them.

Neonatal teeth

Figure 15-11 Epstein's pearls. (*Courtesy of Dr. W. G. Young, Department of Oral Biology and Oral Surgery, University of Queensland, Australia.*)

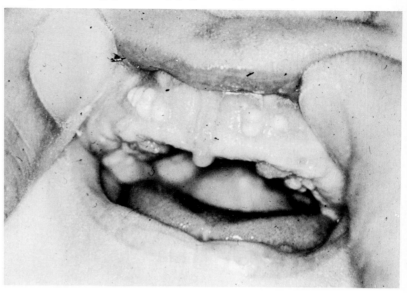

Epstein's pearls

Type II Type II neonatal teeth, sometimes called Epstein's pearls (Figure 15-11), are not really teeth. They can be mistaken for erupting teeth but in fact are gingival cysts filled with keratin. They are usually located in the front of the mouth or the maxilla and present no physical problems in terms of feeding or development. They reabsorb spontaneously and therefore require no treatment.

Teething The most effective ways of treating pain are "natural" rather than pharmacological methods. It may help to give the child lots of liquid or a hard food (carrot or apple) to chew on. If the child permits, the mother may be able to massage the gum or give the child a safe teething rattle or ring to chew on. Dental experience has been that drugs such as Orajel are of little use in controlling teething pain.

If teething is accompanied by generalized fever, aspirin or acetaminophen is appropriate. If the pain cannot be managed by natural means, the child should be examined by a dentist, who can provide topical anesthesia or incise the often cystlike tissue over the erupting tooth.

Thumb sucking Dentists do not see thumb sucking up to age 6 as harmful to teeth. Between 6 and 10 years, it will affect the position of erupting adult teeth and should be stopped. If thumb sucking persists after age 10 years, considerable orthodontic problems are likely to occur.

Thumb suckers fall into two categories. Children in the first group suck their thumbs as a harmless habit. Mothers can stop the practice by talking to the child or by applying an unpleasant-tasting material (e.g., Thumbs) to the thumb or fingers before bedtime. Such preparations are available over the counter. The second category of thumb suckers have deeply based psychological reasons for the habit. Merely stopping the thumb sucking will almost certainly cause antisocial behavior to appear. Professional psychological management may be necessary.

PREVENTION AND PATIENT EDUCATION

Dental Checkups

Despite the fact that dental disease afflicts 95 percent of those living in the western world, it is nevertheless possible to retain the natural teeth throughout a long life. Regular checkups give the dentist a chance to detect and correct decay before radical treatment becomes unavoidable. The recommended frequency for checkups is once a year for adults and twice a year for children and adolescents.

Frequency of checkups

Encouragement of Good Oral Hygiene

Our teeth and gum tissues are genetically programmed to handle a caveman-like diet, i.e., rough bulky food with grains of sand sometimes embedded in it. The mechanical action required to masticate such material keeps the gums and teeth in excellent physiological health.

Today's diet of soft, processed food, frequently loaded with refined sugar, denies our mouths the opportunity for adequate physiological work. It also creates a fertile environment for oral bacteria to produce acid and cause decay. Dentists use the term *plaque* to describe the transparent scum of saliva, bacteria, and carbohydrate covering teeth. Daily brushing and flossing of teeth is necessary in order to remove plaque, which, if left, will generate tooth decay and soft tissue inflammation.[3] (See Figure 15-12.)

Oral hygiene

Diet and Decay

Refined sugar is the greatest killer of teeth, and children's teeth are the most susceptible.[4] It is a good idea to encourage the substitution of fruit for sticky sweets and to promote the consumption of high-fiber foods.

Diet

Figure 15-12   "Plaque" on decaying tooth of 14-year-old girl. (*Courtesy of Dr. D. P. Cunningham, Dental Faculty, Dalhousie University, Halifax, N.S., Canada.*)

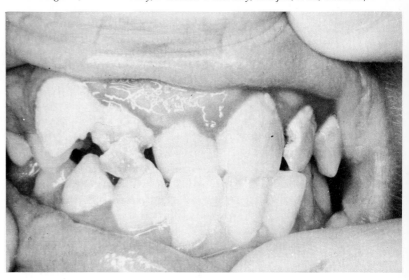

Supplementary Fluoride

Fluoride

Sodium fluoride is a trace element that makes teeth hard and dramatically reduces the incidence of decay in children's mouths, an effect that continues throughout adult life.[5] It is most conveniently obtained through a fluoridated public water supply. Children living in areas which do not have such a system can benefit from prescribed fluoride tablets or drops. Treatment for an individual family is best worked out in collaboration with the family dentist.

REFERENCES

1 *Accepted Dental Therapeutics,* 36th ed., American Dental Association, Chicago, 1975–1976.
2 American Heart Association, "Prevention of Bacterial Endocarditis: A Committee Report of the American Heart Association," *Journal of the American Dental Association,* **95:**600–605, 1977.
3 A. E. Nigel, *Nutrition in Preventive Dentistry: Science and Practice,* W. B. Saunders, Philadelphia, 1972.
4 J. Spouge, *Oral Pathology,* C. V. Mosby, St. Louis, 1973.
5 *Fluorides and Human Health,* World Health Organization Series 59, World Health Organization, Geneva, 1970.

SOURCES OF MATERIALS

Dental health brochures on brushing, flossing, gum disease, nutrition, etc., are available from the following sources:

The American Dental Association
211 East Chicago Avenue
Chicago, IL. 60611

The British Dental Association
64 Wimpole Street
London, W1M 8AL, United Kingdom

The Canadian Dental Association
1815 Alta Vista Drive
Ottawa, Ontario K1G 3Y6, Canada

Chapter 16

High-Risk Pregnancy

D. C. Brown, M.D.

PRINCIPLE

No patient in family medicine is more susceptible to behavioral modification and education than the expectant mother. A pregnant patient may change her high-risk behavior out of concern for her child's and her own health.

Family physician's role

As the physician of first contact and because of a continuing relationship with the patient, the family physician is in an excellent position to identify and manage the high-risk pregnant patient. Knowledge about all members of the family and their interrelationships and about the many strings of attachment improves the family physician's ability to help a couple or a single mother cope with the stress of a high-risk pregnancy and, possibly, with a sick or deformed child, a stillbirth, or a perinatal death.

DEFINITION

A *high-risk pregnancy* is one in which the fetus is at increased risk for stillbirth, neonatal morbidity, or death and/or the expectant mother is at increased risk for morbidity or mortality.

PREVALENCE

Perinatal mortality in North America has declined dramatically in the last 35 years.[1] In an average family practice, approximately 10 to 20 percent of obstetric patients will fall into the category of high risk. In the average family physician's practice (35 deliveries per year), four to six high-risk pregnancies are encountered yearly.[1]

ETIOLOGY

High risks may be predicted before conception in certain women, especially those with serious renal, liver, or heart disease. Risk factors considered at the first prenatal visit include "extremes" of maternal age, parity (first delivery or more than four), strong family history of diabetes, low social class, previous obstetric performance (a perinatal death increases the risk, as do two or more abortions or a previous cesarean section), and specific medical disorders such as essential hypertension, pyelonephritis or glomerulonephritis, diabetes, and rheumatic or congenital heart disease.

Causes of hi-risk

NATURAL HISTORY AND RECOGNITION

The outcome of a high-risk pregnancy varies considerably with each risk factor and with the physician's skill in management. The more adept the physician is in getting the expectant couple to modify their habits in order to reduce their risks and the more pertinent the anticipatory guidance given by the physician and/or health-care team, the more likely a happy outcome will be.

The most efficient way to recognize and appropriately manage a high-risk pregnancy is to have an organized approach, which can be facilitated by a high-risk scoring system built into the prenatal record. Numerous risk-scoring systems have been devised to bring attention to risk factors so that problems can be identified, treated, and/or prevented. The most useful of the indexes developed to date (1985) appears to be that of Goodwin et al.,[2] which groups 27 factors into three categories. The great value of this index is its high sensitivity and predictability. Only 14 percent of the test population was defined as being at risk, and these patients accounted for 77.8 percent of perinatal deaths and 67.3 percent of low Apgar scores.[3]

Organized approach

Risk-scoring methods

A fetal risk project was carried out in Nova Scotia from 1971 to 1975. Thirty percent of family physicians delivering obstetrical care in the province participated. They used the Goodwin, Dunne, and Thomas fetal risk scoring system. Patients scoring 4 to 10 on the scale accounted for 60 percent of stillbirths and 68 percent of neonatal deaths. Further analysis revealed that these patients accounted for 10 percent of the total of 17,270 patients.[4]

An example of a multicopy prenatal record is that produced by the Medical Society of Nova Scotia. Page 1 of this form (Figure 16-1)[5] goes to the hospital as part of the patient's record, and the back of the page has the prenatal scoring form shown in Figure 16-2. Page 2 remains with the family physician's record. On the back of page 2 there is a delivery record and a form to record the postpartum examination, as shown in Figure 16-3. This could prove helpful if the patient moves her residence during pregnancy or changes physicians; she can take the top sheet to her new physician. This facilitates communication as well as patient care.

MANAGEMENT

The most important visit with a pregnant patient is the first. Perhaps the best predictor of the fetal outcome of pregnancy is the mother's medical history, from which two-thirds of high-risk pregnancies can be identified.

Previous obstetrical history

Do a reproductive history. Prior fetal compromise or neonatal loss may indicate undiagnosed maternal disease or structural abnormality. A woman who has had a stillbirth is twice as likely as other women to have another. Determine the reasons and duration of gestation for any elective abortion.[6] Assess previous births in regard to length of labor, route of delivery, closeness to due date, and maternal well-being. Ask the primigravida about her mother's and grandmothers' reproductive history and determine whether there is a family history of diabetes. Ask the patient to describe her menstrual cycle and give the date of her last *normal* menstrual period and any prior use of birth control pills.

Socioeconomic history

Take the socioeconomic history. Assess possible prenatal risks, including poor nutrition, alcohol or drug abuse, and cigarette smoking. Rule out sexually transmitted disease. Consider age. A teenager may not cope well with the physical and emotional demands of pregnancy; a woman age 35 or older is at higher risk for Down's syndrome or complications caused by preexisting medical problems. Find out whether the pregnancy is wanted and evaluate stress in the patient's daily life.[7]

Of course, if you have been the patient's family physician for years, you will already have most of this information, especially if you have delivered her before. Don't trust your memory; check the record!

At the first prenatal physical examination, look for evidence of hypertension, cardiopulmonary insufficiency, and renal, circulatory, or thyroid disorders. Establish baseline weight and reflexes,

Figure 16-1 Medical Society of Nova Scotia Prenatal Record.

THE MEDICAL SOCIETY OF NOVA SCOTIA PRENATAL RECORD (REVISED 1982)

FOR COPIES CONTACT · REPRODUCTIVE CARE PROGRAM, 5821 UNIVERSITY AVENUE, HALIFAX, NOVA SCOTIA B3H 1W3

NAME	ADDRESS	PHONE	
DOCTOR	HOSPITAL	MED INS NO	
AGE MENSTRUAL CYCLE PILL STOPPED LNMP		EDC	

OBSTETRICAL HISTORY

GRAV _____ PARA _____ ABORT _____ ALIVE _____ SB _____ NND _____

PREM _____ IUGR _____ CONG ABN _____ C/S _____

YEAR	WT	GEST	COMPLICATION	HOSPITAL OF DELIVERY

HOSPITAL COPY — Prenatal Score on Flip Side

	YES	NO	HIGH RISK SCORE
BREASTFEEDING			1st VISIT 36 WEEKS
PRENATAL CLASSES			☐ ☐
ADEQUATE DIET			
ALLERGIES			
MEDICATIONS			
PREV. TRANS			

FAMILY HISTORY	e.g. DIABETES HYPERTENSION TWINS HEREDITARY DISEASE	SOCIAL HISTORY (OCCUPATION, SPECIAL PARENTING NEEDS, ETC.)
PAST HEALTH	e.g. DIABETES EPILEPSY U.T.I SURGERY	
FUNCTIONAL ENQUIRY	HYPERTENSION RENAL DIS SMOKING ALCOHOL	

EXAMINATION	DATE PRE-PREG WEIGHT B.P HEIGHT	LAB DATA
HEAD AND NECK	BREASTS PELVIC	HGB. RUBELLA TITRE
HEART	LUNGS CX.	VDRL BLOOD SUGAR
ABDOMEN	EXTREMITIES CORPUS	GROUP Rh
	ADNEXA	HUSBAND'S Rh
		ANTIBODIES _____

OBSTETRIC PELVIC ASSESSMENT

URINE	P . S	MICRO	C AND S	PREG. TEST DATE
CERVIX	PAP.		G.C. C AND S	QUICKENING DATE

28 WEEK Rh IMMUNE GLOBULIN DATE:

DATE	WT	BP	URINE P / S	GESTATION WEEKS	FUNDAL HEIGHT cm 1SYMPH	PRESENTATION	FH	RISK SCORE	RETURN IN	HGB AND REMARKS

**Examination of
uterus**

confirm the pregnancy by means of pelvic examination, and do a thorough pelvimetric evaluation. If gestation is less than 4 months, estimate the uterine size.[6] This is a *very* important part of the examination; estimation of current gestation should be stressed for the first and subsequent visits. X-ray pelvimetric evaluation now has almost no place in obstetrical management. The best pelvimeter is previous vaginal delivery, and the next best is a trial of labor, since only an adequate trial can you tell *in retrospect* whether the pelvis was adequate.

**Laboratory
tests**

First-visit laboratory investigations should include a Pap smear if one has not been done within the previous 6 months. Do a Venereal Disease Research Laboratories (VDRL) and rubella titer, complete blood count (CBC), ABO blood type, Rh, and antibodies. Check the urine for sugar, acetone, and protein and obtain a urine culture. These tests will help identify possible diabetes, poor nutrition, renal disorder, or bacteriuria. If the patient is a teenager or if gonorrhea is endemic in your population, obtain a cervical culture. Follow up a finding of glycosuria with a 2-hour postprandial blood sugar.[6]

Bacteriuria

Asymptomatic bacteriuria occurs in 4 to 7 percent of pregnant woman. Up to 50 percent of patients with asymptomatic bacteriuria or cystitis may have silent pyelonephritis and may be at increased risk for frank pyelonephritis. Unless treated, these women have a much greater chance of giving birth prematurely.[6] As many as 30 percent of woman who have asymptomatic bacteriuria will progress to acute pyelonephritis if untreated, while only 3 percent will progress to acute pyelonephritis if adequately treated.[6]

If you find a tender unilateral swelling on examination during the first trimester as you palpate the ovaries and if the uterus seems less than 6 weeks in size, suspect ectopic pregnancy, particularly if the patient has a previous ectopic history and has vaginal spotting. If the uterus extends above the symphysis, ectopic pregnancy is unlikely. Rule out or confirm ectopic pregnancy by means of serum pregnancy tests (BHCG), ultrasound examination, and operative intervention as indicated.

At the end of the prenatal patient's first visit, calculate her high-risk score using the form shown in Figure 16-2. Then enter her score on page 1 of your prenatal record in the appropriate box. Patients with preexisting hypertension are monitored more closely. The antihypertensive therapy is continued unless there is a good reason not to do so, such as orthostatic hypotension or a pressure consistently lower than 120/80 mm Hg and no sign of end organ problems (i.e., normal fundus and electrocardiogram).[7] In addition to putting the patient on a diet that includes 90 g per day of protein, ask her to rest on her side for 30 minutes at least three times a day. If more convenient, suggest an afternoon rest of 1 to 1½ hours plus a good night's rest. The antihypertensive recommended during pregnancy is methyldopa (Aldomet).[8] If the patient has been on diuretic therapy, continuation is usually necessary.[7]

Low-risk prenatal patients should be seen monthly until the twenty-eighth week, then biweekly to 36 weeks, then weekly until delivery. At each visit, the patient is weighed, blood pressure is recorded, and a urine sample is taken for protein and sugar and microscopic examination. (With each visit ask whether her dates correlate with the estimate of gestation.) Fundal height is recorded in centimeters above symphysis pubis. The patient is asked to record the date when she first feels the baby kicking (i.e., the date when she feels it for 2 days in a row). One can expect the first fetal movement at 17 to 20 weeks in a first pregnancy and 16 to 19 weeks in subsequent pregnancies. Another way to verify gestational age is by listening with an unamplified fetal stethoscope; in most cases, the fetal heart tones are audible at 18 to 20 weeks.

If these two data corroborate the expected date of confinement (EDC) calculated at the first visit, your estimate of gestational age is reasonably accurate. If there is a discrepancy, consider confirming the date by means of ultrasound. The biparietal diameter (BPD) of the fetal skull sonographic measurement provides an accurate assessment of gestational age during the first 15 to 25 weeks of pregnancy, with an accuracy of ±10 days. Crown–rump measurement between 10 and 14 weeks has an accuracy of ±5 days. Another useful assessment of gestation is uterine size in the second trimester:

Estimating gestation

@ 12 weeks: symphysis
@ 16 weeks: midway symphysis to umbilicus
@ 20 weeks: at umbilicus.

For example, at 20 weeks, the patient has felt movement for 2 weeks, the fundus is at the umbilicus, and you can hear the fetal heart with fetoscope.

INAPPROPRIATE GROWTH

Analyze inappropriate growth. You may not suspect intrauterine growth retardation (IUGR) until the early weeks of the third trimester. In addition to being secondary to hypertension or insufficient renal function, IUGR can also result from poor nutrition, fetal malformation, heavy smoking, high alcohol intake, or vascular insufficiency resulting from diabetes. Confirm suspected IUGR by means of ultrasound, BPD, abdominal circumference, and femur length.

Figure 16-2   Medical Society of Nova Scotia Prenatal Scoring Form.

NOVA SCOTIA PRENATAL SCORING FORM

1) SCORE EACH QUESTION AS INDICATED   2) TOTAL EACH CATEGORY SCORE AT 1st VISIT   3) REPEAT

AT 36 WEEKS   4) RECORD ON P / N SHEET

I REPRODUCTIVE HISTORY

AGE <16 : 1
     16 - 35 : 0
     >35 : 2

PARITY 0 : 1
        1 - 4 : 0
        5+ : 2

PAST OB HISTORY

HABITUAL ABORTION/ INFERTILITY   . 1

P. P. H. /MANUAL REMOVAL   . 1

BABY >9 LBS. (4082 gm)   . 1

BABY <5.5 LBS. (2500 gm)   . 1

P.E.T. /HYPERTENSION   . 1

PREVIOUS CAESAREAN   . 2

STILLBIRTH OR NEONATAL DEATH   . 3

PROLONGED LABOUR OR DIFFICULT DELIVERY   . 1

CATEGORY SCORE   . _____

II ASSOCIATED CONDITIONS

PREVIOUS GYNECOLOGICAL SURGERY   . 1

CHRONIC RENAL DISEASE   . 2

GESTATIONAL DIABETES   . 1

DIABETES MELLITUS   . 3

CARDIAC DISEASE   . 3

OTHER MEDICAL DISORDERS

(CHRONIC BRONCHITIS. LUPUS, ETC.)

SCORE ACCORDING TO SEVERITY (1 TO 3)

CATEGORY SCORE   . _____

III PRESENT PREGNANCY

	1st VISIT	36 WEEKS
BLEEDING < 20 WEEKS . 1	☐	☐
> 20 WEEKS . 3	☐	☐
ANEMIA < 10 GM % . 1	☐	☐
PROLONGED PREGNANCY (42 WEEKS) . 1	☐	☐
HYPERTENSION . 2	☐	☐
PREMATURE RUPTURE MEMBRANES . 2	☐	☐
POLYHYDRAMNIOS . 2	☐	☐
SMALL FOR DATES . 3	☐	☐
MULTIPLE PREGNANCY OR BREECH OR MALPRESENTATION . 3	☐	☐
RH ISOIMMUNIZATION . 3	☐	☐

CATEGORY SCORE   _____

TOTAL RISK SCORE

1st VISIT ☐   TOTAL AT 36 WEEKS ☐

(RECORD SCORES IN BOX ON PRENATAL SHEET)

NOTE :

LOW RISK   • 0 - 2

HIGH RISK   • 3 - 6

EXTREME RISK   • >7

IUGR   Urge the patient with IUGR to undertake home bed rest on
her side for as much of the day as possible during the remainder
of the pregnancy. This will increase blood flow to the uterus and
fetus. If this fails, consider hospitalization. In the meantime, consider the IUGR fetus to be at very high risk for birth complications
such as meconium aspiration, asphyxiation, and acidosis, along
with neonatal hypoglycemia, developmental inadequacy, and difficulty in controlling body temperature.[8]

Larger than normal uterine size may signal hydramnios, which
can be confirmed by ultrasound. The underlying cause may be unknown or may be related to multiple pregnancy, gestational or
overt diabetes, Rh or other hematologic sensitization, or fetal
anomaly.

DIABETES

Do a 2-hour postprandial blood sugar test on all patients at 28 to
30 weeks of pregnancy in order to check for gestational diabetes
and at 18 weeks in the high-risk group. If the findings lead to a
diagnosis of gestational diabetes, try to maintain the patient's fasting glucose level within a range of 60 to 100 mg per 100 ml and
take a fasting and postprandial blood sugar at every visit. Also ask
the patient to check her second voided morning urine for sugar
and acetone each day. For mild patients, moderate exercise and
carefully controlled diet may help keep a diabetic within normal
range, but insulin supplements may be necessary in some cases.
Oral hypoglycemic drugs are contraindicated in pregnancy because they may be teratogenic and may produce hypoglycemia in
the neonate. During the third trimester, watch for ketoacidosis,
which can appear rapidly but is very rare in the gestational
diabetic.[8]

Hypoglycemia   In patients with diabetes mellitus, symptomatic hypoglycemia
may be the prominent early symptom of pregnancy. The fetus is a
successful parasite; its requirements will be adequately met, even at
the mother's expense.

Diabetic control   Because of the tendency to fasting hypoglycemia and hypoami-
noacidemia and to food-induced hyperglycemia even in normal
pregnancies, all pregnant patients should be urged to adopt a diet
of the type recommended by the American Diabetic Association,
with frequent small feeds as opposed to less frequent large meals.
(See Chapter 35.) The diagnosis and management of diabetes during pregnancy requires regular measurements of blood glucose.
Fortunately, modern technology allows women to test their levels
of blood glucose at home simply, reliably, and frequently so that
regulating insulin doses becomes a relatively simple task. Since

pregnancy is a 24-hour-a-day affair, blood glucose control should also be a 24-hour-a-day affair, and most diabetic patients will require insulin twice daily. Maternal hyperglycemia for only 6 or 8 hours a day seems to be sufficient to produce fetal macrosomia.

Good control of blood glucose makes for better babies and healthier mothers. During pregnancy we want the patient to gain weight, and we expect her insulin doses to change dramatically, not because she is failing to comply but because she is pregnant.[7] Failure to comprehend the magnitude of this change can cause serious psychological as well as metabolic distress.

Plan to see the patient with chronic disease, particularly diabetes or hypertension, twice a month until the third trimester and twice a week after that, unless her condition warrants more frequent visits.

PREGNANCY-INDUCED HYPERTENSION

Several reports in the literature confirm the reliability of the supine pressor test (the rollover test) as a reliable predictor of nulliparous pregnant women at increased risk for gestational hypertension, preeclampsia (PET), or eclampsia.[9] A high-risk group can be easily identified with the rollover test between 28 and 32 weeks of gestation. This test involves taking two upper arm readings of blood pressure 5 minutes apart. The first is taken with the patient lying on her side, and the second is taken with the patient lying on her back. The test is considered positive if the diastolic pressure increases more than 20 mm Hg, and these patients are at higher risk of PET if they are not treated with rest.[9]

In your ongoing evaluation of the degree of risk for pregnancy-induced hypertension (PIH), consider compliance with nutritional recommendations, bed rest, and medical appointments as well as blood pressure readings.

If a patient at risk for PIH (e.g., positive rollover test at 22 to 32 weeks)[8] begins to show elevated blood pressure or fails to experience the expected drop during the second trimester (up to 20 mm Hg systolic and 10 mm Hg diastolic), suggest that she increase bed rest to at least an hour three times a day. Ask her to monitor her blood pressure at home. Urge her to call you if she has an elevated reading and to do so *immediately* if she notices swelling in her hands and face, frequent headaches, or disturbances in vision; these are signs of rapidly increasing PIH which dictate immediate hospitalization. Do not rely on standard figures for high blood pressure in diagnosing PIH. Rather, make that diagnosis and hospitalize the patient if there is an increase in diastolic blood pressure of 15 mm Hg or more or an increase of 30 mm Hg or more in

"At risk" management

systolic pressure.[8] In reliable patients with minor levels of elevated blood pressure, you may wish to observe closely at home first, with increased rest.

If the patient does not respond to bed rest and proper diet, consider the indications for delivery and determine the need for magnesium sulfate to prevent convulsions. If the pregnancy is of less than 35 weeks' duration, transfer the patient to a tertiary care center.[8]

PREMATURE RUPTURE OF MEMBRANES

Amniotic fluid examination

If the patient reports that she is leaking fluid vaginally, determine whether she has had a premature rupture of the membranes (PROM) and/or a prolapsed umbilical cord. On sterile speculum examination, you can observe whether fluid is draining from the cervical os or pooling in the posterior fornix. With Nitrazine paper, measure the pH of the posterior fornix or the midvaginal fluid; readings from these locations are more reliable than readings taken from the os. Amniotic fluid is likely to be pH 7.0 to 7.5, while the vaginal fluid is usually pH 4.5 to 5.5. A fern test may be more reliable than Nitrazine paper analysis; microscopically look for arborization or ferning in a dried sample of vaginal fluid. Ferning is an indication that amniotic fluid is present. You should also take a culture from the central vaginal wall for identifying beta-hemolytic streptococci.

Amnionitis and prematurity are the most worrisome side effects of PROM. Consultation and referral are recommended unless circumstances require you to continue care.

PREMATURITY

Prematurity continues to be the major cause of perinatal mortality in North America. Testing of high-risk patients is routine at 28 to 30 weeks of pregancy. The primary screening test for assessing fetal well-being is a weekly nonstress test (NST), which measures fetal neurocardiovascular status by monitoring continuous fetal heart rate. This test, which is done on an outpatient basis, checks acceleration of fetal heartbeat normally accompanying fetal activity.[8]

Biophysical profile

A more up-to-date method of antepartum fetal evaluation is based on the fetal biophysical profile developed by Manning et al., in which five physical variables are determined: fetal breathing movements, fetal movements, fetal tone, qualitative amniotic fluid volume, and the nonstress test. Available data suggest that the biophysical profile is more accurate in predicting fetal well-being than any other method of evaluation.[12]

Figure 16-3 Medical Society of Nova Scotia Delivery Record and Post-Partum Examination Form.

DELIVERY RECORD

	TYPE OF LABOUR	INDUCTION	ANAESTHESIA
DATE OF BIRTH	SPONTANEOUS	FORCEPS	THIRD STAGE
HOUR OF BIRTH	WEIGHT	L.B./S.B./N.N.D.	EPISIOTOMY
PRES. POS.	BLOOD LOSS		NURSING
BABY-SEX	ASPHYXIA NEONATORUM		

COMPLICATIONS:

_____
DOCTOR'S SIGNATURE

POSTPARTUM EXAMINATION

DATE

	LOCHIA	PELVIS	PERINEUM
WEIGHT	MENSES	CERVIX	CORPUS
B.P.	NURSING		
HAEMOGLOBIN	BREASTS		
URINE			
FAMILY PLANNING			

4 HIGH-RISK PREGNANCY

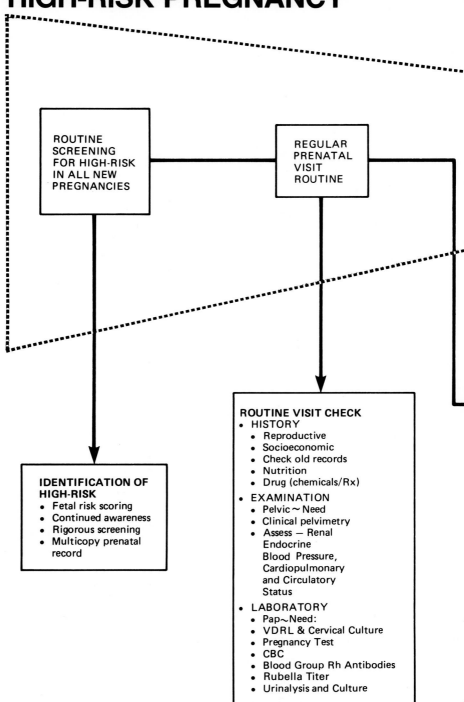

ROUTINE
SCREENING
FOR HIGH-RISK
IN ALL NEW
PREGNANCIES

REGULAR
PRENATAL
VISIT
ROUTINE

**IDENTIFICATION OF
HIGH-RISK**
- Fetal risk scoring
- Continued awareness
- Rigorous screening
- Multicopy prenatal
  record

ROUTINE VISIT CHECK
- HISTORY
  - Reproductive
  - Socioeconomic
  - Check old records
  - Nutrition
  - Drug (chemicals/Rx)
- EXAMINATION
  - Pelvic ~ Need
  - Clinical pelvimetry
  - Assess — Renal
    Endocrine
    Blood Pressure,
    Cardiopulmonary
    and Circulatory
    Status
- LABORATORY
  - Pap~Need:
  - VDRL & Cervical Culture
  - Pregnancy Test
  - CBC
  - Blood Group Rh Antibodies
  - Rubella Titer
  - Urinalysis and Culture

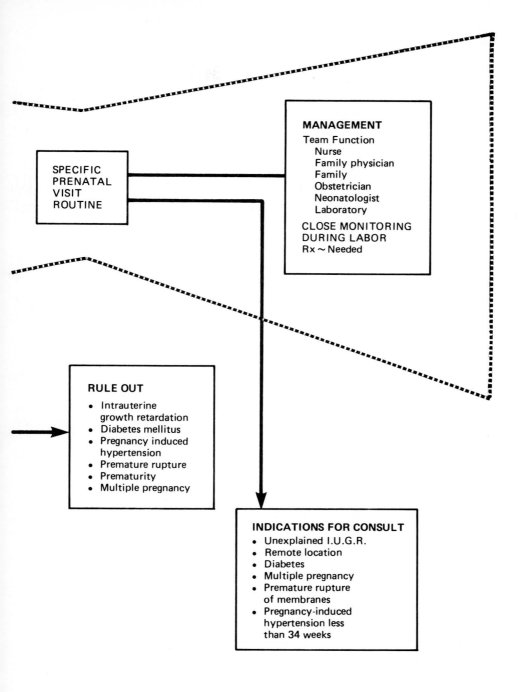

SPECIFIC
PRENATAL
VISIT
ROUTINE

MANAGEMENT
Team Function
    Nurse
    Family physician
    Family
    Obstetrician
    Neonatologist
    Laboratory

CLOSE MONITORING
DURING LABOR
Rx ~ Needed

RULE OUT
- Intrauterine
  growth retardation
- Diabetes mellitus
- Pregnancy induced
  hypertension
- Premature rupture
- Prematurity
- Multiple pregnancy

INDICATIONS FOR CONSULT
- Unexplained I.U.G.R.
- Remote location
- Diabetes
- Multiple pregnancy
- Premature rupture
  of membranes
- Pregnancy-induced
  hypertension less
  than 34 weeks

MULTIPLE PREGNANCY

There is considerable evidence that bed rest can maintain a twin pregnancy. Proponents believe that it can also increase birth weight and decrease IUGR, thereby promoting an overall decrease in perinatal mortality. All patients with triplets or quadruplets should be hospitalized at 26 weeks.[10]

SUMMARY

A high-risk patient must be monitored from the onset of labor until delivery not only by nurses but also by the physician responsible for her care. The care of such patients requires teamwork, with the family physician coordinating the other team members, including the obstetrician, the perinatologist, and the neonatologist. Naturally, the composition of the team varies with the size of the community.

Identifying the high-risk pregnancy early, along with proper team management throughout the prenatal period, does make a difference in neonatal morbidity and mortality. It is important that family physicians, obstetricians, perinatologists, neonatologists, and nurses all cooperate and work as a team.

Between 1971 and 1980, the perinatal mortality rate in 28 community hospitals in Nova Scotia fell from 18.7 to 7.0 per 1000 births. With regionalization of perinatal services, it is possible to reduce the perinatal mortality rate in small community hospitals to levels that approximate those of a sophisticated tertiary care hospital.[11]

In order to make this system work, it is important that family physicians (the primary care obstetricians) have an efficient screening system for identifying high-risk pregnancies and arrange early consultation and referral as indicated by the clinical status of the patient and the community resources available.

REFERENCES

1 D. P. Zoller, "Principles of Managing the High-Risk Pregnant Patient," *American Family Physician,* **27**(1):216–221, 1983.

2 J. W. Goodwin, J. T. Dunne, and B. W. Thomas, "Antepartum Identification of the Fetus at Risk," *Canadian Medical Association Journal,* **101**:57–67, 1969.

3 J. A. Fortrey and E. W. Whitehorse, "The Development of an Index of High-Risk Pregnancy," *American Journal of Obstetrics and Gynecology,* **143**(5): 501–508, 1982.

4 M. Hebb et al., "Nova Scotia Fetal Risk Project," *Canadian Family Physician,* **26**:1664–1673, 1980.

5 *The Medical Society of Nova Scotia Prenatal Record,* revised 1982. Reproductive

Care Program, 5821 University Avenue, Halifax, Nova Scotia, Canada, B3H 1W3.

6 S. G. Gabbe et al., "High-Risk Pregnancy: Trimester I: Assessing Risk and Options," *Patient Care*, **15**(12):76–109, 1981.

7 R. V. Lee, "A Bull in the China Shop—The Internist and the High-Risk Pregnancy," *New York State Journal of Medicine*, **83**:304–310, 1983.

8 S. G. Gabbe et al., "Trimester 2 & 3: Taking the High-Risk Pregnancy to Term," *Patient Care*, **15**(13):132–192, 1981.

9 R. X. Spinopolice, S. Feld, and J. T. Harrigan, "Effective Prevention of Gestational Hypertension in Nulliparous Women at High Risk as Identified by the Rollover Test," *American Journal of Obstetrics and Gynecology*, **146**(2): 166–168, 1983.

10 C. T. Shaw, "High Risk Obstetrics: Multiple Gestations," *Family Practice Recertification*, **4**(7):91–104, 1982.

11 L. J. Peddle et al., "The Nova Scotia Reproductive Program," *American Journal of Obstetrics and Gynecology*, **145**(2):170–176, 1983.

12 F. A. Manning et al., "Antepartum Fetal Evaluation: Development of a Fetal Biophysical Profile." *American Journal of Obstetrics and Gynecology.* **136**(6): 787–795, 1980.

Chapter 17

Sexually Transmitted Diseases

F.S.S. Crombie, M.D.

PRINCIPLE

The family physician must consider the health of the community as well as that of the patient. Sexually transmitted diseases are endemic in North America, and the physician has a legal and moral duty to help control their spread. Diagnosis of these diseases may be complicated by the absence of symptoms, especially in women. Prompt and effective treatment is essential.

ETIOLOGY

Importance of reporting

Sexually transmitted diseases (STDs) are currently out of control. Twenty-five different STDs have been identified, including hepatitis B and acquired immune deficiency syndrome (AIDS).[1] Family physicians are extremely important in the control of STDs because they represent the patient's first contact with the health care system. While 80 percent of reportable STDs are treated by family doctors,[2] only 30 percent of these cases are actually reported.

Young women bear the greatest burden of STD complications,

since pelvic inflammatory disease (PID) is a major sequel.[2] The frequency of PID is increasing, as are its consequences (ectopic pregnancy and infertility). Women are four times more likely than men to acquire an STD when exposed to an infected partner. Many of these women remain asymptomatic.

Given the magnitude of the problem, family doctors need to develop an understanding of and an approach to STDs which can help control the spread of these diseases.

PREVALENCE

Accurate data on true prevalence of STDs are difficult to obtain. Only five types of STDs are "reportable" in most countries: gonorrhea, syphilis, lymphogranuloma venereum, granuloma inguinalae, and chancroid. In general, nonreportable STDs are far more common than reportable ones. For example, nongonococcal urethritis (NGU) is three to five times as common as gonorrhea. Fewer than 3000 cases of syphilis per year are recorded in Canada, and the disease is thought to be under control.[3]

Approximately 1 in 20 North Americans is infected by an STD. Estimated cases exceed 1 million per year, with the annual cost of treating both complicated and uncomplicated STDs estimated at more than $200 million.[2]

Widespread importance

The major age group affected by STDs is 15- to 29-years-old.

HISTORY TAKING

Taking a complete and detailed history is essential to the treatment of STDs, since it determines the nature of the ensuing examination. Patients often report a symptom which may indicate an STD but are reluctant to discuss their worry directly with a physician. For this reason, it is important that the physician establish a relaxed, communicative, and nonjudgmental rapport with the patient. The patient may not volunteer important information, but if the physician asks the right questions in the right way, the patient will usually answer truthfully. Questions should be open-ended but detailed: Is there discharge? What type? Is there dysuria, rash, growth or ulcer, abdominal pain or fever?

Asking the right questions

The most difficult part of history taking and one which is often neglected is establishing the patient's sexual orientation. This is essential, since it determines what further questions the physician should ask, what examination or laboratory tests will be needed, and what counseling the patient should receive. The physician

Sexual orientation

must take care not to seem judgmental and to phrase such questions in a nonoffensive way. Whether the patient is homosexual or heterosexual, the physician should determine the precise type of sexual activity in which the patient engages: oral sex (receptive and/or insertive), anal sex (receptive and/or insertive, oral), etc.

The physician should also determine the number of partners and contacts, dates of contacts, contraception, history of pregnancy, menstrual history, previous STDs, drug allergy, and recent treatments.

The following discussion will focus on two common problems in family medicine: urethritis in men and vaginitis and cervicitis in women.

URETHRITIS IN MEN

Definition

Urethritis is an inflammation of the urethra which clinically can produce symptoms of dysuria or discharge. The severity of symptoms ranges from clinically unapparent to disabling. Patients in the former group, who are culture-positive only, may not be diagnosed or treated.[4]

Etiology

A number of infective agents can cause urethritis, including *Neisseria gonorrhoeae, Chlamydia trachomatis, Ureaplasma urealyticum,* and *Trichomonas vaginalis.* (See Table 17-1.)

Clinical Examination

Specimen
taking

This should include a complete examination of the external genitalia, including retraction of the foreskin if present, as well as examination of the scrotum, pubic hair, and regional lymph nodes. If the patient's sexual orientation indicates, the physician should also examine the pharynx and rectum. If no urethral discharge is present, the urethra should be milked by pressure between the thumb and forefinger on the ventral surface. A calcium alginate swab should be inserted 1 to 2 cm into the urethra. An inoculum for culture and a glass slide for Gram's stain can be prepared directly from the swab, or the swab can be placed in transport medium. A rectal culture can be done by inserting a cotton-tipped swab into the anus (but not into the stool). Normally, smears from the rectum or pharynx are not Gram stained but are prepared for culture.

Table 17-1   Causes of Urethral Discharge

A   Infective types
    1   Gonococcal urethritis
    2   Nongonococcal urethritis
        a   *Chlamydia trachōmatis*
        b   *Ureaplasma urealyticum*
        c   *Herpes simplex*
        d   *Trichomonas vaginalis*
        e   *Candida albicans*
        f   Genital warts
B   Noninfective types
    1   Physiological discharge
    2   Trauma or foreign body
    3   Metabolite (e.g., calculi, oxalemia)
    4   Allergies
    5   Chemicals (e.g., antiseptics)

Epidemiology

Nongonococcal urethritis is the most common form of urethritis and may be three to five times more common than gonorrhea. The causative organism is *C. trachomatis* in approximately 30 to 50 percent of cases. *Chlamydia* is present in 20 to 30 percent of patients who also have gonorrhea.[4] Gonococcal urethritis is the most commonly reported infectious disease in Canada.[2] It is important to remember that up to 50 percent of patients exposed to gonorrhea may be asymptomatic carriers.[4] *Chlamydia* infections are often asymptomatic as well and may coexist with gonorrhea.

NGU most common

Diagnosis

In gonorrheal infections symptoms usually occur within 7 days of exposure, and the discharge is usually quite purulent and copious. Culture of the exudate on specific media such as Thayer-Martin and Gram's stain for intracellular gram-negative diplococci will give the diagnosis. In cases of NGU, the discharge is usually less abundant and more mucoid and the dysuria is usually not as severe. Symptoms usually appear 7 to 21 days after contact and tend to last longer. These clinical differences are not, however, sufficiently reliable to differentiate NGU from gonococcal urethritis. In some centers, *C. trachomatis* can be cultured in hospital or government laboratories, but the transportation of specimens to the laboratory can be difficult since specimens need to be kept at 4°C (at −70°C if more than 24 hours must elapse in transport).

Some facilities now use an antigen identification technique which can be done rapidly and without the need for culture. This method makes the transportation of specimens less of a problem,

Culture methods

and testing may become more widely available. Until this happens, the diagnosis of *Chlamydia* may have to be made by exclusion, that is, by a culture negative for gonorrhea.

Treatment

Immediate
treatment

Bacteriological culture must be done in order to determine disease prevalence and antibiotic sensitivity patterns, institute appropriate treatment and contact tracing, and advise patients.[4] Once cultures have been obtained, however, the practitioner should institute treatment immediately, without waiting for laboratory results (Table 17-2).

Follow-up
important

In a practice where gonorrhea is rare, the practitioner should choose a medication effective against both gonorrhea and *Chlamydia*. If follow-up treatment of a patient is difficult (e.g., in emergency departments), guidelines recommend treatment for gonorrhea in the form of a single dose of ampicillin and probenecid followed by 7 days of tetracycline; this regimen should deal with both gonorrhea and *Chlamydia*.

The patient should have a follow-up examination with cultures done 7 to 10 days after the first treatment. Until follow-up results are available, the patient should be advised to refrain from sexual activity.

Contact Tracing

It is essential that every effort be made to treat the sexual contacts of the patient. When possible, cultures should be obtained from the contacts before they are treated, but treatment should not be withheld until the results are available. If the spread of STDs is to be curbed, treatment of contacts is essential, since up to 80 percent of infected women may be asymptomatic.[4]

Contact tracing often creates difficult situations. For example, a patient may have a regular partner but contract gonorrhea from a casual partner. Both partners must be contacted and treated, and the physician must emphasize the importance of this to the patient. The diagnosis may create difficulties in the couple's relationship, and supportive counseling for one or both partners may be necessary at some point during therapy.

Contact-tracing

Another common problem in contact tracing is anonymous partners. If the patient is unable or unwilling to inform a contact, the public health department may be helpful in tracing a casual partner. Such a situation provides an opportunity to educate the patient about the public health problems and increased risk of infection which result from having multiple sexual partners. If the patient is likely to continue to have multiple sexual partners, he or

Table 17-2   Treatment of Urethritis

1   *Neisseria gonorrhoeae*

Probenecid 1 g + Ampicillin 3.5 g PO* *or*
+ Amoxicillin 3 g PO* *or*
+ Procaine penicillin G 4.8 million units IM

Tetracycline 500 mg PO, qid for 5 days

Spectinomycin 2 g IM (for penicillinase-producing gonococci)

Cefoxitin 2 g IM

Cefotaxime 1 g IM   } (for penicillinase-producing and non-
penicillinase-producing gonococci)

Ceftriaxone 250 mg IM

2   Nongonococcal urethritis (presumed to be *C. trachomatis* or *U. urealyticum*)

Tetracycline 500 mg PO, qid for 7 days *or*

Doxycycline 100 mg PO, bid for 7 days *or*

Erythromycin 500 mg PO, qid for 7 days†

*Not effective for pharyngeal gonorrhea.
†May also be used to treat gonorrhea.
Source: Adapted from Bowmer.[4] For complete treatment guidelines, see reference 5.

she should be advised about the use of condoms to protect against contracting or spreading disease.

VAGINITIS AND CERVICITIS

Definition

Vaginitis is a superficial infection of the vaginal epithelial cells without significant tissue invasion. The infection may be asymptomatic or may cause a fair amount of discomfort. Serious long-term consequences are unusual.[6] *Cervicitis,* an infection of the cervix, may be completely asymptomatic, with an apparently normal cervix. The term *mucopurulent cervicitis* describes an endocervical mucopus and/or area of ectopy (i.e., the extension of columnar epithelium onto the exocervix) that is erythematous, edematous, and friable.[6]

Causes

The major causes of these problems are listed in Table 17-3. With the exception of yeast infections and trichomoniasis, which occasionally can be contracted from an inert surface, these organisms are spread by oral or penile contact with the external genitalia.

Diagnosis

The diagnosis of vaginitis requires a combination of symptoms and signs. The physician must ask about the amount, color, consistency,

Table 17-3   Causes of Vaginitis, Vulvitis, and Cervicitis

Vaginitis	1	Yeasts
	2	*Trichomonas vaginalis*
	3	Nonspecific vaginitis (mixed *Gardnerella vaginalis* and anaerobic infection)
	4	Chemical causes
Cervicitis	1	*Chlamydia trachomatis*
	2	*Neisseria gonorrhoeae*
	3	Herpes simplex virus
	4	*Mycoplasma hominis*
Vulvitis	1	Yeasts (*Candida albicans* and *Torulopsis glabrata*)
	2	Herpes simplex virus

Source: Adapted from Bowie.[6]

Culture

and odor of discharge; itch; dysuria; and lesions on the labia (Table 17-4).

The three organisms responsible for most vaginitis (yeast, *Trichomonas,* and *Gardnerella vaginalis*) can be cultured. However, diagnosis does not depend on this. In infections caused by yeast or *G. vaginalis,* a positive culture without the appearance of other symptoms does not necessarily indicate a need for treatment. The diagnosis of nonspecific vaginitis does not depend on culture. Cervical cultures for gonorrhea and *Chlamydia* should be done in most cases of vaginitis if culture services are available.

Treatment

Treatment failure

Treatment of yeast infections and nonspecific vaginitis is indicated only if a woman is symptomatic. In cases involving either infection, one should consider treating the partner only if the initial treatment fails. With yeast infections, treatment of an asymptomatic partner is not usually helpful. There are a variety of therapies for yeast infections, but recurrences are frequent regardless of the regimen. (See Table 17-5.)

Treatment of recurrent yeast infections with oral nystatin provides no benefit.[6] Sexual intercourse may continue during therapy for either of these infections.

T. vaginalis should be treated when present whether or not it is symptomatic. Initially, both partners should be treated with a single dose of metronidazole. If this fails, a 1-week course of metronidazole should be used.

CERVICITIS

Danger of PID

Very often cervicitis is diagnosed only when a partner becomes symptomatic. If symptoms are present, they may include a dis-

Table 17-4 Diagnosis of Vaginitis

	Normal	Nonspecific vaginitis	Yeasts	*T. vaginalis*
Symptoms				
Discharge	±	+	±	+ +
Itch	−	−	+ +	+ +
Fishy odor	−	+ +	−	−
Wet mount				
Epithelial cells	+ +	Clue cells	+ +	+ +
Polymorphonuclear leucocytes	±	+	+ +	+ +
Trichomonas vaginalis	−	−	−	+ +
Potassium hydroxide preparation				
Fungi	−	−	+	−
Fishy odor	−	+ +	−	−
pH	< 4.5	> 4.5	< 4.5	5.5–6.0
Gram's stain	GPR*	GVR†	Fungi	*T. vaginalis*

*Gram-positive rods.
†Gram-variable rods.
Source: Adapted from Bowie.[6]

Table 17-5 Initial Treatment of Vaginitis

Organism	Drug and dose	Number of doses per day	Treatment duration, days	Failure at 1 month, %
Yeasts	Nystatin 100,000 units	1	14	30–40
	Clotrimazole 100 mg	1	6	10–20
	Miconazole 100 mg	1	7	10–20
	Econazole 150 mg	1	3	25–30
	Boric acid 600 mg	1	14	10–20
Gardnerella vaginalis and anaerobes	Metronidazole 500 mg	2	7	15
	Ampicillin 500 mg	4	7	40
Trichomonas vaginalis	Metronidazole 2 g	1	1	10–20
	Metronidazole 250 mg	3	7	5–10

Source: Adapted from Bowie.[6]

Table 17-6   High-Risk Groups Needing Treatment for *Chlamydia trachomatis*

1   Mucopurulent cervicitis with or without gonorrhea
2   Gonorrhea or contacts of gonorrhea (30–60 percent *C. trachomatis*–positive)
3   Contacts of men with NGU (30–60 percent *C. trachomatis*–positive)
4   Pelvic inflammatory disease
5   Contacts of men with Reiter's syndrome or acute epididymitis not due to coliforms
6   Mothers of infants with *Chlamydia* infections

Source: Bowie.[6]

charge (rare) or postcoital or mid-cycle bleeding. Symptoms of painful intercourse, abdominal pain, and heavy periods may indicate that the infection has spread to the upper reproductive tract. Undiagnosed and untreated infection may cause PID with all its known complications (e.g., infertility and ectopic pregnancy) and neonatal infection. It may also spread the disease to other partners. Approximately 10 percent of patients with chlamydial or gonorrheal cervicitis will develop PID, but the infection may be present for long periods before this occurs.[6]

Diagnosis

Cultures
necessary

Data for diagnosis may include signs of infection in the partner and clinical signs and symptoms in the patient as well as culture. Samples for culture and Gram's stain for gonorrhea should be taken from the cervical os. If the probable diagnosis is gonorrhea, samples for culture should also be taken from either the urethra or the anus. Other sites should be cultured depending on the sexual history. The sensitivity of cervical culture is 80 to 90 percent. A cervical Gram's stain can be useful in diagnosing gonorrhea; in experienced hands, it will be positive in 60 percent of infected cases with high specificity.[6]

Culture for *Chlamydia* should be done if available. The sample should contain epithelial cells, not mucus; therefore, mucus should be removed by swab, and a calcium alginate swab should be rotated in the cervical os several times after the mucus has been removed. Chlamydial culture may be positive in only 40 to 60 percent of infected patients; problems with transportation have already been discussed in this chapter.

Herpes can often be diagnosed clinically, with confirmation by culture.

Treatment

Cultures for *Chlamydia* are often not available. You must therefore decide whether to treat certain high-risk groups (Table 17-6). As has already been discussed, treatment of partners with or without symptoms is mandatory.

If your patient is compliant, you may wish to treat gonorrhea with tetracycline for 7 days, as *Chlamydia* often coexists (30 to 60 percent of cases).

SUMMARY

Sexually transmitted diseases are endemic in every community and present a daily challenge to family physicians.

Good management begins with prevention through patient education as well as good interviewing and examination skills to detect the variety of STDs. The application of up-to-date diagnostic tests and therapeutic procedures is essential if the spread of these diseases is to be brought under control.

REFERENCES

1 K. K. Holmes et al., "Epidemiology of Sexually Transmitted Diseases," *Urologic Clinics of North America*, **11**(1):3–13, 1984.
2 A. G. Jessamine, R. Mathias, and R. Sutherland, "Epidemiology and Control of Sexually Transmitted Diseases," *Canadian Journal of Public Health*, **74:** 163–166, 1983.
3 M. Steben and J. Yelle, "Sexually Transmitted Diseases and the Family Physician," *Canadian Family Physician*, **29:**621–623; April 1983.
4 M. I. Bowmer, "Urethritis and Epididymitis," *Medicine North America*, **6:** 499–505, 1983.
5 "Treatment of Sexually Transmitted Diseases," *Medical Letter*, **26**(653):5–10, 1984.
6 W. R. Bowie, "Vaginitis and Cervicitis," *Medicine North America*, **6:**506–511, 1983.

Chapter 18

Sexual Dysfunction

H. C. Still, M.D.

PRINCIPLE

The management of sexual dysfunction involves three concepts important to the practice of family medicine:

1 Sexuality is as important to health as any other "clinical" matter.

2 Sexual dysfunction may be primarily psychogenic in the young and multifactorial in older patients, but the interrelation between psyche and body is a complex and delicate one.

3 The family physician can do much to aid a patient with such a disorder but must recognize his or her limitations.

INTRODUCTION

"Hidden" problem

The identification of sexual dysfunction plays an important role in the day-to-day practice of family medicine. It has been stated that 10 to 15 percent[1] of patients seen by family physicians express some kind of sexual concern without specific inquiry or history taking. If one includes patients who make specific inquiries, the figures are much higher. Masters and Johnson[2] suggest that at least

50 percent of married couples have a significant sexual problem at some time during their relationship. Vincent[3] has made the point that every physician is a consultant in sexual and marital health by choice or by default. If a physician chooses to ignore patients' sexual or marital problems and makes no effort to refer such patients, the implication being suggested is that such problems are unimportant to the patient's health and well-being.

DEFINITION

Sexual dysfunction may be broadly defined as any situation or symptom relating to sexual behavior, interaction, or functioning which causes distress or concern to the patient and/or to a partner.

CONCEPTUAL MODELS

A conceptual scheme helpful in dealing with sexual dysfunction in a family practice has been described by Annon.[4] He outlines a four-level approach to dealing with sexual concerns and problems which he calls the PLISSIT model. The levels are as follows:

Management model

1 P: permission giving
2 LI: limited information giving
3 SS: specific suggestions
4 IT: intensive therapy

Some of the problems at the third level and almost all the complex and difficult to manage problems at the fourth level will require referral for sex therapy or counseling. Problems at the first two levels and many third-level problems can be dealt with by an interested, competent, properly trained, and sympathetic family physician.

Permission giving involves "demythologizing" patients' ideas about their own, their partners', or their families' sexuality. Infants and children should be allowed to touch their genitals. People of any age, sex, or marital status should be permitted to masturbate or to have sexual fantasies without guilt and should be comfortable with individual sexual preference, frequency of arousal, and level of sexual activity. Conversely, some people may need to be allowed not to enjoy sex or to be celibate.

Permission giving

Providing limited information deals with such concerns as penis size, breast size and shape, vaginal adequacy, frequency of intercourse, sexual variations, coital practices, oral-genital contact, orgasmic response, and masturbation. Sexuality during pregnancy, the effects of aging, common medications (including alcohol and

Providing limited information

Specific
therapeutic
suggestions

street drugs), and the effects of illness and surgery on sexual performance are areas requiring specific instruction and counseling.

Specific suggestions, which may involve brief therapy, include counseling for uncomplicated and selected cases of erectile dysfunction and premature ejaculation in men and secondary anorgasmia in women. However, most cases of significant erectile dysfunction, premature ejaculation, and retarded ejaculation in men and all cases of primary anorgasmia and many cases of secondary anorgasmia and vaginismus in women, require referral for more intensive therapy. The increasingly common sexual dysfunction of inhibited sexual desire, which is predominantly seen in women, with its associated relationship problems, is usually very difficult to manage and will also require referral for skilled counseling and intensive therapy.

Because male erectile dysfunction or impotence is very common and because its etiology interconnects with so many medical, social, and psychological problems, the author has chosen to discuss the diagnosis and management of this major sexual problem in detail.

ERECTILE DYSFUNCTION

The most common major male sexual dysfunction and the most distressing and devastating to the patient is erectile dysfunction. The word "impotence," like "frigidity," has unfortunate connotations and is considered by many to be pejorative; it should be avoided.

Prevalence

Definition

The incidence of erectile dysfunction in 60-year-old men has been found to range from 10 percent[5] to over 18 percent.[6] It is consistently more prevalent in men receiving medical treatment than in age-matched healthy men. For clinical purposes, erectile dysfunction may be defined as "the inability to obtain or maintain an erection of sufficient firmness to permit coitus to be initiated or completed."[7] It is said to be primary if the individual has never had an adequate erection and secondary if previously existing erectile competence has been lost. Primary erectile dysfunction is so rare that for all practical purposes it is never encountered in routine clinical practice.

Etiology

The causes and contributing factors are so numerous and variable (Table 18-1) that a systematic approach is required in order to con-

Table 18-1   Erectile Dysfunction: Etiology and Contributing Factors

1	Psychogenic
2	Aging
3	General debility and/or obesity
4	Alcohol
5	Drugs, prescription medications
6	Neurological
7	Endocrine and/or metabolic
8	Vascular
9	Urogenital
10	Multifactorial

sider the many possible etiologic factors. In many cases, especially in the older age group, the causes are often multifactorial and unclear.

Psychogenic   The largest group, accounting for about 80 percent of all patients with erectile dysfunction seen by the primary care physician, have a predominantly psychogenic etiology. With increasing age, however, the frequency of organic causes become much higher, approaching 50 percent or more in men 50 years old or older. Even when the patient suffers from an organic problem, his sexual anxiety may complicate the problem. Younger men without any health problems may report loss of erectile function as a result of fatigue, overindulgence in alcohol, or an anxiety-producing sexual encounter. Many of these patients need reassurance and explanation; otherwise, their anxiety and fear of failure may lead to a self-perpetuating sexual problem.

Psychogenic causes are most common

In a man under 50 years of age with a short history and no obvious organic illness or drug abuse (medications or drugs, including alcohol) whose nocturnal or early morning erections are normal, it is always worth instituting a trial of counseling and therapy before beginning major investigative procedures. If the patient has normal nocturnal erections and can obtain a good erection through masturbation or erotically stimulating books or pictures, a major organic cause is unlikely. If there is some question about the adequacy of the patient's nocturnal erections, the use of a simple snap gauge made by Dacomed can be helpful. This is placed around the base of the shaft of the penis before the patient retires and is examined in the morning for the breaking of one or more of three colored snaps.

The physician should look for evidence of sexual boredom, overwork and fatigue, stress, depression, obesity, heavy smoking and overindulgence in alcohol (acute or chronic) or other drugs,

Explore causes of anxiety

and aging. Above all, anxiety resulting from many causes—including performance anxiety and fear of failure, loss of self-esteem, and relationship problems may lead to psychogenic erectile failure.

Aging   "To maintain masculinity is a life-long biological struggle."[8] Masters and Johnson[9] have given us a clear understanding of the physiological changes in sexual performance and response which may occur as a man moves into his middle fifties and beyond. If he does not anticipate or understand the nature of these changes, he is very likely to worry about his sexual performance and develop erectile failure. If his wife is also ignorant of the changes, she may misinterpret them, leading to relationship problems and an even greater likelihood of avoidance or failure. More recently, Masters has described the *widower's syndrome*. The typical patient is a man in his middle fifties or older whose spouse has died or has been in failing health. As a result, he has been sexually inactive for more than a year. When a subsequent opportunity for sexual activity occurs, he finds that he cannot achieve or maintain an erection, although he had never had such a problem in his marriage. Unless he has a very understanding and cooperative partner or receives adequate counseling and support, he may continue to have erectile failure for the rest of his life. A similar situation may occur after a divorce.

Masters recently stated that the old saw "I'm too old for sex" can be translated into "I'm too anxious about my current level of sexual performance as judged against remembered functional facility in my 20's rather than realistically from the perspective of my 60's."[10]

General Debility   General debility can reduce libido and potency either temporarily or permanently. Fatigue resulting from overwork, day-to-day tensions of living, or lack of sleep may cause temporary erectile dysfunction that often can be relieved by means of a change in lifestyle or a vacation. Severe malnutrition from any cause, severe anemia, uremia, and generalized atherosclerosis are examples of debilitating illnesses that can cause erectile dysfunction. *Gross obesity* leading to reduced plasma testosterone levels and increased estrogen levels may cause erectile dysfunction.

Alcohol   Alcohol is a significant cause of erectile dysfunction; virtually all young men have had the embarrassing experience of failing to achieve or maintain an erection after too many drinks. If the cause is recognized, there should be no further difficulties. If it is not, anxiety and fear of failure can lead to problems. Chronic

Widower's syndrome

alcoholism, with or without hepatic cirrhosis, can be a major cause of organic erectile dysfunction.

Drugs Drugs, prescribed or not, may be a leading cause of erectile dysfunction. Physicians' prescribing habits must be regarded as one of the major factors contributing to erectile dysfunction. Approximately 75 prescription drugs which may cause sexual dysfunctions, principally erectile failure, have been identified.[11] The most common offenders among prescribed medications are the antihypertensives [except hydralazine (Apresoline) in doses of 100 mg per day or less], antipsychotics, sedatives and minor tranquilizers (in large doses), and most antidepressants. Antihistamines, cimetidine, and metoclopropamide are also offenders. Street drugs such as marijuana in large amounts, heroin, and methadone may also cause erectile dysfunction.

Common drug causes

Neurological Causes Penile erection can be considered a hemodynamic phenomenon controlled by a neurological mechanism. In diabetes and multiple sclerosis, the neuropathy which may occur early in the disease can lead to erectile failure. Other neurological causes include cord transection and tumors.

Endocrine or Metabolic Factors Endocrine or metabolic factors are among the major organic causes of erectile dysfunction and may include diabetes, hypoandrogynism (including primary testicular failure), hyperprolactinemia, Addison's disease, Cushing's syndrome, Klinefelter's and Turner's syndromes, and (rarely) hypothyroidism or hyperthyroidism.

Vascular Causes It has been known for years that obstruction of the lower part of the aorta or its major branches causes erectile failure (Leriche syndrome). During the past 10 years, a great deal of research has demonstrated that obstruction of the smaller arteries supplying the penis can be a significant cause of organic erectile failure.

Urogenital Causes Urogenital causes can be structural, including severe phimosis, Peyronie's disease, and amputation of the penis. Chronic priapism leading to painful or abnormal erections can be a cause of erectile dysfunction, as can trauma secondary to abdominoperineal surgery or radical surgery for cancer of the prostate or bladder. A recently described condition causing abnormal leakage from the venous drainage system of the corpus cavernosum may lead to erectile failure in otherwise healthy teenage boys.[12]

5 SEXUAL DYSFUNCTION

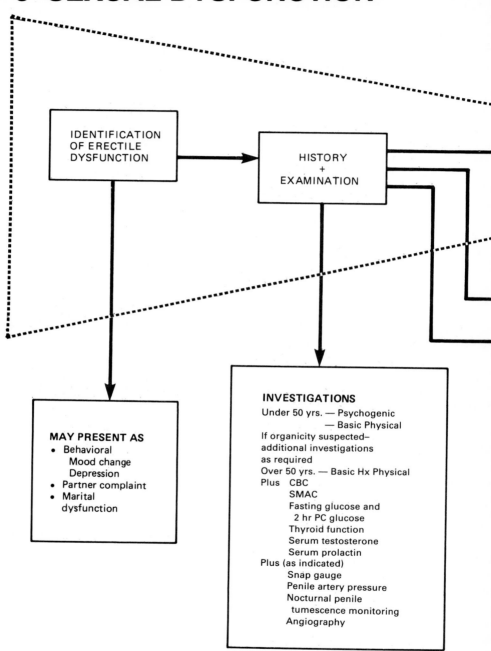

IDENTIFICATION
OF ERECTILE
DYSFUNCTION

HISTORY
+
EXAMINATION

MAY PRESENT AS
- Behavioral
  Mood change
  Depression
- Partner complaint
- Marital
  dysfunction

INVESTIGATIONS
Under 50 yrs. — Psychogenic
— Basic Physical
If organicity suspected–
additional investigations
as required
Over 50 yrs. — Basic Hx Physical
Plus   CBC
       SMAC
       Fasting glucose and
        2 hr PC glucose
       Thyroid function
       Serum testosterone
       Serum prolactin
Plus (as indicated)
       Snap gauge
       Penile artery pressure
       Nocturnal penile
        tumescence monitoring
       Angiography

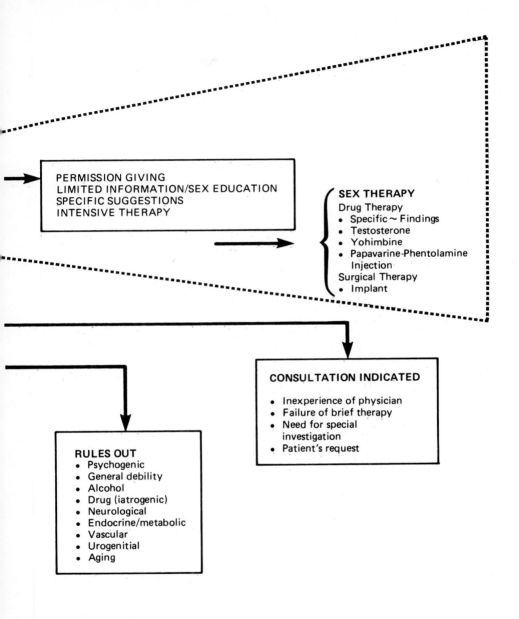

PERMISSION GIVING
LIMITED INFORMATION/SEX EDUCATION
SPECIFIC SUGGESTIONS
INTENSIVE THERAPY

SEX THERAPY
Drug Therapy
- Specific ~ Findings
- Testosterone
- Yohimbine
- Papavarine-Phentolamine
  Injection
Surgical Therapy
- Implant

CONSULTATION INDICATED

- Inexperience of physician
- Failure of brief therapy
- Need for special
  investigation
- Patient's request

RULES OUT
- Psychogenic
- General debility
- Alcohol
- Drug (iatrogenic)
- Neurological
- Endocrine/metabolic
- Vascular
- Urogenitial
- Aging

EVALUATION AND ASSESSMENT OF ERECTILE DYSFUNCTION

Laboratory
investigations

All patients require a careful history and physical examination, including general assessment and a detailed urogenital examination and urinalysis. This may be all that is required for younger patients who have no symptoms of an underlying organic problem.

In all other cases, especially in patients 50 years old or older, a complete laboratory workup including complete blood count (CBC), SMAC, a.c. and 2-hour p.c. blood sugars, T_4, T_3, thyroid-stimulating hormone (TSH), luteinizing hormone (LH), follicle-stimulating hormone (FSH), serum testosterone (morning specimen), and serum prolactin. Other special investigations may include measurement of systolic blood pressure in penile arteries and assessment of nocturnal erections using the snap gauge mentioned earlier in this chapter or a portable nocturnal penile tumescence monitor, now available for use at home as well as in hospital sleep laboratories. More specialized and sophisticated investigations include x-ray angiography, with selective angiography of the pudendal and penile arteries, and infusion cavernosography with a radiopaque dye.

Treatment I: Psychogenic Erectile Dysfunction

Counseling

The management of psychogenic erectile dysfunction consists of a series of therapy sessions with the patient and his partner, with the object of relieving performance anxiety and increasing all aspects of their communication skills. Psychotherapeutic suggestions may improve all aspects of the relationship. At the outset, any direct sexual activity is prohibited; instead, the couple is instructed in methods which focus on sensual awareness without the need for sexual performance. These assignments are practiced at home and discussed at the couple's next visit to the therapist. In some centers, behavioral therapy, biofeedback training, and hypnotherapy have also been used.

Treatment II: Organic Erectile Dysfunction

The essential point here is to arrive at an accurate etiologic diagnosis if possible. However, because the etiology is often multifactorial, this may be a difficult process. Where the problem is reversible, the chances of recovery are good although sex therapy often may be necessary to allay performance anxiety or relationship problems.

Drug therapy

A small group of men with clearly demonstrated endocrinopathy and subnormal early morning testosterone levels will benefit from testosterone replacement therapy. If no medical contraindications exist, this should be tried for 3 or 4 months and continued if effective.

Yohimbine hydrochloride (an alpha$_2$-adrenergic antagonist) in doses of 6 to 12 mg per day has been tried in some cases of organic erectile dysfunction. Patients with a peripheral neuropathy (e.g., diabetes) are the most likely candidates for success. More recently, erectile dysfunction has been treated with local intracorporeal injections of a papaverine phentolamine preparation, using a fine hypodermic needle. This produces a good sustained erection sufficient for vaginal intromission and may become an alternative to a penile prosthesis for some patients.

At the present time, the only option for obtaining satisfactory penile intromission for long-term cases of erectile dysfunction caused by organic or multifactorial causes which are not medically reversible or amenable to sex therapy is the use of a surgically implanted penile prosthesis or, when indicated, either corrective surgery on the arterial supply to the penis or corrective surgery for the rare cases of drainage failure of the corpus cavernosum. Candidates for a penile prosthesis should always be adequately counseled before such an operation is undertaken.

REFERENCES

1 D. K. Kentsmith, and M. T. Eaton, *Treating Sexual Problems in Medical Practice,* Arco, New York, 1979.
2 W. H. Masters and V. E. Johnson, *Human Sexual Inadequacy,* Little, Brown, Boston, 1970.
3 C. E. Vincent, *Sexual and Marital Health,* McGraw-Hill, New York, 1973.
4 J. S. Annon, *Behavioral Treatment of Sexual Problems: Brief Therapy,* Harper and Row, 1976. Hagerstown, MD.
5 A. C. Kinsey et al., *Sexual Behavior in the Human Male,* W. B. Saunders, Philadelphia, 1948.
6 E. Pfeiffer et al., "Sexual Behavior in Middle Life," *American Journal of Psychiatry,* **128**:1262–1267, 1972.
7 J. B. R. McKendry et al., "Erectile Impotence: A Clinical Challenge," *Canadian Medical Association Journal,* **128**:653–662, 1983.
8 B. Hudson, "Virility and Sterility: Some Aspects of Endocrine Function in the Male," Royal College of Physicians and Surgeons of Canada, *Annals,* **15:** 209–215, 1982.
9 W. H. Masters and V. E. Johnson, *Human Sexual Response,* Little, Brown, Boston, 1966.
10 "AGS Conference Discusses Improving the Quality of Later Life," *Canadian Medical Association Journal,* **124**:1636–1638, 1981.
11 *Medical Letter,* "Drugs that Cause Sexual Dysfunction," **25**:73–76, 1983.
12 J. Ebbehoj and G. Wagner, "Insufficient Penile Erection due to Abnormal Draining of Cavernous Bodies," *Urology* **13**:507–510, 1979.

Chapter 19

Fatigue

B. K. Hennen, M.D.

PRINCIPLE

Some symptoms lead directly to a straightforward inquiry, after which we can diagnose and manage the patient's problem with dispatch. More undifferentiated symptoms offer no such immediate solution but instead demand evey ounce of our skill, experience, resources, and time. Such symptoms may represent a patient's inability to deal with the problems of everyday life, a specific component of a major psychiatric syndrome, or the first subtle evidence of a serious physical disease. Fatigue or tiredness is one such undifferentiated symptom.

DEFINITION

Fatigue is defined as "weariness on exertion, continuous tiredness, or inability to get going." Patients do not often use the word "fatigue." They say, "I'm tired all the time," "I feel weak," or "I am just pooped," or they request "something to pick me up" or ask "to have my blood checked." They may also be more specific: "When I do this, my arms get tired."

PREVALENCE

About 1 of 10 patients in family practice presents with fatigue as a primary symptom. The peak ages are from 15 to 24 and over 60, and two-thirds of these patients are women. No more than one-half of cases have a proven physical cause, but persons over 40 are twice as likely to have physical causes as those under 40.[1,2]

ETIOLOGY

Psychological causes include clearly recognized psychiatric problems, among which anxiety is by far the most frequent, with depression and other neuroses following (Table 19-1). Psychological causes also include day-to-day problems and undue stress which goes beyond the normal person's coping abilities. Some people suffer from fatigue simply because they work too hard.

The physical causes of fatigue are usually disorders found in four body systems: endocrine, cardiovascular, respiratory, and hematologic. Table 19-2 summarizes the common physical causes of fatigue.

PRESENTING FEATURES

Symptom Complexes

When the symptom is difficult to describe, when the tiredness is present on arising, when it is accompanied by a vague headache or muscular aches and pains (without weight loss), or when the symptom is improved by distractions ("not so bad over the weekends"), the likelihood is that the fatigue is due to a functional or emotional problem. However, if the patient can describe specific muscular weakness, an urge to sleep, inability to maintain performance, or worsening of the fatigue with usually nontiring activities, a physical or organic cause is more likely.

Associated symptoms

In approaching the symptom inquiry under the traditional categories, the following considerations may be helpful.

1 *Duration*: A very short duration tends to make one think of acute infection, acute blood loss, or acute cardiovascular or pulmonary insult. A more moderate duration with a gradual increase in awareness of the symptom may indicate underlying malignancy, the wearing effect of chronic pain, or smoldering infection. Life-long duration of fatigue is more likely to be found in people who have difficulty coping generally or who have a basic personality disorder.

2 *Onset*: It is often helpful to know whether the onset has been acute or gradual. For example, a death in the family may

Table 19-1 Associated Features of Psychological Causes

Problem of living	Psychiatric disorder	Workaholic
Irritability	Reduced appetite	Aggressive
Tearful	Sleep disorder	Unresolved guilt
Loss of concentration	Previous mental symptoms	Open-ended profession
Reduced libido	Abnormal personality patterns	Own conscience monitor
Muscle aches and pain	Specific features of anxiety or depression	Work used as solution to life's problems
Tension headaches*		
Life-change score over 100†		No inner governor to recognize needs for recreation and rest‡

*See Hargreaves.[4]
†See Holmes.[3]
‡See Rhoads.[5]

Table 19-2 Common Physical Causes of Fatigue

Endocrine	Diabetes mellitus Hyperthyroidism Hypothyroidism
Cardiovascular	Hypertension Arteriosclerotic heart disease Undifferentiated congestive heart failure
Respiratory	Acute viral illnesses, aftermath Chronic bronchitis
Hematologic	Iron deficiency anemia

precede an acute onset of fatigue. On the other hand, recent dental extraction precipitating subacute bacterial endocarditis is an example of the gradual onset of an organic problem.

3 *Periodicity*: If the fatigue is constant, it suggests a structural or physical problem. If the symptom is fluctuating, especially in relation to mood, stress, and anxiety, a functional etiology seems more likely.

4 *The worst time of the day*: Knowing the worst time of day for the symptom may provide a helpful clue. A person who wakes up feeling tired after apparently adequate sleep is more likely to have a functional problem, especially if things improve as the day goes on. On the other hand, a person whose fatigue worsens as activity proceeds during the day is more likely to have a physical cause.

5 *Precipitating and relieving factors*: The effects of exertion and sleep on the symptom are worth exploring. Fatigue related to specific events during the day may be either functional or physical, depending on the nature of the event. An afternoon class in a disliked subject may be sufficient to tire a worried student; a basketball game that unusually tires a youngster who has played a lot of basketball is more likely to represent a physical problem. Finally, a careful exploration of the patient's daily routine in terms of rest and physical activities is often useful.

APPROACH TO THE PATIENT

An early and unexplained exploration of psychological factors may confuse or even irritate patients who have come with the expectation of finding a physical and treatable cause for fatigue. It does not follow, however, that such an early review of psychological factors should be reserved until physical causes have been ruled out. On the contrary, it deserves an early place in the interview, but with an adequate explanation to the patient. Consider the following example.

Rule out physical causes

> For someone of your age, the most common cause of fatigue is a buildup of too many things happening at once, which wears you down. I am going to ask you some questions which at first may not appear to be related to your problem, and I hope you will answer them as frankly as possible.

This may make it less difficult to explain a subsequent diagnosis that does not involve a physical (and perhaps a more socially acceptable) cause. Such a diagnosis should be made only after you have completed the examination and ordered whatever tests seem necessary.

At this point, it is also important to identify patients who do not have a psychiatric illness but are simply overburdened by a series of life events which, by occurring simultaneously, have been more than they can deal with. An accurate analysis of life-change events is worth doing, and the list identified by Holmes[3] should be reviewed.

Overburdened life situation

In his practice, Hargreaves identified what he called the *new town neurosis,* a neurosis characteristic of young married housewives in a newly established town that involved transplanted people.[4] We have observed a similar syndrome in our practice, which we call *new-in-town fatigue syndrome,* in which the family has moved to a new town, usually because of the husband's new job. The move often means a promotion about which the husband is pleased and a job in which he is happily engaged with new colleagues in a new setting. The wife, however, is at home with the children in an unfamiliar neighborhood, has lost previous neighborhood support, and is trying to deal with new schools, a new house, and so on. Needless to say, the wife is the one affected by the syndrome.

New-in-town syndrome

Table 19-3   Workaholic Attitudes toward Work

1   A reaction against or an incorporation of parental and cultural attitudes
2   A basis of self-evaluation ("Work is good, I work to be considered good, and the more work I do, the better I am")
3   A convenient vehicle for displacement or sublimation of certain drives

Source: Rhoads.[5]

Table 19-4   Some Reminders for Less Common Physical Causes of Fatigue

If present	Think of
Paralytic episodes or progressive muscular weakness	Hypokalemia, myasthenia gravis
Pigmentation and gastrointestinal complaints	Addison's disease
Kidney stones and gastrointestinal complaints	Hyperparathyroidism
Episodes with sweating, palpitations, peculiar behavior	Hypoglycemia
Fever	Subacute bacterial endocarditis, blood dyscrasia, lymphoma
Diarrhea and weight loss	Malabsorption
Uncontrollable urge to sleep	Narcolepsy
Muscle weaknes	Cushing's syndrome
Joint pain or swelling	Disseminated lupus erythematosus or rheumatoid arthritis

Source: Goldberg.[6]

Table 19-5   Drugs Which Cause Fatigue as a Common Side Effect

Alcohol

Antihistamines

Antihypertensives: thiazides, propranolol, reserpine, methyldopa, guanethidine, clonidine, prazosin

Corticosteroids

Digitalis

Narcotic analgesics

Sedatives and hypnotics

Sodium valproate

Tranquilizers

Tricyclic antidepressants

Source: Rockwell and Burr[7] and Meyler.[9]

Table 19-6 Initial Investigation of Fatigue with Normal Examination

Fatigue only	Other symptoms but no weight loss
Hemoglobin	Blood sugar
White blood count	Blood urea nitrogen
Differential smear	Thyroid screen
Sedimentation rate	Serum calcium
Urinalysis	

Rhoads[5] describes another group of fatigued patients—the workaholics—whom he identifies as busy professionals or executives who share a personality type which appears to lack an inner governor "and for various reasons prevents them from recognizing the commonplace signs that inform us of the need for rest or recreation" (see Table 19-3).

Workaholics

Goldberg[6] has listed some specific examples of system review questions which he found particularly discriminating in identifying less common physical disorders causing fatigue. It is, of course, not a complete list (see Table 19-4).

Commonly used drugs are associated with fatigue as a significant side effect.[7] These drugs are listed in Table 19-5.

Drugs

The family history is obviously important, particularly for conditions such as diabetes, anemia, thyroid disorders, and depression.

INVESTIGATIONS

We have found the approach to investigation suggested by Goldberg[6] to be practical, although in persons under age 40 in whom psychological and stress problems are clearly involved we may do none of these tests initially. In one group of patients presenting in family practice with fatigue, an average of 4.4 tests were done per patient.[8] We would also almost certainly have a consultation for a patient before conducting carotene, edrophonium bromide (Tensilon), or other tests requiring particular interpretation (Table 19-6).

Tests

MANAGEMENT

The management of specific organic problems is related to the specific diagnosis. The management of functional fatigue or the fatigue syndrome may involve the following.

At the first meeting, if the diagnosis is primarily functional, if the patient seems receptive, and if time allows, one can proceed

6 FATIGUE

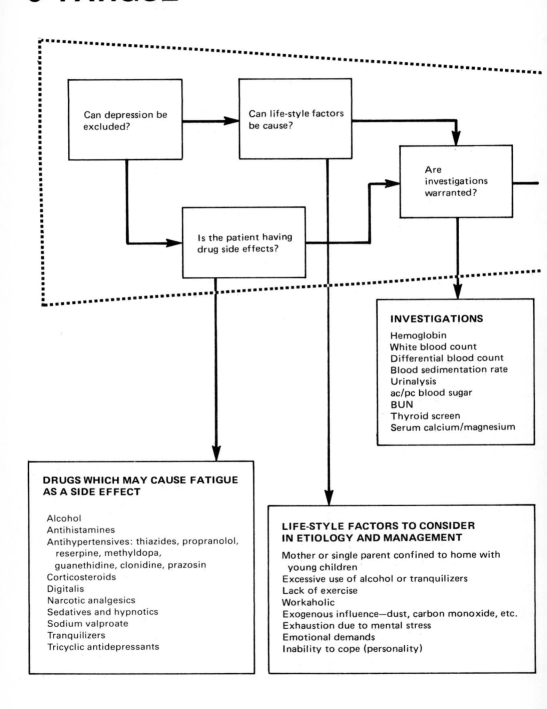

Can depression be excluded?

Can life-style factors be cause?

Are investigations warranted?

Is the patient having drug side effects?

INVESTIGATIONS

Hemoglobin
White blood count
Differential blood count
Blood sedimentation rate
Urinalysis
ac/pc blood sugar
BUN
Thyroid screen
Serum calcium/magnesium

DRUGS WHICH MAY CAUSE FATIGUE AS A SIDE EFFECT

Alcohol
Antihistamines
Antihypertensives: thiazides, propranolol,
 reserpine, methyldopa,
 guanethidine, clonidine, prazosin
Corticosteroids
Digitalis
Narcotic analgesics
Sedatives and hypnotics
Sodium valproate
Tranquilizers
Tricyclic antidepressants

LIFE-STYLE FACTORS TO CONSIDER IN ETIOLOGY AND MANAGEMENT

Mother or single parent confined to home with
 young children
Excessive use of alcohol or tranquilizers
Lack of exercise
Workaholic
Exogenous influence—dust, carbon monoxide, etc.
Exhaustion due to mental stress
Emotional demands
Inability to cope (personality)

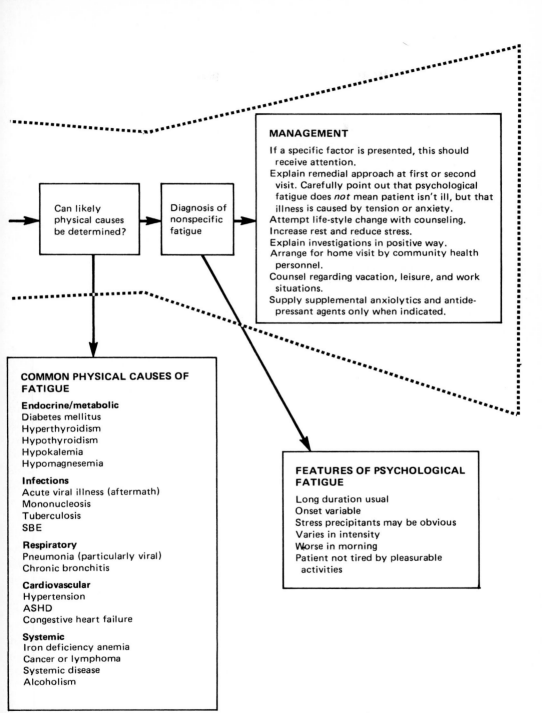

Can likely physical causes be determined?

Diagnosis of nonspecific fatigue

MANAGEMENT

If a specific factor is presented, this should receive attention.

Explain remedial approach at first or second visit. Carefully point out that psychological fatigue does *not* mean patient isn't ill, but that illness is caused by tension or anxiety.

Attempt life-style change with counseling.

Increase rest and reduce stress.

Explain investigations in positive way.

Arrange for home visit by community health personnel.

Counsel regarding vacation, leisure, and work situations.

Supply supplemental anxiolytics and antide-pressant agents only when indicated.

COMMON PHYSICAL CAUSES OF FATIGUE

Endocrine/metabolic
Diabetes mellitus
Hyperthyroidism
Hypothyroidism
Hypokalemia
Hypomagnesemia

Infections
Acute viral illness (aftermath)
Mononucleosis
Tuberculosis
SBE

Respiratory
Pneumonia (particularly viral)
Chronic bronchitis

Cardiovascular
Hypertension
ASHD
Congestive heart failure

Systemic
Iron deficiency anemia
Cancer or lymphoma
Systemic disease
Alcoholism

FEATURES OF PSYCHOLOGICAL FATIGUE

Long duration usual
Onset variable
Stress precipitants may be obvious
Varies in intensity
Worse in morning
Patient not tired by pleasurable activities

immediately to a discussion of remedial approaches aimed at altering the patient's lifestyle, reducing the amount of stress, enabling the patient to have more rest, etc.

Expressing confidence with diagnosis

It is important that the physician present a confident opinion to the patient, e.g., that the problem is due to stress, depression, a postflu syndrome, or iron deficiency anemia. "I don't think it is anything serious, but I am just going to do a few tests to make sure" is not quite as supportive a statement as "I am confident that your fatigue is due to the stress that you have been under recently because of your recent move. I am going to do a few tests to see if there are any physical factors involved, but whatever the tests show, I believe that the stress is the most significant cause for your fatigue."

When patients do not seem receptive to the idea that they have a functional or stress cause for fatigue, they may be right. If the patient is wrong, however, such lack of receptiveness may make management more difficult. In this case, it is probably wiser to await the results of the tests and use them to reassure the patient about the etiology of the problem.

It is important to explain to the patient why he or she is feeling fatigued. In particular, it is necessary to clearly separate patients who suffer from depression or anxiety from those who are basically normal but are not coping with excessive stress so that treatment can be specific.

Situational awareness

In his plan of management for young housewives with fatigue, Hargreaves stressed rest and encouraged the women to stay in bed longer (up to 12 hours a day) for at least 3 weeks.[4] He tried to talk to the spouses in order to explain and solicit their support. We have found that simply making the spouse aware of the problem and suggesting a regular evening out together without the children aids considerably in such a program. Asking relatives to help in child care and trading child care responsibilities with neighbors are other possible ways of securing one or two half days a week for oneself.

Home visits for follow-up and to gain better understanding of the home situation are useful. Such visits may help the doctor ascertain the necessity of rest. A home visitor or community health nurse may be a more appropriate person than the physician for making such a visit.

Anxiolytics

Hargreaves felt that one could anticipate reasonable improvement within 6 weeks. He would supplement his advice with anxiolytics or antidepressants but cautioned against using either of these as the sole method of treatment.[4] We have used short-term (2 weeks) diazepam on occasion but reserve antidepressants for clearly identifiable depression.

In his study of overwork, Rhoads emphasized the importance of evaluating the patient's attitudes toward work[5] (see Table 19-3) as part of the management, which may also include a vacation and counseling about future work, recreation, and rest.[9]

The symptom of fatigue requires an approach which takes account of the social, psychological, and physical aspects of the patient's health. Given the various probabilities and considering the importance of the initial interview in setting the stage for the ultimate management, we would caution that an approach of ruling out serious physical causes first may not be the most effective one in dealing with such an undifferentiated problem.

REFERENCES

1 D. W. Marsland, M. Wood, and F. Mayo, *Content of Family Practice: A Statewide Study in Virginia with Its Clinical, Educational, and Research Implications*, J. Geyman (ed.), Appleton-Century-Crofts, New York, 1976.
2 S. T. Bain and W. B. Spaulding, "The Importance of Coding Presenting Symptoms," *Canadian Medical Association Journal*, **97**(16):953–959, 1967.
3 T. Holmes, *Journal of Psychosomatic Research*, Pergamon Press, New York, 1976, vol. II, pp. 213–218.
4 M. Hargreaves, "The Fatigue Syndrome," *Practitioner*, **218**:841–843, 1977.
5 J. M. Rhoads, "Overwork," *Journal of the American Medical Association*, **237**:2615–2618, 1977.
6 W. M. Goldberg, "The Management of Chronic Fatigue," *Canadian Family Physician*, **15**(1):31–33, 1969.
7 D. A. Rockwell and B. D. Burr, "The Tired Patient," *Journal of Family Practice*, **5**:62–65, 1977.
8 J. D. Morrison, "Fatigue as a Presenting Complaint in Family Practice," *Journal of Family Practice*, **10**(5):795–801, 1980.
9 *Meyler's Side Effects of Drugs: An Encyclopedia of Adverse Reactions and Interactions*, M. N. G. Dukes (ed.), Elsevier, New York, 1984.

Chapter 20

Depression

B. K. Hennen, M.D.

PRINCIPLE

Family
supports

Appropriate involvement of a patient's family can often provide invaluable diagnostic information and make a substantial contribution to therapy. Caring for and about an ill family member is part of a healthy family's function and is usually willingly performed when the need is made clear.

The physician who is willing to involve family input when approaching an individual patient facilitates the use of a valuable resource. While this is true for any patient, a patient who is depressed is particularly likely to benefit if family resources are called upon.

DEFINITION

Depression, or a *depressive syndrome,* involves a predominantly depressed mood persisting for a month or more and including at least four of the following: poor appetite, sleep disturbance, energy loss, physical agitation or psychomotor retardation, loss of interest in usual activities, reduced sex drive, self-reproach or guilt, impaired thought processes, thoughts of death or suicide and wishing for death. This definition by Cadoret and Coble serves as a useful guide but does not take account of patients who present with symptoms that last less than a month.[1]

A depressed patient may be demonstrating a normal but exaggerated response to unresolved conflicts and stresses, a response that will probably vary according to basic personality. Such a patient is said to have a *reactive* or *neurotic* depression. On the other hand, patients who demonstrate an apparently unexplainable but clearly established depression are probably suffering from what is variously called an *endogenous, organic,* or *primary* depression. Such patients are usually divided into those who demonstrate primarily depressive features (the greatest proportion) and those who show the manic-depressive characteristics of cyclical swings of mood. When a primary depression coincides with midlife changes, it is felt by some to have specific enough characteristics to be separately labeled as an *involutional* depression.

PREVALENCE

Hodgkin reported 20 cases of depression in 1000 British National Health Service patients; of these patients, 1 had a manic-depressive syndrome and 19 had endogenous depression. He cited an attempted suicide rate of 1.4 per 1000 in which one of six attempts was successful.[2]

Data on the frequency of depression based on doctors' diagnoses must generally be considered underestimates. They do not take account of all the patients who present in doctors' offices with symptoms of depression.

NATURAL HISTORY

Patients who are depressed can generally expect improvement without specific intervention. Most depressions remit spontaneously, and the average duration is 2 to 3 months.

If one drew up a scale from normal with depressed mood to reactive depression to endogenous and manic-depressive syndrome, most patients with depressed feelings seen by the family physician would fall into the normal range.

In family practice, the individual at greatest risk for depression can be characterized as a woman over 30 with three or more children under age 14 still at home who has no interests outside the home, who has a low family income, who lost her own mother before the age of 11, who does not have an extended family, who is

At-risk population

without a confidant such as a receptive spouse, who has low self-esteem, and who has recently (within 2 years) lost a close friend or relative.[3]

Suicide risk

At highest risk for suicide among depressed patients are men, those who live alone, patients with a family history of suicide, patients on psychopharmacologic agents, alcoholics, persons with primary depressions as opposed to reactive depressions, and persons with a history that includes previous attempts at or gestures of suicide.[4]

ETIOLOGY

Anticipatory intervention

A depressed mood is a significant factor in many illnesses either as part of the pathogenesis or as a result of the particular illness. Chronic illnesses such as rheumatoid arthritis and chronic anxiety, life-threatening illnesses such as cancer and coronary heart disease, and frustrating illnesses such as a young athlete's fracture and an adolescent's acne may all contain significant elements of depression. It is well known that the sequelae of relatively common acute illnesses include depression; depressions tend to follow influenza, infectious hepatitis, and mononucleosis in particular. Other at-risk groups that deserve special attention are patients undergoing major surgical procedures and patients who have suffered acute and serious illnesses such as myocardial infarction.

Associated causes

In addition, iatrogenic problems are created by poor doctor-patient relationships and inappropriate medical advice, although these problems are harder to identify.

Specific illnesses, particularly of the endocrine group, classically include depressive features, for example, hypothyroidism and Cushing's syndrome.

Specific mechanisms of inheritance may be responsible for the manic-depressive syndrome.

APPROACHING THE PATIENT WITH
SUSPECTED DEPRESSION

Recognize clues

The problems the family physician faces in dealing with depression include recognizing the major clues, connecting vague presenting complaints, determining when a physical complaint is really an excuse for getting into the doctor's office and is in fact masking a depression, identifying the complications of alcohol and drug misuse and the relation of those behaviors to depression, finding practical ways to prevent or anticipate depression by becoming familiar with high-risk groups, knowing how to assess quickly and effectively a patient suspected of being depressed, and dealing with particularly difficult age groups such as the very young and the very old.

Depressed patients may present with tiredness, headache, changes in appetite, backache, or gastrointestinal symptoms. They may come in because they have been sent by a relative ("My daughter insisted that I see you, but I don't know why"). Often the first presentation of the depressed patient is a suicidal gesture or attempt.

When a patient presents with an undifferentiated symptom which has a high likelihood of being part of a depression (for example, fatigue) or with indications of being unable to cope or to "get going," or when a patient is looking for a physical reason for the way he or she feels ("I think my blood must be down"), there is a strong possibility that the patient is depressed. Such physical complaints must be taken seriously, but the major part of the interview should be directed toward the most likely diagnosis and the elements which constitute the greatest risk to the patient.

The doctor should consider the extent to which he or she is surprised to see a familiar patient presenting in such a way. Are there obvious reasons for the mood change, such as recent illness with chronic pain, frustration, or disability? Has the patient lost a friend or a close relative? Is the patient unemployed or in financial trouble? If such factors are present, the physician should try to determine how they may be affecting the patient's mood. Holmes's guideline for stress factors, which can be found in Table 4-1, may be helpful in your assessment. **Relative stress factors**

Often the first clue to a depressive illness is reported by another family member during an office visit ("Mom isn't herself, Doctor"). Once depression has become a recurrent or cyclical problem, a family member may take on the job of watching for signs of exacerbation ("He seems to be getting high again; he's restless, doesn't sleep, and works at his desk for hours").

The extent to which the classic depressive symptoms are present should be explored. They are fatigue, feelings of unworthiness and hopelessness, changing sleep patterns, physical and mental slowing down, and certain physical complaints (headache, backache, anorexia, gastrointestinal disturbance, and amenorrhea).

The patient should be asked specifically about suicide intent and thoughts of death. If there is suicide intent, ask what methods have been considered. The previous history should be discussed with the patient and also with relatives or friends, who may be able to cite examples of previous mood changes of which the patient may be unaware. A family history is particularly significant for manic-depressive kinds of illnesses.[5] **Ask about suicidal thoughts**

According to Cadoret and Coble,[1] the manic-depressive patient demonstrates a relatively sudden onset of increased activity during

Table 20-1   Drugs Causing Depressed Mood

Diuretics

Steroids

Atropine/belladonna group

Estrogens

Bromides and iodides

Vitamin D excess

Diazepam

Haloperidol

Physostigmine

Levodopa

Antihypertensives: reserpine, methyldopa, hydralazine, propranalol, clonidine

Antineoplastics: vinblastine, vincristine

Source: Cadoret and Coble[1] and Opie.[6]

manic phases, accompanied by a loss of insight. Also, 40 percent of full-blown anxiety attacks present for the first time in patients with serious depressions. Symptoms such as hyperventilation, palpitations, chest pain, and fear may be part of an anxiety syndrome and may be the first sign of serious depressive illness the doctor sees.

Hodgkin[2] reminds us that most emotional problems have two basic components: the cause and the patient's personality. He also believes that most psychoneurotic behavior has two common factors—the existence of unresolved conflicts and the fact that the conflicts are usually related to role or status—and finds it more helpful to think of "unresolved conflicts" rather than simply of "elements of stress."

Social supports

Hodgkin[2] encourages us to explore the four major sources of self-confidence in patients: marriage, family, friends, and job. He feels that family practitioners have the advantage of being able to objectively observe changes in the roles of patients in their practice, for example, the well person who becomes sick, the married person who becomes single, or the individual who is promoted or fired. This makes it easier for family physicians to anticipate and prevent problems.

Medication list

It is important to determine what medications the patient takes, both physician-prescribed and over the counter.[1] A list of drugs which may affect mood is given in Table 20-1. One should also determine whether the patient has recently been withdrawn from certain drugs, particularly narcotics, barbiturates, or amphetamines. The specific history of recent and past alcohol intake is also relevant.

EXAMINATION

The physical signs of depression include depressed facies, obvious reduction in physical mobility, readiness to cry and actual crying, and difficulty in maintaining attention.

The examination of mental status should stress in particular thought processes, delusions, feelings of unworthiness, and suicidal intent. Some patients may appear more anxious than depressed. In others, anger or hostility may be predominant. If the doctor feels sad after a few moments of the interview, the patient is probably sad also.

Examination of mental status

MANAGEMENT

Major factors that should be assessed early in the management include the following:

1   The risk of suicide
2   The availability of family and community resources
3   The family doctor's counseling skills
4   The need for consultation
5   The need for hospitalization

The Risk of Suicide

If a patient reports thoughts of suicide—especially if he or she has considered (or even chosen) a method—one must immediately consider preventive measures. Can the patient be watched around the clock? Will he or she enter a care facility willingly or will the doctor have to complete a commitment paper for involuntary admission?

The Availability of Resources

The next step in management is to make the most of the resources available to patients. These resources will probably be found within the family and to a varying extent in the community at large. It will save time if a resource list for the family is available (see Table 6–1).

A supportive family may cooperate by getting rid of potential suicide weapons such as guns, sharp knives, and unused medications. Or family members may take turns staying with a patient who is at risk while he or she awaits a hospital bed or the beneficial results of medication.

Family support

Stresses can be temporarily removed if family members are able to care for the children or the elderly or sick dependents of the depressed patient. Care may take the form of lending money, listening, simply being available, and discussing interpersonal conflicts, among many other types of involvement.

The Family Doctor's Counseling Skills

Contractual
counseling

Given the personal and physical resources available to the patient, the family physician should consider whether he or she is willing or able to provide supportive or directive psychotherapy to depressed patients. The physician should know how to prescribe himself or herself.[7] What are the indications? How frequent should the visits be? How long should they last? What are the risks and potential side effects of therapy? The physician should look on his or her own skills as a medication and prescribe them accordingly. At the same time, a clear contractual arrangement should be made with any other professionals whom the physician or the patient may wish to involve in the management of the problem.

The family physician may have the advantage of familiarity with the patient and the family and a relationship of preexisting trust. The psychological support provided by the family physician should be based on previous experience with the patient and on the patient's current circumstances.

A careful explanation of how depression can be both a cause and an effect of the patient's feelings and reassurance about the self-correcting nature of depression and the likelihood of future improvement are important elements of support. The physician can help take the pressure off a depressed patient while being careful not to make the patient completely dependent. Exploring ways to increase a patient's confidence and self-esteem and to improve his or her social contacts, in particular by finding a reliable confidant, are other important elements of management.

The Need for Consultation

Psychiatric
consultation

Local laws may require a psychiatric consultation before involuntary admission is permitted. Other reasons for consultation exist. A psychiatrist may have access to resources such as a hospital unit that are not available to the family physician, or a psychiatrist's special skills may be required for complicated medical assessment or for psychological management. If the patient is not responding to attempts at management or if the family physician is unable or unwilling to deal with the illness, consultation is indicated.

Professionals other than psychiatrists may complement the continued involvement of the family physician. The family practice nurse, the social worker, and the marriage counselor are examples.

The Need for Hospitalization

The main indications for hospitalization include suicidal risk, impairment of the patient's ability to care for himself or herself, lack of patient compliance in taking medication or making behavioral changes at home, and the patient's need simply to unload stresses and get some rest on a temporary basis. If the depression involves the possibility of a concomitant nonpsychiatric illness, the necessary investigations may require hospitalization.

MEDICATION

Probably the greatest errors in the pharmacotherapeutic management of depressed patients are excessive dependence on medication as the mode of treatment and the prescribing of inadequate doses of antidepressants.

The mainstay of pharmacotherapeutic management of the depressed patient remains tricyclic antidepressants.[8] The initiation of such therapy includes a trial period of at least 2 weeks to ensure that the drug is tolerated and is appropriate. A period of treatment of 3 to 6 months with a gradual tapering off toward the end is appropriate for most depressions. Prescribing amitriptyline and/or imipramine 150 mg daily is reasonable. Small doses of 10 to 15 mg may be tried as an initial test for extreme sensitivity. Ordinarily, start with 50 mg a day, increasing the dose at 3- to 7-day intervals until improvement is noted. One should be careful in prescribing these drugs for patients with recent myocardial infarction, those who are at high risk for glaucoma, and those who have degrees of prostatism.

Tricyclic antidepressants

Monoamine oxide (MAO) inhibitors are reserved as a second line of treatment. They should never be initiated without special dietary precautions that are clearly understood by the patient. The patient should not have been on tricyclic antidepressants for at least 1 week before taking the MAO inhibitor. Very good diet lists which specify the restrictions required for patients on MAO inhibitors are available.[1]

MAO inhibitors

For patients with a manic-depressive syndrome with recurrent episodes, lithium has a very specific effect. Precautions should be taken to monitor kidney, liver, and cardiac function; these functions should be assessed before therapy and then every 3 months during therapy. Lithium carbonate 600 to 1200 mg daily resulting in a serum level of 1.0 ± 0.2 mg/liter is a reasonable goal. Lithium can be combined with either tricyclics or MAO inhibitors.

Lithium

Whether or not one adds tranquilizers and/or hypnotics to the antidepressants depends on the extent to which symptomatic relief is required for superimposed symptoms of anxiety or sleeplessness. Usually the tricyclics provide a hypnotic effect from the beginning of therapy.

The effects of the antidepressants may not be felt for 10 days.

7 DEPRESSION

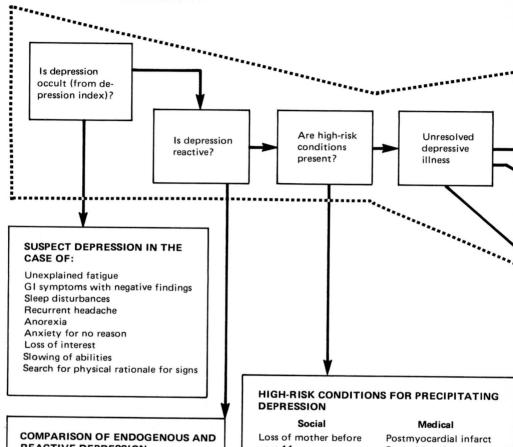

Is depression occult (from depression index)?

Is depression reactive?

Are high-risk conditions present?

Unresolved depressive illness

SUSPECT DEPRESSION IN THE CASE OF:

Unexplained fatigue
GI symptoms with negative findings
Sleep disturbances
Recurrent headache
Anorexia
Anxiety for no reason
Loss of interest
Slowing of abilities
Search for physical rationale for signs

COMPARISON OF ENDOGENOUS AND REACTIVE DEPRESSION

Endogenous	Reactive
Gradual onset, no precipitating factors	Identifiable precipitating factors
Feels worse in morning	Feels worse when tired
Persistent pattern	Variable pattern
Somatic effects—GI, sexual, musculoskeletal	Less somatic effect
Functions impaired	Functions relatively well
Sleep disturbance	Problems in getting to sleep
Early wakening	
Self-absorbed and egocentric	

HIGH-RISK CONDITIONS FOR PRECIPITATING DEPRESSION

Social	Medical
Loss of mother before age 11	Postmyocardial infarct
Three children under 14 at home	Postsubtractive surgery
No outside job	Postpartum or abortion
Low income	Postviral illness (e.g., infectious mononucleosis)
Absence of confidante	Drugs
Low self-esteem	Diuretics
Recent loss of friend or relative	Steroids
Aging	Estrogens (BCP)
Absence of extended family	Bromides
	Haloperidol
	Atropine group
	Levadopa
	Antineoplastics
	Antihypertensives
	Reaction to diagnosis of chronic or life-threatening illness

DEPRESSION

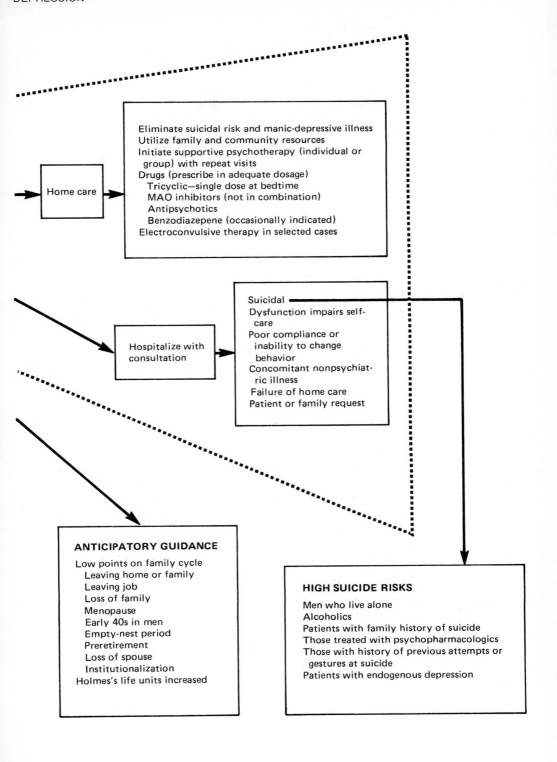

Home care

Eliminate suicidal risk and manic-depressive illness
Utilize family and community resources
Initiate supportive psychotherapy (individual or
  group) with repeat visits
Drugs (prescribe in adequate dosage)
  Tricyclic—single dose at bedtime
  MAO inhibitors (not in combination)
  Antipsychotics
  Benzodiazepene (occasionally indicated)
Electroconvulsive therapy in selected cases

Hospitalize with
consultation

Suicidal
Dysfunction impairs self-
  care
Poor compliance or
  inability to change
  behavior
Concomitant nonpsychiat-
  ric illness
Failure of home care
Patient or family request

ANTICIPATORY GUIDANCE

Low points on family cycle
  Leaving home or family
  Leaving job
  Loss of family
  Menopause
  Early 40s in men
  Empty-nest period
  Preretirement
  Loss of spouse
  Institutionalization
Holmes's life units increased

HIGH SUICIDE RISKS

Men who live alone
Alcoholics
Patients with family history of suicide
Those treated with psychopharmacologics
Those with history of previous attempts or
  gestures at suicide
Patients with endogenous depression

CONTINUED CARE

The frequency of visits depends on the severity of the problem, the type of therapy used (supportive, directive, or counseling), the familiarity of the physician with the patient, and the available family resources. Follow-up should monitor changes in the patient's behavior and feelings of well-being as well as compliance in taking medication or in following the behavioral changes suggested. Initially weekly visits are generally appropriate, with a subsequent reduction in visits when the major symptoms are obviously resolving. Longer term follow-up depends on the severity and duration of symptoms, previous episodes, available resources, and continued use of medication.

Note anniversaries

When the depression is related to a particular loss, it is worthwhile to note the anniversary of that loss, particularly if it was a death or a divorce. It is also useful to check on the patient on subsequent anniversaries either directly or through the family practice nurse, social worker, or other outreach professional.

In patients in whom depression may be compounding a physical problem, it is reasonable to initiate treatment for the depression while investigating that problem. Often the investigation of an organic illness (e.g., a suspected malignancy) takes 4 to 6 weeks; so long as treatment does not interfere with the investigation, the patient should be treated symptomatically. Treatment may also be initiated while the physician is assessing possible dementia or pseudodementia.[9]

THE YOUNG AND THE OLD

Special problems involving both recognition and management exist at the extremes of age.

Children

In children before puberty, depression does not present in the classical way. Tantrums, truancy, running away from home, and self-destructive behavior are often the first signs of depression in a child. Accident-proneness is another clue.

Particularly at risk are children who are hospitalized for other than short-term problems and children whose parents are hospitalized. Spending time helping such youngsters understand what is happening to them or to their parents in the hospital and encouraging and facilitating frequent family visiting are worthwhile preventive practices.

Teenagers

Teenagers may present with the same symptoms as adults. However, they may also exhibit acting-out behavior such as episodes of drunkenness, running away from home, switching friends frequently, and poor school performance. The latter may be associated with acting-out behavior or may be part of a syndrome of boredom, restlessness, withdrawal, impaired concentration, and unusual interest in trivia.

Increasing one's availability to teenagers and demonstrating to them one's intention to maintain absolute confidentiality are two steps that may be of preventive value. [One experienced physician told me that except for the obvious emergencies, the only patients he saw in the office without appointments were teenagers who dropped in with an apparently small problem.] The introduction from about the age of 8 or 9 of short private interviews with a youngster is another way of emphasizing that the physician takes the youngster's concerns seriously.

At the other end of the human life cycle are the elderly. When depressed, they may present with dementia, including agitation, memory problems, confusion, and disorientation. Such symptoms should never be set aside as senility before careful consideration has been given to the possibility of depression and a thorough investigation has been made.

The elderly

EFFECT ON THE FAMILY

Spouses and children of depressed patients have been noted to visit the doctor more frequently for infection, painful conditions, and anxiety during the period of the spouse or parent's illness. Often a relative's presentation to the doctor precedes the patient's presentation with depression. Being alert to what's going on in the family may improve our ability to achieve early detection of depressive illness.[10]

REFERENCES

1 R. Cadoret and R. J. Coble, "Depression," in H. F. Conn and R. E. Rakel (eds.), *Family Practice II*, W. B. Saunders, Philadelphia, 1978.
2 K. Hodgkin, *Towards Earlier Diagnosis in Primary Care*, 4th ed., Churchill-Livingstone, Edinburgh, London, New York, 1978.
3 A. M. W. Porter, "Depressive Illness in a General Practice: A Demographic Study and a Controlled Trial of Imipramine," *British Medical Journal*, **1**: 773–778, 1970.
4 R. Steel, "Suicide, Attempted Suicide and Depression," *Update*, **9**(3):343–350, 1974.
5 J. Price, "The Genetics of Depression," in *Depression* (monograph), Medcom, New York, pp. 21–23.
6 S. L. Opie, "Antidepressant Chemotherapy," *Drugs and Therapeutics for Maritime Practitioners*, **2**(3):9–12, 1979.

7 M. Balint, *The Doctor, the Patient and His Illness,* International Universities Press, New York, 1972.

8 "Drugs for Depression," *Medical Letter on Drugs and Therapeutics,* **20**(11):49, 1978.

9 F. Post, "Dementia, Depression, and Pseudodementia," in D. F. Benson and D. Blumer (eds.), *Psychiatric Aspects of Neurological Disease,* Grune & Stratton, New York, 1975, pp 190.

10 R. B. Widmer, R. J. Cadoret, and C. S. North. "Depression in Family Practice: Some Effects on Spouses and Children," *Journal of Family Practice,* **10**(1): 45–51, 1980.

Chapter 21

Wheezing

D. B. Shires, M.D.

PRINCIPLE

Patients with chronic or recurring illness, as well as their families, must come to terms with the disorder and try to live as normal a life as possible. However, people with chronic disorders may fail in this aim for a number of reasons. They may not be aware of available resources or public education or may not understand the nature of the disorder. They may lack self-esteem. They may be overprotected by the family and become unnecessarily dependent. The family physician has a responsibility to try to remedy these problems as well as to treat the disorder and keep up with medical advances. *Asthma* is a chronic disorder which is often accompanied by such problems.

Chronic disability

DEFINITION

Wheezing can be defined as audible, musical, expiratory rhonchi. It is generally assumed to be part of asthma; however, all wheezing is not due to asthma, nor is asthma always characterized by wheezing.

All wheezing is not asthma

Wheezing in the lower respiratory tract may be caused by (1) a foreign body, (2) obstructing tumors, (3) congenital vascular rings, (4) pulmonary edema, (5) angioneurotic edema, (6) transient respiratory infection (acute bronchitis), (7) infection (chronic bronchitis), (8) cystic fibrosis (rarely), and (9) asthma.

Stridor versus wheezing

The sound of upper airway obstruction is sometimes mistaken for wheezing. Such a sound is more properly termed *stridor* and is a coarser, harsher sound than the higher-pitched and more musical rhonchi of wheezing. Upper airway obstruction may be due to a nasal tumor, a laryngeal tumor, or a congenitally floppy larynx.

Difficulties exist with the definition of terms such as asthma, asthmatic bronchitis, bronchitis with wheezing, acute bronchitis, chronic bronchitis with or without emphysema, chronic obstructive lung disease, and chronic obstructive pulmonary disease, leading to problems in accurate diagnostic labeling. As a result, epidemiologic surveys are fraught with inaccuracies.

PREVALENCE

The prevalence of "asthma" in the United States has been estimated at 5 percent of the general population.[1] The Virginia study identified 6 patients per 1000 patient visits as having "asthma" and 26 per 1000 as having "acute bronchitis."[2] A morbidity survey done in Australia in 1974 indicated that asthma constituted some 2 percent of visits to the general practitioner in that country.[3]

Asthma is more common in males than in females before age 3, but it is seen predominantly among females in adolescence. Otherwise, there are no apparent sex differences. The incidence of asthma peaks in adolescence and in midlife.

ETIOLOGY AND NATURAL HISTORY OF ASTHMA

Asthma is defined as hyperreactive airway disease, or reversible obstructive airway disease, and is usually divided into extrinsic and intrinsic asthma.

Extrinsic asthma

Extrinsic asthma usually begins in childhood and is associated with other allergic tendencies such as eczema, hay fever, and positive family history. Skin tests (for grass or tree pollen, mold, dander, mites, and house dust) are positive; the asthma is usually mediated by IgE and is part of a type I allergic reaction. Some cases of extrinsic asthma are mediated by IgG with a delayed (by 6 to 12 hours) type III reaction that is usually triggered by industrial exposure.

Intrinsic asthma

Intrinsic asthma more often presents in adulthood, often following a lower respiratory viral infection. Nasal polyposis is com-

Figure 21-1 The asthmatic cycle.

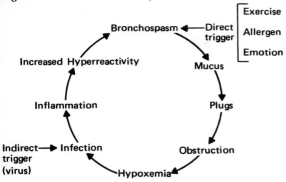

mon, and the usual skin tests for allergens are negative. However, most adults presenting with wheezing recall childhood wheezing, and some have an allergic family history. More than likely a basic defect is present, which can be triggered by various stimuli. The stimuli are more easily identified in extrinsic asthma and include inhaled allergens or irritants, air pollutants, cold air, changes in the weather, infection, exercise, and emotional upsets. Sometimes asthma is triggered by ingestion of salicylates, indomethacin, or tartrazine (a colored dye).

The pathophysiology of an asthmatic attack is illustrated in Figure 21-1. A trigger enters the cycle either directly by causing bronchoconstriction (allergen) or indirectly by leading to bronchoconstriction (viral infection).

A time study of asthmatic children showed that most had established a pattern of severity by age 14. In severely persistent asthmatics, the onset of illness had occurred before age 3, followed by a high frequency of attacks in the first year of illness, persistent airway obstruction and hyperinflation, chest deformity, and growth retardation. Most were clearly severe cases by age 7. Mild or "recovered" asthmatics experienced the onset after age 3 and had episodic illness with little evidence of airway obstruction between attacks. In these patients, attacks were rare after age 10.[4]

The extent to which mild to moderate asthma affects respiratory health in adults has not been established, but it is suspected that pediatric respiratory disease may be a contributing factor in adults who develop chronic airway disease.[5]

Prognosis

SYMPTOMS AND SIGNS

The usual symptoms include a tight feeling in the chest, cough productive of white sticky sputum, wheezing, and dyspnea. Anxiety in the patient, or in the parents if the patient is a child, is often part of the picture.

The signs include increased respiratory and heart rates, prolonged expiration, wheeze, and an air-trapped chest (expanded and poorly moving). The patient may lean forward, and the use of accessory muscles may be apparent.

Absence of wheeze may be danger signal

Intercostal indrawing, shallow respiration, restlessness, and cyanosis are signs of worsening. When obstruction is advanced, air movement is reduced so far that wheezing stops. From this, the physician may incorrectly assume that the treatment is working. Asthma is thus not always characterized by wheezing; however, when wheezing is absent during an attack, the patient may be in severe trouble.

APPROACH TO THE PATIENT

Alerting symptoms

When a patient presents for the first time with wheezing, one must ascertain that the problem is not stridor associated with serious upper airway obstruction. Listening to the lung bases and over the open mouth with the stethoscope usually clarifies the source of the obstructive sound.

Cyanosis, restlessness, or confusion may indicate a degree of hypoxia that warrants the administration of oxygen during initial assessment.

The history nearly always rules out a foreign body, but if a foreign body is present high up in the airway, it is sometimes difficult to distinguish wheezing from stridor. Foreign bodies usually require bronchoscopy or surgical removal.

Pulmonary edema is accompanied by other signs of heart disease. Pulmonary edema responds best to oxygen, morphine, and intravenous diuretics. Intravenous aminophylline and/or digitalis may also be indicated.

Angioneurotic edema with wheezing is usually associated with a very recent contact with an allergen (for example, overdose of desensitization serum, insect sting, penicillin injection, intravenous injection of radiopaque medium). Facial edema and pruritis are often present before or coincidentally with wheezing. Angioneurotic edema with asthma responds best to subcutaneous epinephrine (0.001 aqueous epinephrine 0.01 ml per kilogram of body weight to a maximum dose of 0.5 ml).

If the usual bronchodilation and symptomatic treatment do not eliminate the wheeze, the possibility of obstructive lesions such as tumors, foreign bodies, and vascular rings should be considered.

Bronchitis, as well as asthma, usually improves with bronchodilator and symptomatic treatment. Fever, colored sputum, and recent symptoms of upper respiratory infection suggest a diagnosis of bronchitis, although an upper respiratory infection can trigger an asthmatic episode.

MANAGEMENT

Initial Management of the First Acute Wheezing Episode

If the other alternatives have been ruled out, a patient who first presents with acute wheezing can normally be expected to respond favorably to the management approach outlined below.[6,7]

First attack

    1 Prescribe a sympathomimetic, such as *(a)* an inhaler, one to two puffs immediately of a β_2 stimulant such as albuterol (salbutamol), orciprenaline, terbutaline, or fenoterol (this can be repeated every 6 hours for as long as the wheeze persists) or *(b)* subcutaneous 0.001 aqueous epinephrine 0.01 ml per kilogram of body weight to a maximum of 0.5 ml.[8]

    2 Give theophylline orally as *(a)* aminophylline (80% aminophylline), starting with an oral dose of 16 mg/day per kilogram of body weight to a maximum of 400 mg (administered in divided doses every 4 hours) and increasing to 25 mg/day per kilogram of body weight to a maximum of 900 mg in children, or 15 mg/day per kilogram of body weight (administered in divided doses every 6 hours) for adults or *(b)* choline theophyllinate (64% aminophylline), with an oral dose of 24 to 37 mg/day per kilogram of body weight for children (every 4 hours) or 23 mg/day per kilogram of body weight for adults (every 6 hours). Either regimen can be continued for 10 days.

Broncho-
dilators

    3 Alleviate anxiety. This is especially important when anxious parents are making their concern unnecessarily evident to the child.

General
measures

    4 Ensure that hydration is adequate. This is most important in a child who has been wheezing for a long time and is apt to be dehydrated. Frequent oral fluids (juices, Popsicles, or oral rehydration formula) and a vaporizer to maintain humidity are important.

    5 Do a chest x-ray. This should always be done at the first presentation of wheezing in order to rule out some of the other possibilities which may be identifiable on x-ray, such as a foreign body. For subsequent episodes, an x-ray is not routinely indicated.

    6 Make follow-up plans within the week. It is important to know whether the wheezing has virtually disappeared within 48 hours and to assess the child just prior to discontinuation of medication following the initial episode.

Follow-up

    Patients with a first episode who worsen in spite of this initial management and patients who fail to improve with initial management after 48 hours should be reviewed for assessment of compli-

Hospitalization

ance and proper administration of medications. The next step might be to admit the patient to the hospital and repeat the management program under supervised conditions or to begin intravenous aminophylline (a loading dose of 5.6 mg/kg administered over 15 to 20 minutes and a maintenance dose of 0.9 mg/kg per hour is advised for all patients who have not had previous aminophylline and who are otherwise healthy). Patients with other diseases, in particular liver disease, should start with one-tenth the doses of aminophylline.

An alternative to intravenous aminophylline for the worsening patient is subcutaneous epinephrine. Ultimately, steroids may be required before complete resolution is obtained.

A word of warning about theophylline is necessary, as it is a stimulant and may increase anxiety and activity and cause abdominal pain in the child.

After the First Episode

Subsequent management

In a patient who has infrequent asthmatic episodes (fewer than three per year) and whose first episode occurred after age 3, repeated episodes can be managed in much the same way as the initial episode. If a no-smoking rule is established for the patient's room and items that harbor dust are removed, a relatively trigger free environment can be created. These precautions and the removing of pets to the backyard are reasonable initial measures for treating mild asthma.

For a patient who is having more frequent episodes (three or more a year) or whose first episode occurred before age 3, it is advisable to make a definitive diagnosis of reversible airway disease by means of pulmonary function tests in order to demonstrate the physiological abnormality along with evidence of its reversibility. This type of patient probably needs continuous maintenance medication, using theophylline in the oral dose as recommended above, a sympathomimetic inhaler if theophylline alone is not effective, or disodium cromoglycate aerosol inhalations of 20 mg four times a day. Steroids may be needed for the long-term maintenance of a patient subject to recurrent episodes. If steroids are necessary for long-term maintenance, alternate-day oral prednisone or beclomethasone by inhaler should be considered. With persistent symptoms or in a more severely affected patient, more extreme measures may be required, including changing furniture, rugs, and drapes; removing all feathered or furry pets; and installing special dust-removing air conditioners and hot air furnaces.

A patient with recurrent asthma is often best controlled when the medication is used prophylactically against known triggers. In

Table 21-1   Known Triggers to Wheezing in Asthmatics

1   Ingested drugs, in particular aspirin
2   Known allergens inhaled: pets, dander, grasses, pollens, house dust
3   Tobacco smoke
4   Inhalants: perfumes, toiletries, cleaning agents in the home, paints and
    shellacs
5   Exercise
6   Emotion
7   Cold
8   Dietary ingestants

Source: Canadian Family Physician.[10]

order to identify such triggers, it is useful for the patient to keep a wheezing record to be reviewed with the physician.

This approach leads to measures aimed at the avoidance of known triggers of wheezing attacks, which are listed in Table 21-1. When the history makes one suspect that common allergens are responsible, skin testing may help. Skin tests are not, however, infallible; if the patient wheezes after contact with pollen, dust, or animal dander, these items should be considered causal and avoided even when skin tests are negative. Smoking in the home should be stopped. Strongly perfumed irritants that are suspect can be tested by temporary removal. The effects of cold air, if not avoidable, can be lessened through the use of a scarf over the mouth. Allergens that may have been ingested, especially aspirin, should be looked for. Emotional pressures should be dealt with intelligently so that the patient does not have the opportunity to make the family give in to his or her demands for fear of an attack. *(Avoiding triggers)*

Exercise deserves special mention. Exercise-induced asthma is well recognized. As a result, however, many young asthmatics have been deprived of participation in normal games and athletic endeavors without a careful assessment of their condition. Most asthmatics can learn to undertake all physical activities if these are introduced gradually and accompanied by the intelligent use of prophylactic medication. Swimming has been proved to provoke the least amount of exercise-induced bronchoconstriction and can be recommended with caution for even severe asthmatics. Fitch has shown that older child asthmatics who were enrolled in a 5-month swimming program improved their posture, rid themselves of excess body weight, reduced their need for medication and lowered the rate of their wheezing attacks, improved their functional expiratory volume and functional vital capacity, and derived the emotional benefits of decreased dependence and less protective parents.[9] Prophylactic doses of disodium cromoglycate or salbutamol immediately before exercise help protect the patient. *(Exercise)*

8 WHEEZING

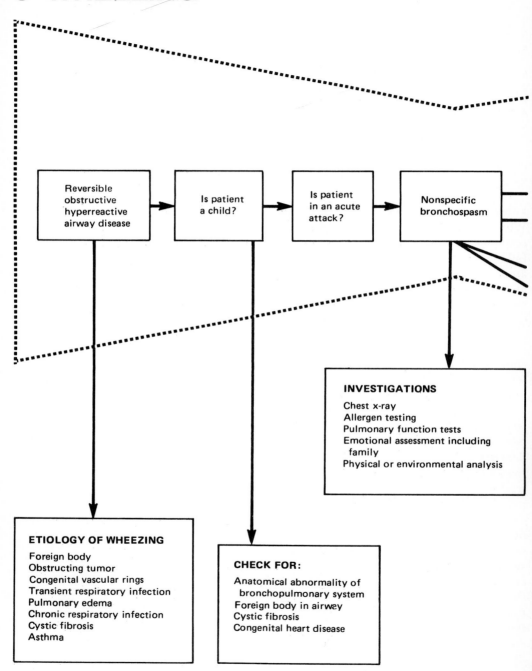

Reversible obstructive hyperreactive airway disease

Is patient a child?

Is patient in an acute attack?

Nonspecific bronchospasm

INVESTIGATIONS

Chest x-ray
Allergen testing
Pulmonary function tests
Emotional assessment including
 family
Physical or environmental analysis

ETIOLOGY OF WHEEZING

Foreign body
Obstructing tumor
Congenital vascular rings
Transient respiratory infection
Pulmonary edema
Chronic respiratory infection
Cystic fibrosis
Asthma

CHECK FOR:

Anatomical abnormality of
 bronchopulmonary system
Foreign body in airway
Cystic fibrosis
Congenital heart disease

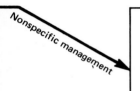

Specific therapy

Nonspecific management

ACUTE ATTACK

1 Break cycle of trigger factor→spasm→anxiety→spasm (see text).
2 Provide adequate ventilation.
3 Treat intercurrent infection.
4 Treat nonidentified patients, e.g., family.
5 Watch for danger signals, i.e., shock, ventilatory decompensation, and dehydration.

GENERAL MANAGEMENT AND PREVENTION

1 Identify trigger factor: allergy testing→avoidance of allergen; diet trials.
2 Ensure environmental purity: dust-free, frequent vacuuming, air conditioner, temperature control, no pets in bedroom, humidifier or dehumidifier.
3 Provide adequate recreational opportunity: introduce gradual exercise program.

INDICATIONS FOR CONSULTATION

Inadequate response to therapy in acute attack
Increase in number or severity of attacks despite adequate therapy
Patient or family request

PROGNOSTICATORS

Minimal
Onset after age 3; less than three wheezing episodes per year; ended by age 10

Mild
Usually ended by age 10; less than five episodes in last 5 years.

Moderate
Still episodic wheezing by age 14, though reducing in frequency.

Severe
Unremitting or severe up to age 14; more than 10 episodes in 3 months. Many wheezing episodes before age 1. Physically under-developed.

ANTIBIOTICS

Most asthma and bronchitis in otherwise healthy children does not involve bacterial infection, and the routine use of antibiotics in such wheezing children has no proven benefit.[11] Children who suffer from recurrent severe asthma or who have other clinical illnesses (e.g., cystic fibrosis) and adults with recurrent or chronic bronchitis may benefit from broad-spectrum antibiotics during acute episodes. Prophylactic use of antibiotics is likely to be of little benefit.

DESENSITIZATION

The efficacy of desensitization in treating asthma is doubtful at best. Weinberger and Hendeles suggest that it be attempted only in patients in whom allergic rhinitis is part of the allergic syndrome.[7]

GENERAL MEASURES

Normalizing lifestyle

In managing a patient with recurrent asthma, it is particularly important to focus on the potential for leading as normal a life as possible. Emphasis should be placed on the individual's worth, and the limitations created by the illness should be approached with honesty.

Some medical centers have special asthma units with both outpatient and inpatient resources and play a significant role in family education. Special summer camps for asthmatics have been successful.[12] Some community resource associations have parent education programs, such as the family asthma program of the American Lung Association of Hennepin County in Minnesota.

Teachers of asthmatic children require advice and support. In particular, a teacher needs to understand that these children may be unable to participate fully in athletic activities, that the attention span of a child on medication may on occasion be affected, that there may be extra absences from school, and that such children may have problems with peer rejection.

A patient with severe recurrent asthma has a serious and probably lifelong disability, but many of these problems can be alleviated by means of careful attention to community supports. An example of such a program in New York City illustrated how family education for home management of asthma could improve a child's school performance.[13]

Thus, asthma is a multifactorial problem involving all the skills of the well-trained family physician.

REFERENCES

1 T. Godar, A. Beyer, and J. Donnelly, "Pulmonary Medicine," in H. F. Conn and R. E. Rakel (eds.), *Family Practice,* W. B. Saunders, Philadelphia, 1978, p. 891.
2 D. W. Marsland, M. Wood, and F. Mayo, *Content of Family Practice: A Statewide Study in Virginia with Its Clinical, Educational, and Research Implications,* J. Geyman (ed.), Appleton-Century-Crofts, New York, 1976.
3 P. P. Bateman, "The Prevalence of Asthma in General Practice," *Australian Family Physician,* **5:**102–110, 1976.
4 K. N. McNicol and H. B. Williams, "Spectrum of Asthma in Children. I: Clinical and Physiological Components," *British Medical Journal,* **4:**7–11, 1973.
5 B. Burrows, M. D. Lebowitz, and R. J. Knudson, "Epidemiological Evidence That Childhood Problems Predispose to Airway Disease in the Adult (an Association between Adult and Pediatric Respiratory Disorders)," *Pediatric Research,* **2:**218–220, 1977.
6 J. Gray, "What's New in the Therapy of Asthma?" *Drugs and Therapeutics of Maritime Practitioners,* **1**(6):1–4, 1978.
7 M. Weinberger and L. Hendeles, "Management of Asthma," *Postgraduate Medicine,* **61:**85–100, 1977.
8 A. M. Harvey, R. J. John, A. M. Owens, and R. R. Ross, "Obstructive Pulmonary Disease," in *The Principles and Practice of Medicine,* Appleton-Century-Crofts, New York, 1976, p. 474.
9 K. D. Fitch, "Effects of Exercise on Asthma," *Australian Family Physician,* **6**(6):592–597, 1977.
10 N. Epstein, "The Glue Ear and What to Do About It," *Canadian Family Physician,* **19**(5):52–54, 1973.
11 A. Goldbloom, "Antibiotics in Children with Asthma," *Drugs and Therapeutics for Maritime Practitioners,* January-February 1979, pp. 3–4.
12 P. D. Phelan, "The Victorian Asthma Camp", *Australian Family Physician,* **5**(2):207–209, 1976.
13 N. W. Clark, C. H. Feldman, et al., "Changes in Children's School Performance as a Result of Education for Family Management of Asthma," *Journal of Occupational and School Medicine,* **54:**143–145, 1984.

Chapter 22

Hypertension

D. B. Shires, M.D.

PRINCIPLE

Habits are hard to change, and patients who feel well find it difficult to take medication regularly. However, the management of hypertension is based on lifestyle changes combined with medication. Although the literature is inconclusive, it appears that patients who keep in close and continuous touch with a personal physician are more successful at managing illness.

Patient labeling Medicine must, above all, do no harm. Careless, premature, or unwarranted labeling of persons with any disease is never justified. Patients who are told that they have hypertension suffer from more headaches than hypertensive patients who do not know about their condition, and patients with asymptomatic hypertension who are told about the diagnosis take more time off from work for sickness than those who are not told. Insurance companies scrutinize with extra care patients who report hypertensive histories and those who have ever had a higher than normal blood pressure reading.

Range of normality Hypertension is a condition in which inappropriate labeling commonly occurs and, in our opinion, does immeasurable harm.

Hypertension is also a physiological condition which has a wide normal range. There is growing evidence that pharmacological treatment is effective only for patients whose blood pressure is above a certain range. Yet risks remain for those whose blood pressure readings are higher than "normal" even though they are not in the pharmacologically "treatable" group.

The physician must carefully prescribe advice about diet and exercise for those with high blood pressure readings and medication for those with hypertension in the pharmacologically responsive group and must balance the advantages of treatment against the risks of labeling a patient "sick" for life. It is difficult to decide what constitutes good management and to justify professional intrusion into the lives of persons who feel well but have "above-average" blood pressure. Family doctors must use their understanding of human behavior as well as their medical skills to meet the needs of every individual who seeks their professional guidance.

DEFINITION

The definition of hypertension, like that of diabetes, is based on a normal curve. A normal range of blood pressure, variable and increasing with age, has been defined, and an arbitrary level has been set above which the diagnosis of hypertension is made. High blood pressure is a sign, not a disease.

We would define *hypertension* in adults under 65 years of age as the recording of blood pressures of 160 mm Hg or above systolic and/or 100 mm Hg diastolic on three consecutive occasions, with the appropriate-size cuff being applied to the arm in the sitting position. We would define an elevated blood pressure reading as any recording over 140 mm Hg systolic and/or 90 mm Hg diastolic.[1]

PREVALENCE

It has been estimated that 10 to 20 percent of Americans are hypertensive. Half of these cases have not been detected, and only one in five is adequately treated.[2] It is a common problem in Europe and Australasia as well as in the developing world.[3]

Benign and nonspecific hypertension was the top-ranked diagnosis in family practice according to the Virginia study, with women predominating 2 to 1 over men and with half the identified patients being over age 55.[4]

NATURAL HISTORY

Risk factor

Hypertension is generally accepted as a significant risk factor for stroke, congestive heart failure, and renal failure.

Fry followed 704 hypertensives for 20 years and observed an incidence of complications in 9 percent and a death rate of 46 percent.[5,6] He noted that 30 percent of the patients identified as hypertensive (which he defined as diastolic over 100 mm Hg in the sitting position on three readings) became normotensive without treatment. In 18 percent of cases blood pressure remained at the original level, and in 52 percent blood pressure readings continued to increase. (Fry was treating pharmacologically only 35 of the 704 patients who were initially diagnosed.)

Fry also found that a stroke was four times as likely to occur in hypertensives than in normotensives and that the risk of coronary heart disease was 2.4 times greater for hypertensive women than for normotensive women. He noted that hypertensive women were more likely to suffer dementia than normotensive women.

DETECTION OF HYPERTENSION BY SCREENING

Population screening

Silverberg reported a study in which 9591 adults were screened in a shopping center program.[7] The study found that 185 of the subjects had abnormally high blood pressure and that 85 percent had visited a doctor in the previous 6 months. Follow-up on those patients who were found to have persistent hypertension showed that over 90 percent complied with treatment for a period of 18 months.

In another study of 15,594 high school students aged 15 to 20, Silverberg found that 350 (2.2 percent) had systolic readings over 150 mm Hg or diastolic readings over 95 mm Hg or both.[8] After 6 months, 232 of the 350 had been followed; 19 of them had had the diagnosis of hypertension confirmed by the doctor, 1 had had a surgical cause corrected, 4 were on drug therapy, and 8 were under observation. However, in no case did a doctor use a cuff smaller than the standard size for taking blood pressure, even though this was indicated for two-thirds of the students.

ETIOLOGY

Primary and Secondary Hypertension

Nine of ten hypertensive patients do not have a specific identifiable cause for the disease and are said to have *primary,* or *essential,* hypertension.

Secondary hypertension accounts for about 10 percent of all hypertensive patients. The causes include pheochromocytoma, aldosteronism, unilateral renal problems, Cushing's syndrome, coarctation of the aorta, polycythemia, birth control pills, and toxemia of pregnancy.

Secondary hypertension

HISTORY

Most patients with hypertension do not have initial symptoms. Important elements of past history to be considered include previous hypertension, having been refused insurance after examination, pregnancy, family history, amount of exercise taken, and smoking habits. The significant symptoms are impaired vision, unexplained congestive heart failure, and symptoms of renal disease. Although frequently cited as hypertensive symptoms, headaches, nosebleeds, and dizziness are of little diagnostic value, since it is difficult to distinguish hypertension from the more common causes of these symptoms.[9] Moreover, there is little evidence to suggest that the frequency of these symptoms is any greater in hypertensives than in the normal population.

Associated symptoms

PHYSICAL EXAMINATION

Blood pressure should be taken with the cuff width equal to two-thirds the distance from elbow to shoulder. Too wide a cuff gives low readings, while too narrow a cuff gives high readings. For obese patients, readings may be more accurate when the cuff is placed on the forearm, putting the stethoscope at the radial pulse.

Readings showing elevation on three separate occasions and with reasonable consistency are required for a diagnosis to be made. A resting reading (taken after 5 minutes of rest) and a prone reading should be done at least once each. Both arm readings should be compared at least once and should be within 10 mm of each other. At least one leg reading is desirable. The diastolic pressure should be recorded as both the muffling and the disappearance of the Korotkoff V sound. In 10 percent of normals the diastolic sound may not disappear entirely.

Technical definition

Patients with a diastolic blood pressure below 100 and a systolic pressure below 140 are classified as having mild hypertension, those with a diastolic of 100 to 114 or a systolic above 160 are considered to have moderate hypertension, and those with a diastolic pressure above 114 are characterized as having severe hypertension. [10,11]

The patient's weight should be recorded, and retinal abnormalities should be identified by means of funduscopic examination. Central nervous system and cardiovascular examinations should focus on arterial obstructions, evidence of congestive heart failure, and left ventricular hypertrophy. The retina, heart, blood vessels, kidneys, and brain are the "target organs" of hypertension; thorough assessment of these areas is necessary in deciding on the form of therapy.

INVESTIGATION

Baseline tests

Basic investigations in a new patient with hypertension should include the following.

1   Urinalysis with a midstream urine being collected and tested for albumin, sugar, and microscopic. If abnormal albumin is found or microscopic examination is abnormal, the urine should be sent for a culture and a sensitivity test. If there is sugar in the urine, a 2-hour pc blood sugar test should be done.
2   Hemoglobin.
3   Creatinine and blood urea nitrogen.
4   Electrolytes, particularly potassium.
5   Cholesterol.
6   Thyroxine.
7   Electrocardiogram.
8   Chest x-ray.
9   Hypertensive intravenous pyelogram (IVP) is seldom required in primary care practice and should be reserved for acutely hypertensive patients with symptoms, patients under 50 with a diastolic pressure of 130 or more, and patients under 25 with a diastolic pressure over 110. Patients with the likelihood of renal disease should also have an IVP.

Specific tests

10   Depending on the history, age, and sex of the patient and on other factors, blood sugar, lipids, uric acid, 24-hour vanillylmandelic acid, catecholamines, renal arteriogram, adrenal CT scan, and basal split renin tests might be considered. However, the last three procedures should probably await the consultant's assessment.

Children

In young children, secondary causes of hypertension, especially renovascular, are most likely.[12] The age of 3 is suggested as appropriate for a routine blood pressure recording in the well-child check. An investigation of hypertension in the young child should include urinalysis, a urine culture, and hemoglobin, electrolytes, and creatinine tests. Higher ranges (for example, a diastolic pressure over 90 mm Hg in 3- to 12-year-olds) indicate the need for an IVP or a renal arteriogram.[13]

In adolescents, essential hypertension is more likely and arteriography is rarely indicated.

MANAGEMENT

Successful management will depend on the patient's understanding of the condition and willingness to undertake a program which may involve the care indicated below, depending on the severity of the condition.

Blood pressure reading	Level of care
Under 140/90	Level 1: Simple, regular monitoring of slight elevations of blood pressure; obvious lifestyle changes.
Under 160/100	Level 2: If no target organ damage, level 1 plus a program of nonpharmacological management; lifestyle reinforcement by follow-up.
160/100 or over	Level 3: Levels 1 and 2 plus pharmacological management. Also applies to level 2 if target organ damage is present.
160/100 or over with failure to respond adequately to level 3	Level 4: Levels 1, 2, and 3 plus more extensive consultation for investigation and/or management.

Examples of two different approaches to management follow.

A slightly obese, out-of-shape housewife with readings of 140/90 may choose not to diet or exercise but may agree to come for a visit every 3 months for a blood pressure reading and a chat about a stressful home situation (level 1). On the other hand, she may be willing to undertake a gradual weight-reducing diet and an exercise program three times a week and may agree to be seen every 2 weeks until a desirable weight and exercise level are established and a measurable improvement in blood pressure is noted. At that point she can be returned to a program requiring monitoring and reinforcement every 3 months. This patient may never need to be labeled hypertensive.

A 40-year-old executive who is overweight, overworked, and sedentary and has readings of 160/115 should be diagnosed and investigated as a hypertensive. Such a patient should be encouraged to start at level 3 and offered reasonable expectations of ultimately needing only the level 2 program.

Hypertension in pregnancy is a management problem in its own right and cannot be adequately dealt with in this chapter. The

Table 22-1   Expected Effects of Nondrug Therapy

Technique	Expected systolic reduction (mm)	Expected diastolic reduction (mm)
Weight reduction	20–30	15–20
Na⁺ restriction*	10	5
Exercise	15	10
Biofeedback	20	15

*Salt restriction includes the elimination of condiments, salty pickles, salty snacks, instant drinks, kosher foods, sauerkraut, and prepared meats, all of which have a high sodium content.
Source: Dodek and Wilkins.[2]

Table 22-2   Hypertensive Emergency

That state of severe arterial pressure elevation which demands rapid reduction:

Immediately (within minutes or hours)
   Hypertension with acute left ventricular failure
   Hypertensive encephalopathy
   Hypertension with aortic dissection
   Hypertension with cerebral (or subarachnoid) hemorrhage

Promptly (within hours or days)
   Malignant hypertension
   Accelerated hypertension

Source: Frohlich.[15]

diagnosing of women patients as hypertensive should be delayed until high readings persist beyond 6 weeks postpartum or beyond 6 months after the discontinuation of the contraceptive pill.

Nonpharmacological Management

Sodium restriction

Nonpharmacological management has been shown to be effective in producing moderate reductions in blood pressure (Table 22-1). Sodium restriction to 150 mmol/day, which is achieved by removing discretionary use of salt from the diet, can be recommended as an ancillary measure in mild hypertension; severe sodium restriction to 80 mmol/day using professional nutritional guidance can be effective in reducing blood pressure in some patients with mild hypertension.[11]

The Hypertensive Emergency

Frohlich differentiates between hypertensive emergencies and nonemergencies.[15] He defines the hypertensive emergency as a state of severe arterial pressure elevation which demands rapid reduction (Table 22-2).

Table 22-3 The Stepped Care Approach

Step 1	Step 2	Step 3	Step 4
			Other alternatives Guanethidine Bethanidine Minoxidil
		Add vasodilator	
	Add beta blocker	Hydralazine Prazosin	
Advice on lifestyle	Other options Methyldopa Prazosin Clonidine		
Diuretic			

Source: Modified from Abbott et al.[19]

FOLLOW-UP

Initial management of hypertension may require visits weekly or twice a week. These visits should include patient education regarding the nature of the disease and the effects of therapy. Patient handouts such as the PMI series of the American Medical Association are useful. Once the disease begins to be under control, the follow-up should include visits every 3 months, when blood pressure recordings should be taken, weight recorded, and compliance evaluated. Potassium levels can be measured every 6 months after initial therapy has been stabilized, and uric acid tests can be repeated on a yearly basis. Annual blood sugar readings are probably appropriate for patients on thiazides. At this time the doctor should watch for end organ damage, focusing in particular on the patient's funduscopic, urinary, cardiovascular, and cerebrovascular status.

Maintenance

Potassium monitoring

Pharmacological Management[11,16–19]

The stepped care approach has been advocated and found useful in practice (Table 22-3).

Thiazide diuretics and beta blockers are equally effective in reducing blood pressure in patients with mild hypertension.[19] The choice of agent should be based on the risk of either therapy in the particular patient and the success or failure seen with the initial drug chosen. Black patients may do better with a diuretic, while the reverse may be true of white patients. Beta blockers may be favored as initial therapy in younger patients, especially those with a rapid resting pulse rate and wide pulse pressure, and in patients with ischemic heart disease.[10]

Hypokalemia manifested by fatigue, muscle weakness, and arrhythmias may occur in a significant proportion (25 percent) of patients on thiazide therapy. Thus, potassium supplements should

Thiazides

Potassium supplements

be considered and the serum potassium levels should be monitored regularly.

To reduce the frequency and severity of hypokalemia with thiazide use in mild hypertensives, the recommended dosage of hydrochlorothiazide is 25 to 50 mg once daily or 25 mg chlorthalidone every 1 to 2 days. The maximum doses are 150 mg per day for thiazides and 200 mg per day for chlorthalidone. Step 1 therapy should be continued for at least 4 to 8 weeks while modifying dosages and assessing effectiveness and side effects before proceeding to step 2.

Beta blockers

Beta blockers are usually used as step 2 therapy except in the circumstances mentioned above. They are usually given in the dosage of 40 to 320 mg per day but should not be given to patients with congestive heart failure, enlarged heart, or asthma. Caution should be exercised in treating diabetics since beta blockers mask the symptoms of hypoglycemia. Therefore, if a beta blocker is required, a cardioselective drug should be chosen.

Other effective drugs for reducing blood pressure in step 2 therapy are methyldopa, which may cause biochemical abnormalities and abnormal antinuclear and Coombs' tests; prazosin, a vasodilator; and clonidine, which has an autonomic effect through central action on vasopressor centers.

Step 3 therapy involves the addition of a vasodilator. Hydralazine and prazosin are examples. Hydralazine is recommended in a dosage of 25 to 100 mg per day twice daily.

Step 4 alternatives are guanethidine, which has been associated with elevation of blood urea nitrogen, postural hypotension, and impotence; bethanidine; and minoxidil, which is more potent than hydralazine but can cause hypertrichosis and substantial fluid retention.

Stopping medications

Stepping Down   After blood pressure is reduced to goal level and maintained for a 6- to 12-month period, "stepping down" with reduction of drug doses may be attempted; in this procedure, medications are withdrawn under surveillance but are not stopped abruptly. There is accumulating evidence[20] that patients with successfully controlled hypertension for several years can discontinue antihypertension drug therapy and remain normotensive for extensive periods if they lose weight and restrict sodium intake. This is not true for severe hypertensives.

The Birth Control Pill

Oral contraceptives

Large studies have demonstrated that most patients who have been put on birth control pills show a slight increase in blood pressure at a 6-month follow-up visit. Such an increase is more likely in patients with a history of toxemia or a family history of hypertension.

Most patients who show abnormal blood pressure readings on the pill find that blood pressure reverts to normal 6 months after discontinuation of the pill. Persistent hypertension has, however, been reported in some cases.[21]

Diazepam

Diazepam is not an antihypertensive drug, and it has not been shown to be useful in the long-term treatment of hypertension.[14] Furthermore, there is no evidence that diazepam enhances the hypertensive effect of any blood-pressure drug. Therefore, unless anxiety is a separate problem or is believed to be aggravating hypertension, this minor tranquilizer has no place in therapy.

PROGNOSTICATORS (THE SIGNIFICANCE OF END ORGAN CHANGES)

The 5-year mortality rate of patients with grades 3 to 4 Kimmelstiel-Wilson (KW) syndrome is 80 percent. If there has been a neurological deficit, the mortality rate increases. If renal dysfunction has been demonstrated, the 5-year mortality rate is 76 percent. One seldom sees 3 + retinopathy without impaired renal function.[18]

Mortality

SPECIAL PROBLEMS OF COMPLIANCE

Careful attention should be paid to a patient who is consistently found to have a higher blood pressure reading than expected. This type of patient may say, "I've had a tense month" or "I guess I'd better lose ten pounds fast." It is easy for the physician to be led astray by such statements and let the patient go until the next visit. Podell refers to such patients as "anxiety and obesity cop-outs" and recommends that they not be allowed to cop out.[22]

Podell identified several *doctor factors* in poor compliance, including (1) therapeutic timidity (having too lenient treatment goals), (2) acceptance of the "obesity-anxiety cop-outs," and (3) failure to recognize the labile hypertensive. Once acceptable control has been achieved, one should congratulate the patient, but one must also emphasize the necessity of continuing treatment and follow-up. Patients who are simply told that the problem is "controlled" may discontinue medication.

Doctor-assisted compliance

In cases of labile hypertension in which the blood pressure fluctuates with stresses of living, it is useful to teach patients to take their blood pressure at home. In fact, some physicians recommend that blood pressure be taken by all patients who have hypertension requiring treatment and patients in whom the lability of hyperten-

9 HYPERTENSION

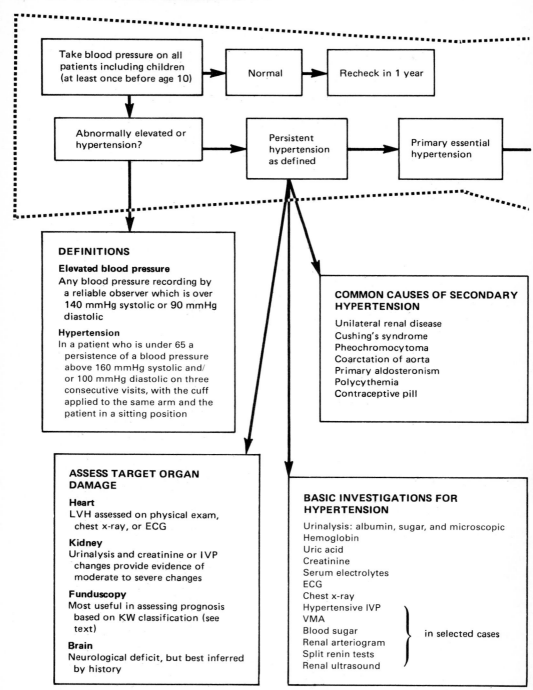

Take blood pressure on all patients including children (at least once before age 10) → Normal → Recheck in 1 year

Abnormally elevated or hypertension? → Persistent hypertension as defined → Primary essential hypertension

DEFINITIONS

Elevated blood pressure
Any blood pressure recording by a reliable observer which is over 140 mmHg systolic or 90 mmHg diastolic

Hypertension
In a patient who is under 65 a persistence of a blood pressure above 160 mmHg systolic and/ or 100 mmHg diastolic on three consecutive visits, with the cuff applied to the same arm and the patient in a sitting position

COMMON CAUSES OF SECONDARY HYPERTENSION

Unilateral renal disease
Cushing's syndrome
Pheochromocytoma
Coarctation of aorta
Primary aldosteronism
Polycythemia
Contraceptive pill

ASSESS TARGET ORGAN DAMAGE

Heart
LVH assessed on physical exam, chest x-ray, or ECG

Kidney
Urinalysis and creatinine or IVP changes provide evidence of moderate to severe changes

Funduscopy
Most useful in assessing prognosis based on KW classification (see text)

Brain
Neurological deficit, but best inferred by history

BASIC INVESTIGATIONS FOR HYPERTENSION

Urinalysis: albumin, sugar, and microscopic
Hemoglobin
Uric acid
Creatinine
Serum electrolytes
ECG
Chest x-ray
Hypertensive IVP
VMA
Blood sugar
Renal arteriogram
Split renin tests
Renal ultrasound
} in selected cases

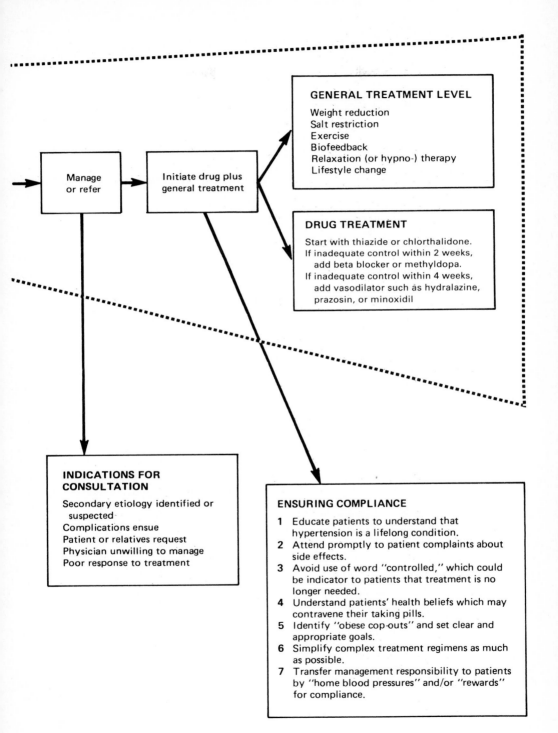

Manage or refer

Initiate drug plus general treatment

GENERAL TREATMENT LEVEL

Weight reduction
Salt restriction
Exercise
Biofeedback
Relaxation (or hypno-) therapy
Lifestyle change

DRUG TREATMENT

Start with thiazide or chlorthalidone.
If inadequate control within 2 weeks,
  add beta blocker or methyldopa.
If inadequate control within 4 weeks,
  add vasodilator such as hydralazine,
  prazosin, or minoxidil

INDICATIONS FOR CONSULTATION

Secondary etiology identified or
  suspected
Complications ensue
Patient or relatives request
Physician unwilling to manage
Poor response to treatment

ENSURING COMPLIANCE

1 Educate patients to understand that
  hypertension is a lifelong condition.
2 Attend promptly to patient complaints about
  side effects.
3 Avoid use of word "controlled," which could
  be indicator to patients that treatment is no
  longer needed.
4 Understand patients' health beliefs which may
  contravene their taking pills.
5 Identify "obese cop-outs" and set clear and
  appropriate goals.
6 Simplify complex treatment regimens as much
  as possible.
7 Transfer management responsibility to patients
  by "home blood pressures" and/or "rewards"
  for compliance.

Table 22-4   Why Hypertensives Don't Take Their Medicine

1 The duration of the treatment is very long.
2 The regimen is often complex, requiring several pills per dose and several doses per day.
3 Most hypertensives are symptomless at the beginning of treatment.
4 Antihypertensive drugs produce side effects.
5 Patients' health beliefs may prevent them from taking their pills.

Source: Sackett.[23]

Patient-assisted
compliance

sion is suspect. Home blood pressure readings taken by the patient are often helpful in diagnosis.

Podell identifies important *patient factors* in poor compliance, including (1) lack of information, especially regarding the asymptomatic nature of hypertension, and (2) a disease denial rationalization in which the patient denies having high blood pressure or needing treatment despite accurate information about his or her condition.[22]

Sackett et al. have identifed five reasons why patients fail to take their medication.[23] These reasons are listed in Table 22-4.

SUMMARY

The management of hypertension has changed dramatically in the past 5 years and continues to change. The medication advice given in this chapter should be considered with this clearly in mind.

REFERENCES

1 W. B. Kannel, M. J. Schwartz, and P. McNamara, "Blood Pressure and Risk of Coronary Heart Disease: The Framingham Study," *Diseases of the Chest,* **56:**43–52, 1969.
2 A. Dodek and G. Wilkins, "A Practical Approach to Hypertension," *Canadian Family Physician,* **22:**61–70, 1976.
3 M. E. Ahmed, "A Blood Pressure Clinic in a Developing Country," *Postgraduate Medical Journal* **59:**632–633, 1983.
4 D. W. Marsland, M. Wood, and F. Mayo, *Content of Family Practice: A Statewide Study in Virginia with Its Clinical, Educational, and Research Implications,* J. Geyman (ed.), Appleton-Century-Crofts, New York, 1976.
5 J. Fry, "Deaths and Complications from Hypertension," *Journal of the Royal College of General Practitioners,* **25:**489–494, 1975.
6 J. Fry, "Long-Surviving Hypertensives—a 15-Year Follow-Up," *Journal of the Royal College of General Practitioners,* **25:**481–486, 1975.
7 D. S. Silverberg, "Long-Term Follow-Up of a Hypertension Screening Program," *Canadian Medical Association Journal,* **114:**425–428, 1976.
8 D. S. Silverberg, C. Van Nostrand, B. Juchle, E. Stuart, O. Smith, and E. Van Dorsser, "Screening for Hypertension in a High School Population," *Canadian Medical Association Journal,* **113:**103–113, 1975.

9 K. V. Rudnick, D. L. Sackett, S. Hirst, and C. Holmes, "Hypertension: The Family Physician's Role," *Canadian Family Physician,* **24:**477–484, 1978.

10 "The 1984 Report of the Joint National Committee on Detection, Evaluation and Treatment of High Blood Pressure," *Archives of Internal Medicine,* **144:**1045–1057, 1984.

11 A. G. Logan, "Report of the Canadian Hypertension Society, Consensus Conference on the Management of Mild Hypertension," *Canadian Medical Association Journal,* **131:**1053–1056, 1984.

12 S. Blumenthal et al., "Report of the Task Force on Blood Pressure Control in Children," *Pediatrics,* **59**(suppl):797, 1977.

13 R. D. Adelman, "Elevated Blood Pressures in Infants and Children," *Journal of Family Practice,* **6:**357–364, 1978.

14 "Diazepam in Hypertension," *Medical Letter on Drugs and Therapeutics,* **16:**96, 1974.

15 E. D. Frohlich, "The Hypertensive Crisis," *Clinician,* Searle, Chicago, 1973, pp. 78–81.

16 R. L. Grissom and P. W. Jewett, "Management of the Patient with Uncomplicated Hypertension: An Update," *Journal of Family Practice,* **3:**135–139, 1976.

17 O. G. Kuchel, W. A. Mahon, J. K. McKenzie, and R. I. Ogilvie, "Approach to Drug Therapy for Hypertension," *Canadian Medical Association Journal,* **120:**565–570, 1979.

18 R. Patterson Russell, "Systemic Hypertension," in A. M. Harvey, R. J. John, A. M. Owens, and R. R. Ross (eds.), *The Principles and Practice of Medicine,* Appleton-Century-Crofts, New York, 1976, chap. 31.

19 C. Abbott et al., *A Handbook of Hypertension,* Hypertension Unit, Camp Hill Hospital, Halifax, Nova Scotia, Canada, 1981.

20 H. G. Langford, "Step-Down Therapy for Hypertension," *Postgraduate Medicine,* **77:**100–110, 1985.

21 R. J. Weir, E. Briggs, and A. Mack, "Blood Pressure in Women Taking Oral Contraceptives," *British Medical Journal,* **11:**533–535, 1974.

22 R. N. Podell, D. Kent, and K. Keller, "Patient Psychological Defenses and Physician Response in the Long-Term Treatment of Hypertension," *Journal of Family Practice,* **3:**145–149, 1976.

23 D. L. Sackett, "Why Won't Hypertensive Patients Take Their Medicine?" *Canadian Family Physician,* **23:**72–74, 1977.

Chapter 23

Diabetes

B. K. Hennen, M.D.

PRINCIPLE

Some chronic conditions require lifelong surveillance by both patient and doctor. The patient understands better than anyone how a chronic condition alters function. A doctor who establishes a continuous relationship with the patient can learn more about the effect of the illness on the patient's function with each contact provided that he or she listens and looks at the problem from the patient's perspective. The patient can also learn more about the illness with each contact provided that both doctor and patient see such learning as integral to better management. Understanding the mechanisms of disease and therapy and preventing or at least recognizing the long-term complications early can help improve the patient's chance for optimal function.

Such mutual learning can be extended to other resources—e.g., family members and other health professionals—so that neither patient nor doctor will have to deal with the problem alone.

Diabetes mellitus is a chronic disease that requires this kind of approach.

DEFINITION

A chronic metabolic disease, diabetes is due to insufficient insulin or inappropriate resistance to its effect.

Type I diabetes, the *juvenile-onset* type, which is caused by failure of insulin production and release, is insulin-sensitive. Type II diabetes, the *maturity-onset* type (also known as the *obese* type), which is caused by impaired peripheral response to insulin, is insulin-resistant.

Several clinical phases have been identified, which commonly include *prediabetes, chemical diabetes,* and *frank diabetes.* However, these are more likely to be etiologically different kinds of diabetes than phases in the same illness.

PREVALENCE

In the Virginia study of family practices, 1 of 40 patient visits was for diabetes. Visits by women predominated 2 to 1 over those by men, and the incidence increased with age.[1] In the United Kingdom, there are 4.8 diabetics per 1000 patients per year under surveillance by general practitioners.[2]

Hodgkin noted one hypoglycemic coma for every six diabetics per year. Diabetic coma, however, did not occur once in 10 years in his practice.[2]

ETIOLOGY

Diabetes is more likely with advancing age. The analysis of complex genetic factors shows no clear mechanisms or patterns of inheritance, but some familial predilection does seem to exist.[3]

Poor nutrition, particularly if it results in obesity, is associated with a higher incidence of diabetes.

Viral infections (mumps and Coxsackie B_4 among others) affecting the pancreas are a factor in some cases. Lack of resistance to such infections depends on immunologic susceptibility, which varies among individuals.[4]

It is now believed that many drugs increase the probability of elevated blood sugar. Among them are diuretics (especially thiazides), oral contraceptives, glucocorticoids, adrenergic blocking agents, diphenylhydantoin, lithium, isoniazid, tricyclic antidepressants, and clonidine as well as caffeine, nicotine, and marijuana.[5]

NATURAL HISTORY AND RECOGNITION

Symptoms   Child-onset diabetics often present with an acute infectious illness of viral or bacterial cause with gastrointestinal symptoms of vomiting and diarrhea.[6] An adolescent who presents with severe ketoacidosis may in retrospect be seen to have experienced undiagnosed polyphagia, polydipsia, polyuria, and weight loss. Sometimes diabetes is suspected in youngsters because of family history and is found either when selective screening is done or when a urinalysis required for camp, school, or insurance shows glucosuria.

Acidosis is associated with a mortality rate which ranges from 1 to 6 percent. Mortality increases if the patient is older and has had impaired renal function, if an acute infection is present, or if the patient is suffering from an acute myocardial infarction.[7]

Hodgkin reported that when diagnosed, half his mature-onset diabetics could retrospectively recall having had symptoms 1 to 5 years before the diagnosis was made. Often a routine urine test provides the diagnostic clue.[2] Fatigue and weight loss may also be problems in the "new" diabetic.

In older persons, perineal pruritus, recurrent infections, visual blurring, obesity, and unusual psychological disturbances may be symptoms.

Complications   The serious complications of diabetes (aside from ketoacidosis or hypoglycemic coma in treated individuals) generally appear 10 to 20 years after the initial diagnosis.[8]

Coronary heart disease is twice as frequent in diabetics of at least 10 years' duration as in the general population. It has a tendency to cause less dramatic chest pain in these patients than in nondiabetics and is associated with higher mortality when myocardial infarction occurs.

Peripheral vascular disease is associated with x-ray evidence of calcification in 15 percent of patients at the time of diagnosis. Patients with severe peripheral vascular disease requiring amputation have a 5-year survival rate of 36 percent.

The renal diseases associated with diabetes are primarily glomerulosclerosis, pyelonephritis, and major arterial occlusion. Proteinuria, hypertension, and full-blown nephrotic syndrome (edema, hypercholesterolemia, and hypoproteinemia) provide evidence of severe involvement.

The eye complications of diabetes are the second most common cause of blindness in North America. Retinal disease, glaucoma, and cataracts are the most frequent causes.

The central nervous system complications of diabetes may involve single-nerve distribution, general peripheral nerve distribution, and autonomic nerves. The usual symptoms are pain, numbness, proprioceptive problems, and skin lesions from trauma or burns. Less frequent are complaints of impotence, peripheral motor weakness, and hypertension.

Findings on physical examination often do not correlate well with the apparent lack of functional impairment. Loss of vibration sense, peripheral sensation, and deep tendon reflexes may be the first indications that the patient has a neurological involvement.

Complications associated with pregnancy will be dealt with later in this chapter.

APPROACH TO THE PATIENT

Until evidence shows that treatment of prediabetes and chemical diabetes alters the long-term outlook, only persons who have frank diabetes should be labeled and treated as diabetic. The others can be considered at risk for diabetes, and reasonable preventive measures can be taken, such as maintenance of ideal weight and exercise programs.[9]

Reducing the high risk

Diagnosis can be difficult, especially for borderline cases in asymptomatic patients. Criteria are changing, and standard diagnostic methods can be affected by many intervening factors. Screening for diabetes in family practice should be directed at high-risk groups: the obese, those with a family history of diabetes, and pregnant women.

EXAMINATION

A functioning and apparently well diabetic will often have no signs of diabetes. A maturity-onset patient is likely to be overweight but will rarely show evidence of end organ disease.

In the acutely ill acidotic patient, signs of dehydration will be present. The skin may be flushed and warm, the patient's breath may smell of acetone, and the level of consciousness may range from drowsy to somnolent. Unless an infection is present, temperature is likely to be normal or even subnormal. Breathing may be deep and rapid.[7] Hypotension may develop, and a rapid, weak pulse may be present.

DIAGNOSIS

Diagnosis depends on the presence of characteristic symptoms (polydipsia, polyphagia, polyuria, or weight loss), strongly suggestive signs on examination (acetone breath, Kussmaul's respiration, retinopathy, or neuropathy), the results of investigations aimed at

Table 23-1   Instructions for Standardizing Glucose Tolerance Testing

300 g carbohydrates should be taken daily for 3 days preceding test.

Discontinue nonessential drugs. Discontinue contraceptive pills for one cycle preceding test.

Eliminate coffee, tea, and smoking on day of test.

Administer standard glucose load, e.g., 1 g per kilogram of body weight up to 100 g.

finding high levels of glucose in the blood or urine, and evidence of classically associated chemical abnormalities.

Glucose in urine is shown by glucose oxidase strip tests (e.g., Clinistix or Testape), which are specific for glucose, or copper sulfate reduction tablet tests, which may be positive for other sugars as well.[10]

Glucose tolerance tests

Measurements of blood sugar are made on whole blood or on plasma, which gives 12 percent higher readings than whole blood. With proper standardization of testing procedures (Table 23-1), diabetes can be diagnosed if

Fasting levels are above 140 mg/dl (plasma)
One-hour pc levels are above 260 mg/dl (plasma)
Two-hour pc levels are above 220 mg/dl (plasma) (162 mg/dl in pregnancy)

Fasting levels below 110, 1-hour pc levels of 184 mg/dl, and 2-hour pc levels of 140 mg/dl are definitely normal.[9]

Two random plasma glucose levels of 250 mg/dl are also sufficient for diagnosis without a glucose tolerance test.

These criteria have been put forward by Siperstein.[11] They are the most lenient criteria for diagnosis but fit with our concern that diabetes is generally overdiagnosed and overtreated.

A reasonable age correction would be to add 7 mg per decade after age 20 to the acceptable threshold level.

In the absence of substantiating clinical findings, we feel that patients in the between or gray zone should be considered at risk but not labeled as diabetics, prediabetics, or clinical diabetics.

The establishment of the renal threshold of glucose in a person who has an abnormal glucose tolerance test should be considered part of the diagnosis. Urine tests done at hourly intervals during an oral glucose tolerance test can be confirmed through coincidental measurements of serum or plasma glucose and double-voided urine glucose before each of the three main meals. To date, this provides the most accurate method of monitoring glucose levels with urine tests.

MANAGEMENT

Educating the Patient

After the initial diagnosis and when the acute symptoms have been resolved, the physician's first task is to help the patient understand and accept the fact that with proper management, diabetes can have relatively moderate adverse effects on his or her life. Establishing routine activites and eating habits is necessary to some extent for all diabetics and is essential for a patient who is on medication (either oral hypoglycemics or insulin). It is important to stress the possibility of leading a normal life; if limitations are explained and justified to the patient, better compliance is likely.

> Patient education can improve compliance

The patient's education should involve the family from the beginning. The family doctor may also need to rely heavily on other resources, in particular the family practice nurse, the nutritionist, and the local diabetic association, to help the patient understand the disease.

Nutrition and Weight Control

Maintaining an ideal weight should be a prime goal for the diabetic. Ideal body weight equals baseline weight (115 lb for men, 100 lb for women) plus 5 lb per inch of height over 5 ft.

The ideal caloric intake equals the ideal body weight in pounds times 10 calories, adding 25 percent for normal activity and 50 percent for heavy, prolonged labor.[12]

> Diet counseling

Weight reduction can be accomplished by subtracting 1000 calories per day until the ideal weight is reached. If the patient is underweight, one can add 500 to 1000 calories per day to the ideal caloric intake.

A combination of 50 to 60 percent carbohydrates, 10 to 15 percent protein, and 30 to 35 percent fat provides a good general balance. High-glucose foods as a part of a general diet should be avoided. Often this is interpreted by patients as "carbohydrates should be avoided," and one should be careful to explain the difference between "straight" glucose and other kinds of carbohydrates.

Most nutritionists find it practical to show people what reasonable quantities of food look like and explain that weighing or measuring quantities is not necessary. "Diabetic" foods are not required and are often expensive.

For patients on oral agents or insulin, regular spacing of meals is important. Harvey[12] demonstrated how one can divide the day's calories into tenths, giving so many tenths per meal and per snack. Six eating times per day are evenly divided by hours during the waking period, with the distribution depending on activity and insulin type. Bedtime snacks should usually be predominantly fat or protein rather than carbohydrate in order to prevent nocturnal hypoglycemia.

MEDICATION

Most type II diabetics can be managed with diet and activity programs alone. For those who cannot be controlled without medications, insulin is the drug of choice, as it is for all juvenile-onset diabetics (Table 23-2).

During the initial adjustment of dosage and during acute illness, regular insulin is usually used alone. Once the total insulin dosage is assessed, the drug can be administered in combinations in order to reduce the number of injections to a minimum. Split insulin doses, one before breakfast and one before the late afternoon meal, are becoming more frequently used.

Oral hypoglycemics

Insulin

For those over age 50 who cannot be controlled by diet and an activity program alone and for whom insulin is impractical or unacceptable, sulfonylureas are worth introducing, particularly if the patient is asymptomatic. If adequate control cannot be obtained with sulfonylureas, insulin may have to be tried. Occasionally a combination of both insulin and sulfonylureas will ultimately result in the smooth control one desires. Another indication for the use of sulfonylureas is a patient who is temporarily diabetic because of maintenance steroid medications given for other conditions.[13] (See Table 23-3.)

The elderly

In the elderly, it is important to watch for prolonged hypoglycemia, which is sometimes associated with the use of oral agents, the long-acting ones in particular. The effect of these agents can be potentiated by drugs such as sulfisoxazole, phenylbutazone, dicumarol (bishydroxycoumarin), alcohol, salicylates, monamine oxidase inhibitors, chlorpromazine, clofibrate, and guanethidine. The drugs mentioned in "Etiology" in this chapter may also interfere with accurate assessment of the effectiveness of treatment.

THE CONCEPT OF GOOD CONTROL

Control

"Therein lies the diabetic dilemma—the perfect control with its inconveniences, restrictions, and even dangers, versus a more relaxed control and life style with its possible (probable) long term complications."[14]

The debate continues about the ideal blood sugar levels for optimal control. There has been little evidence to show that maintaining blood levels very close to the renal threshold results in a

Table 23-2 Peak Action and Duration of Insulins

Type	Maximum effect, hours	Duration, hours
Regular	2.5–5	5–7
Semilente	5–10	12–16
Lente	7–15	18–24
NPH	4–12	18–24
Ultralente	10–30	30–36
PZI	10–30	30–36

Table 23-3 Commonly Used Sulfonylureas: Activity

	Duration of action, hours	Half-life, hours	Usual dose
Tolbutamide	6–10	5	0.5 g tid with meals (maximum 2 g daily)
Chlorpropamide	40–72	32	0.1–0.5 g every morning
Acetohexamide	10–16	7	0.25–1.25 g daily
Tolazamide	10–16	7	0.1–0.75 daily

Source: Bierman.[13]

better prognosis for either complications or longevity. Schaffrin mentions some conditions in which blood sugar levels should be kept close to the renal threshold, including (1) no serious unexpected reactions, (2) the avoidance of constant ketonuria, and (3) the avoidance of chronic excessive hyperglycemia with consequent osmotic diuresis.[15] She goes further in the case of adolescents, accepting the idea that "if a delayed meal results in mildly symptomatic hypoglycemia, and if in a month's time half the urine tests are two percent or greater and half are 0.5 percent or less," optimal control has been achieved. In this case, she indicates, more negative results will result in undue hypoglycemia, which is particularly difficult to manage in an adolescent.

Acute Infections

Management of acute infections by the patient should include (1) notifying the physician, (2) taking an antiemetic if nauseous, (3) taking the usual morning insulin, (4) taking small volumes of carbohydrate-rich foods hourly, (5) testing the urine or blood every 4 hours for sugar and ketones, and (6) taking supplemental or regular insulin on the basis of these tests.

HYPOGLYCEMIA

Prevention

A diabetic control regime that allows showing some urinary sugar or slightly elevated blood sugars, at least on alternate days, will usually prevent any serious periods of hypoglycemia. The patient should know the usual symptoms of hypoglycemia, which may include hunger, sweating, tremor, unusual behavior, excessive irritability, or even convulsion and coma. A patient who experiences any of these symptoms should immediately take some sweet liquid refreshment such as orange juice or soda pop if he or she is able to swallow. If the patient is obtunded or confused, sometimes sprinkling sugar on the tongue or using corn syrup or honey will improve the condition. A diabetic's family should be instructed in the use of glucagon in case of a severe reaction in which the patient cannot swallow. One or two milligrams subcutaneously will usually enable the patient to take glucose orally. The carbohydrate intake should then be maintained until sugar appears in the urine, after which more slowly absorbed carbohydrates should be started.[15]

All diabetics should have a medical alert bracelet indicating their disease and the medication(s) they are taking.

Exercise

Since exercise increases glucose utilization and can cause hypoglycemia, it should be preceded by either an increase in calories or a reduction in the dose of insulin for the time period involved. Dietary adjustment is preferable when the degree of extra activity cannot be predicted.[16]

Maintenance Management

Maintenance

Maintenance management of the diabetic involves continued support and regular visits to review weight, activity, diet, cardiovascular status, funduscopic and eye examination, and neurological assessment as well as monitoring for infections, particularly of the skin and urogenital tract. A special effort should be made to look at the patient's feet. It is always useful to review the patient's urine or blood tests for the previous week, since it is very easy for patients who are doing well to discontinue regular testing of their urine. For an insulin-treated diabetic, urine tests on a double-voided specimen before breakfast, as well as on specimens before meals and before evening snacks, are generally sufficient at first. The before-lunch test may be omitted first, and the test preceding the evening meal may be omitted subsequently as the patient stabilizes and gains control. If urinary glycosuria is 2 percent or greater, if blood sugars exceed 300 mg%, or if the diabetic feels unwell, then urine should be tested for ketones.

Glucose reflectance meters are now more acceptable in terms

of ease of use and cost for self-monitoring. Because of their greater accuracy, they are replacing urine testing as a home measurement method. However, they require educated and careful use and have not yet proved to be as great an improvement in diabetic control as had been hoped.[17]

Glycosolated hemoglobin measures which reflect the blood sugar levels of 6 to 8 weeks ago are useful with type I diabetics who are having unexplained high and low blood sugar swings or diabetics in whom compliance is questionable.

Lane noted that 90 percent of time spent on history taking in routine diabetes visits concerned dietary compliance, medication compliance, and questions about hypoglycemia or hyperglycemia. These areas were the ones nurses focused on in the time spent with patients in an ambulatory setting where the nurses were given responsibility for routine diabetic visits. The following items were also covered: recording weight change, blood pressure, fasting blood sugar, and new problems; asking about compliance with medication and diet, recent infections, skin problems, and hypoglycemia or hyperglycemia; preparing prescriptions for continued medications; and giving instructions about medications, diet, and skin and foot care.[18]

Nurse's role

The patient and family may be referred to the local diabetic association for information about management. Often other diabetics have more practical hints on management than physicians do. The early introduction of the patient and the family to a nutritionist can be of tremendous help to both patient and physician.

Diabetic associations

GENETIC COUNSELING

The family physician may be responsible for genetic counseling. Current opinion varies on the role of genetic factors, and no accurate predictions can be made. As a general rule, however, if one child develops diabetes, about 5 percent of the siblings will probably be affected. If both parents have juvenile diabetes, about 20 percent of their offspring are likely to develop the disease. For an individual who has a brother, sister, or parent with diabetes and is under age 40, the chances are about 1 percent that he or she will develop diabetes. For individuals between 40 and 60 in the same circumstances the risk is 3 percent, and for those over age 60 the risk is 10 percent. The risks double if other siblings or both parents have diabetes.[4]

Counseling parents

COUNSELING REGARDING PREGNANCY

The perinatal mortality rate of newborns of diabetic mothers is about 8 percent. White has classified diabetic mothers into six categories which have some prognostic significance.[19] The six classes can be described as follows:

Class A   Glucose tolerance test abnormality only
Class B   Onset after age 20, duration 0 to 9 years, no vascular disease
Class C   Onset age 10 to 19, duration 10 to 19 years, no vascular disease
Class D   Onset under age 10, duration 20 or more years, vascular disease, calcification of the legs, retinitis
Class E   Calcified pelvic vessels
Class F   Nephritis

Diabetic
mothers

For a controlled young diabetic, fertility can be considered normal. The risks of pregnancy are, however, compounded for both mother and infant. Generally, the younger the mother, the less likely she is to have either advanced diabetes or the complications of pregnancy and diabetes. The exception is, of course, the very young adolescent pregnant girl who is still struggling to manage and accept the disease. Ideally, control without hypoglycemia is preferable in pregnancy, and often it is best to switch to a split dose of insulin in order to maintain optimal control.

The use of biophysical profile assessments and rollover tests have become a routine part of the management of diabetic pregnant women (see chapter 16). Delivery is effected early, usually between 34 and 37 weeks. One must then deal with a premature baby with a high risk of hypoglycemic episodes and, when necessary, the extra risks associated with cesarean section, including respiratory distress.

COMA

For a patient presenting with coma, the physician should have a plan of management that can be quickly put into effect. When a known diabetic presents with coma, immediate blood testing with Dextrostix can show that blood glucose is under 130 mg/deciliters and that ketones are absent, thus ruling out diabetic coma. The patient should be treated immediately with 50% glucose intravenously. Causes of coma in the diabetic include the following: ketoacidosis (3 + glucose, 3 + ketones, decreased CO_2), glucose hyperosmolality (4 + glucose, 0 to 1 + ketones, decreased CO_2), and hypoglycemia (no glucose, 0 to 1 + ketones, and low to normal CO_2).[12]

Management of
coma

A detailed review of the management of ketoacidosis and the much rarer causes of coma (glucose hyperosmolality and lactic acidosis) is beyond the scope of this book. Briefly it involves the immediate establishment of an intravenous line, drawing of blood for blood sugar and potassium and electrolyte values, perfusion of intravenous saline, immediate introduction of insulin in order to maintain a ready circulating quantity, half-hour doctor assessments, hourly blood sugar and urine sugar estimations, consideration of the need for a stomach tube, search for infection and its treatment, cardiogram, and subsequent administration of regular insulin according to urine testing. All these measures should continue until the urine tests are 1 percent or less, when 5% dextrose and water can be started. Sodium bicarbonate can be given slowly intravenously if the CO_2–combining power drops below 8. Potassium should be started at the rate of 15 to 20 mEq per hour to a maximum of 100 mEq intravenously by the fifth hour or when the electrocardiogram shows evidence of hypopotassemia.

SPECIAL PROBLEMS

Surgery

All surgery, including elective dental extractions, should be done before midmorning, as should any x-ray which requires fasting.

A patient going to surgery, even though fasting, still requires insulin. Surgery is usually associated with a reduction in food intake, at least on the day of the surgery, and entails stress to the patient. Sometimes surgical drainage depletes the diabetic patient of important electrolytes.

One approach is to give one-third the daily dose of insulin preoperatively, one-third after surgery, and additional supplements in the form of regular insulin as needed.[20] Blood glucose can be rechecked on the afternoon of the day of the surgery; if it is over 250 mg/decimeters, additional regular insulin can be given. The fasting diabetic is given a continuous slow IV of 5% dextrose and saline or water.

The Contraceptive Pill

The birth control pill affects glucose metabolism and usually results in increased insulin need. There has been no evidence that the birth control pill accelerates the development of diabetes. It does, however, increase vascular risks. If one has a choice of other methods, the pill is probably best avoided. If one feels the pill is still necessary, the pill lowest in estrogen should be used.

Recently diagnosed, young diabetics who do not have evidence of end organ complications, may use oral contraception but should be closely observed.[21]

10 DIABETES

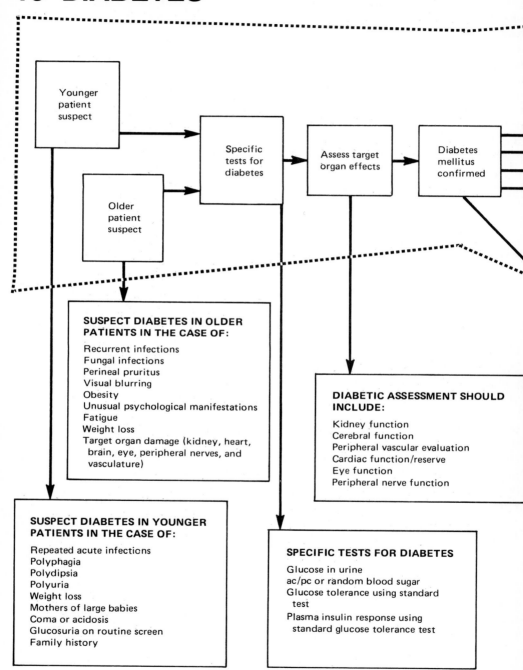

SUSPECT DIABETES IN OLDER PATIENTS IN THE CASE OF:

Recurrent infections
Fungal infections
Perineal pruritus
Visual blurring
Obesity
Unusual psychological manifestations
Fatigue
Weight loss
Target organ damage (kidney, heart, brain, eye, peripheral nerves, and vasculature)

DIABETIC ASSESSMENT SHOULD INCLUDE:

Kidney function
Cerebral function
Peripheral vascular evaluation
Cardiac function/reserve
Eye function
Peripheral nerve function

SUSPECT DIABETES IN YOUNGER PATIENTS IN THE CASE OF:

Repeated acute infections
Polyphagia
Polydipsia
Polyuria
Weight loss
Mothers of large babies
Coma or acidosis
Glucosuria on routine screen
Family history

SPECIFIC TESTS FOR DIABETES

Glucose in urine
ac/pc or random blood sugar
Glucose tolerance using standard test
Plasma insulin response using standard glucose tolerance test

DIABETES

NUTRITION

Appropriate diet—style weight reduction to patient's life habits.
Avoid hypoglycemia—recognize alerting symptoms; carry glucose.
Avoid expensive diabetic foods.

EDUCATION

Avoid precipitant drugs.
Advise regarding Medic-Alert/Diabetic Association.
Counsel on foot and skin care.
Provide patient-oriented literature on diabetes and prevention of
  complications.
Arrange for genetic counseling where indicated.

Life-style changes will depend on severity and presence of other
risk factors.

SPECIFIC TREATMENT

Prime disease
Oral hypoglycemics with sulfonylureas for adult onset diabetics
  who do not have acute complications and in whom control by
  weight reduction or insulin treatment is not feasible.
Insulin.

Complications
Infections; target organ damage should be carefully monitored.

**DRUGS WHICH POTENTIATE
DIABETES**

Diuretics (thiazides)
Oral contraceptives
Glucocorticoids
Adrenergic blockers
Diphenylhydantoin
Clonidine
Caffeine
Nicotine
Marijuana

**AVOID POTENTIATION OF
HYPOGLYCEMIC EFFECT WITH:**

Sulfasuxasole
Phenylbutasone
Bishydroxycoumarin
Alcohol
Salicylates
MAO inhibitors

Driving

Regulations on driving for diabetics vary from region to region. One can apply to diabetics a rule parallel to the one used for epileptics: if the local law indicates that an epileptic may drive if he or she has been free of seizures for 1 to 2 years, it would be reasonable to allow a diabetic to drive if he or she has been free of insulin reactions or coma for 1 or 2 years. One could even argue that a patient who is subject to reactions but is capable of recognizing them early should be allowed to drive unless the early signs of the reaction are of a psychological nature.

Children

Most pediatricians and doctors who deal with child diabetics prefer to have these patients hospitalized for initial management. As a rule, this is warranted only for patients who live at some distance from expert care. Any diabetic who presents with an acute illness will require hospitalization, and initial management can be carried out in the hospital. But a patient (whether child or adult) who is discovered to be a diabetic and is functioning well may be better off as an ambulatory patient at a day care center in a well-staffed and well-serviced medical facility.

After the first few weeks of management, juvenile-onset diabetics sometimes go through a "honeymoon" phase in which their extrinsic insulin requirements approach zero. This happens in less than half of young patients with this disease, usually occurs within 3 months of the initiation of insulin therapy, and may present as increasing numbers of insulin reactions, persistently negative tests, or on rare occasions, coma. Most physicians advocate keeping a minimum dose of insulin for a child going through this phase in order to maintain the habit of giving oneself an injection.

Adolescence

Adolescence is a difficult time for many young people even without a chronic disease such as diabetes. The normal reaction against authority and external controls can create great difficulties for young diabetics. Adolescents need extra support, careful education, and a comfortable relationship with a health professional. Diabetic camps where youngsters can discuss their problems and learn about the disease are helpful for many. Menarche may be delayed in many diabetic girls, and menstrual patterns may be disordered into the teenage years. Some girls also require less insulin at the time of their periods.

Very Old Patients

It is often difficult to initiate insulin therapy in an elderly patient, especially if the patient has other illnesses that affect the vision or the steadiness of the hands required to properly measure and administer insulin. In addition, elderly people often have irregular eating habits and are therefore more vulnerable to hypoglycemic reactions. The signs of impending hypoglycemia are often blurred in the elderly and can be wrongly interpreted as the confusion sometimes attributed to aging.

Often relatives, professional homemakers, or visiting nurses can help elderly diabetics keep the disease under reasonable control. On rare occasions, one must simply accept the fact that the patient is more comfortable running higher levels of blood sugar than one would like. One would then eliminate daily insulin injections or risky sulfonylureas and closely monitor the patient for the acute affects of diabetes through frequent, regular office or home visits.

We have even seen elderly patients come into the hospital to be treated with insulin during an acute illness and go home for reasonable management without continued insulin therapy.

REFERENCES

1 D. W. Marsland, M. Wood, and F. Mayo, *Content of Family Practice: A Statewide Study in Virginia with Its Clinical, Educational, and Research Implications,* J. Geyman (ed.), Appleton-Century-Crofts, New York, 1976.

2 K. Hodgkin, *Towards Earlier Diagnosis in Primary Care,* 4th ed., Churchill Livingstone, Edinburgh, London, New York, 1978.

3 P. H. Forshan, "Diabetes Mellitus: A Multi-Hormonal Disease," *Proceedings of the Eisenhower Medical Center,* International Seminary, no. 3, Fall 1977, p. 15.

4 R. M. Ehrlich, "Is Diabetes Mellitus Preventable?" *Canadian Family Physician,* **24:**680–686, 1978.

5 J. A. Burgess, "Drugs Which Cause Diabetes," *Australian Family Physician,* **5:**1480–1489, 1976.

6 D. G. Eastman, R. A. Guthrie, J. W. Hare, A. Krosmick, J. J. Kristan, C. R. Shurman, and K. E. Sussman, "Young Diabetics in Your Practice" (roundtable), *Patient Care,* **9**(9):12–67, 1975.

7 J. R. Kelly, "Rational Management of Diabetic Ketoacidosis," *American Family Physician,* **15:**119–122, 1977.

8 J. E. Gerich, "Diabetic Control and the Late Complications of Diabetes," *American Family Physician,* **16:**85–91, 1977.

9 C. Reynolds and A. K. Garg, "Who Is Diabetic?" *Canadian Family Physician,* **24:**687–690, 1978.

10 J. A. Burgess, "Methods of Diagnosing Diabetes Mellitus," *Australian Family Physician,* **5:**49–52, 1976.

11 M. D. Siperstein, "The Glucose Tolerance Test: A Pitfall in the Diagnosis of Diabetes Mellitus," *Advances in Internal Medicine,* **20:**297–322, 1975.

12 A. M. Harvey, R. J. John, A. M. Owens, and R. R. Ross, "Diabetes Mellitus,"

in *The Principles and Practice of Medicine,* Appleton-Century-Crofts, New York, 1976, p. 998.

13 E. L. Bierman, "The Oral Antidiabetic Agents," *American Family Physician,* **13:**98–104, 1976.

14 J. E. Smith, "The Diabetic Dilemma—Medical Mode," *Minnesota Medicine,* **67**(2):93–97, 1984.

15 M. Schaffrin, "The Adolescent Diabetic," *Canadian Family Physician,* **23:** 682–686, 1978.

16 A. E. Stocks, "Diabetes and the Sportsman," *Australian Family Physician,* **3:**447–450, 1974.

17 M. M. Mountier, R. S. Scott, and D. W. Beaver, "Use and Abuse of Glucose Reflectance Meters," *Diabetes Care,* **5**(5):542–544, 1982.

18 W. Lane, "Handling the Routine Diabetes Visit," *Patient Care,* **8**(2):121–122, 1974.

19 J. T. Queenan, D. M. Haynes, and W. P. Vanderhaar, "Gynecology and Obstetrics," in H. F. Conn and R. E. Rakel (eds.), *Family Practice,* 2d ed., W. B. Saunders, Philadelphia, 1978, table 41-1.

20 R. A. Currie, "Surgery," in H. F. Conn and R. E. Rakel (eds.), *Family Practice,* 2d ed., W. B. Saunders, Philadelphia, 1978, p. 484.

21 *Report of the Special Advisory Committee on Reproductive Physiology to the Health Protection Branch.* Published by authority of the Minister of National Health and Welfare, Canada, 1985.

Chapter 24

Headache

D. B. Shires, M.D.

PRINCIPLE

A patient who suffers from chronic or recurrent pain needs a comprehensive management program that includes preventive maneuvers, psychological support, physical therapy, pharmacological treatment, and, in selected situations, surgical intervention. Too often, however, the emphasis of both physician and patient is on prescribed medication. Medications should be only one factor in a "whole-person" approach; used in isolation, they are seldom effective over the long run. Unfortunately, they can also become addictive. The risks of psychological and physiological dependence accompany many pain remedies, and these risks tend to make physicians overly cautious in their prescribing habits. The patient is therefore in double jeopardy, faced with either the risk of addiction or the risk of inadequate pain relief.

If pain becomes intolerable, patients and their families are unlikely to be able to cope. Panic often results, and the patient looks for a new doctor. Unnecessary investigations are done and done again to assure patient, family, and physician that nothing has been missed.

Risk of overinvestigation

If it is chronic or recurrent, the pain of headache can lead to such an unsatisfactory situation.

DEFINITION

Any pain or discomfort localized to the head may be designated a "headache."

PREVALENCE

"Headache" (unspecified), "tension headache," and "migraine" are the diagnoses in 1 percent of patients presenting to a family doctor.[1] In addition, patients may present with headache but ultimately may be diagnosed as having other disorders.

ETIOLOGY

Differential
diagnosis

In family practice, patients in the early stages of many systemic and generalized illnesses (particularly depression, chronic anxiety, febrile illnesses, cerebrovascular illness, and hypertension) may report headache. For every 100 patients presenting to the family doctor with headache, about 50 will have the unspecified or combined vascular and muscle-contraction type, 20 will have a headache that is mainly of the muscle-contraction type, 10 will have a vascular type, and the remainder will have headaches associated with intracranial and systemic illnesses, usually acute febrile illnesses.

Serious causes such as meningitis, subarachnoid hemorrhage, brain tumor, acute glaucoma, temporal arteritis, and serious general infections account for about 0.5 percent of all headaches in general practice, with meningitis accounting for half of these headaches and subarachnoid hemorrhage accounting for a quarter.[2]

Defects in visual acuity and ocular muscle imbalance seldom cause headache.[3]

Of headaches with a vascular origin, 85 percent will be common migraine, 10 percent will be classic migraine, 4 percent will be cluster headache, and the remainder will be unusual variants such as hemiplegic, ophthalmoplegic, or basilar artery migraine.[4] (See Figure 24-1.)

The intracranial and systemic group of illnesses includes depression, anxiety, common febrile illnesses, sinusitis, meningitis and encephalitis, trauma, cerebrovascular insufficiency, brain tumors, intracranial bleeds, uncontrolled hypertension, and hypoglycemia.

Illnesses in the vascular and muscular-contraction group are at least twice as frequent in women; the peak seems to be from 15 to

Figure 24-1 Etiology of headache.

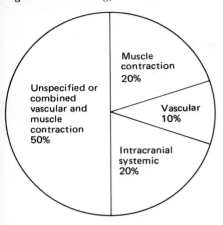

Muscle
contraction
20%

Unspecified or
combined
vascular and
muscle
contraction
50%

Vascular
10%

Intracranial
systemic
20%

45 years of age for vascular-contraction headaches and 25 to 34 years of age for vascular headaches.[1]

DIAGNOSTIC CHARACTERISTICS OF HEADACHE

Tension Headache

Muscle-contraction headaches are usually bilateral, are described as "pressure" or "tightness," do not throb, have a gradual onset with no aura, and often continue steadily for hours or days. Patients are likely to be sensitive, competitive, or perfectionist, and excessive stresses and demands may be taxing their coping abilities. The headache may be an expression of anxiety or may be more complex in origin, arising from unresolved, unconscious conflicts such as repressed hostility, dependency, and psychosexual problems. Patients with occasional tension headaches are usually uptight people, those with frequent headaches are usually people with ongoing stress problems, and patients with constant headache are usually depressed.[5]

Muscular
contraction

Personality
types

Migraine

The criteria for diagnosis of migraine are summarized in Table 24-1. *Classic migraine* has a more specific visual or neurological aura but may not last more than 4 to 6 hours, while *common migraine* usually lasts longer and is more likely to be accompanied by persistent nausea, vomiting, diarrhea, polyuria, weakness, and prostration. Wise says that if two of the four listed criteria are present, one can confidently diagnose migraine.[6] Other factors which substantiate a migraine diagnosis include the following:

Vascular spasm

Table 24-1   Criteria for Diagnosis of Migraine

1 Unilateral thumping headache
2 Nausea and vomiting
3 Visual or CNS aura
4 History of headache in siblings or parents

Note: The presence of two of these criteria is sufficient to make the diagnosis.
Source: Wise.[6]

   1   The occurrence of symptoms such as paresthesias, speech disorders, dizziness, sweating, and other vasomotor disorders during an attack
   2   Relief by ergotamine
   3   Personality characteristics of inflexibility and shyness in childhood, giving rise in the adult to perfectionism, rigidity, resentment, ambition, and efficiency
   4   A constitutional predisposition to sustained emotional stress
   5   A past history of motion sickness during childhood

Cluster Migraine Headache

Cluster headaches are characterized by unilateral sweating and tearing, facial flushing, salivation, and rhinorrhea. They occur six to eight times a day, lasting from a few minutes to 2 hours, for several days or weeks.

Sinusitis

Headache that is due to sinusitis may be localized according to the sinus involved, may be altered by positioning, and has a characteristic periodicity (Table 24-2). Mucopurulent discharge is manifested as postnasal drip, and purulent nasal discharge may be visible in the nasal passages on examination. Sinus x-rays may confirm a clinical impression, but since they may be positive from previous infection or negative in the presence of radiolucent mucopus, they are of little diagnostic use.[7]

Other Causes

Less common
causes of
headache

In any patient, other serious diseases that cause headache must be considered. Though rare, these causes require urgent attention. *Intracranial tumors* may present with a headache that is either unilateral or bilateral. An adult patient who has not been much troubled by headache but develops intermittent headache which progressively becomes persistent, is suspect. If the headache is worsened by activities that increase intracranial pressure, such as

Table 24-2 Sinus Headache

Site of infection	Pain site	Positional effect	Periodicity	Other characteristics
Frontal sinus	Frontal	Relieved in upright position	Onset midmorning with noon peak and late afternoon relief	Frontal percussion tenderness, nasal orbital roof pressure tenderness
Maxillary sinus	Cheek, upper back teeth, radiates to forehead on same side	Increased on bending forward, relieved in supine position	Onset midmorning, peaks late in afternoon	Pain may be referred to ascending ramus of inferior maxilla
Sphenoid	Vertex, forehead, or eye on same side	Aggravated in upright position	Onset morning, increases as day goes on	Reflex otalgia
Ethmoid	Between and behind eyes, temporal region	Relieved in upright position	Diminishes late afternoon	Eye movement aggravates, eyeball pressure painful

straining or lifting, it deserves complete investigation. Cancer patients are always suspect for metastatic cerebral disease.

Constant or intermittent headache weeks to months after head trauma may represent *subdural hematoma,* although this condition is not commonly seen in practice. Changes in mental status or level of consciousness are usual with this condition.

Headaches, nausea and vomiting, and fits, especially after a recent infection (e.g., otitis, sinusitis, chest infection, or acute or subacute bacterial endocarditis), suggest *brain abscess.* This disease is also uncommon in practice.

Subarachnoid hemorrhage causes sudden and severe headache, which is aggravated by movement, and blunting of consciousness may lead to coma. Vomiting and neck stiffness are usual. Blood in the cerebrospinal fluid confirms the suspicion.

Hypertension may be associated with morning occipital headaches, especially with a diastolic pressure over 110 mm Hg. Sudden rises in blood pressure may cause severe throbbing headaches.

Edmeads[8] has identified specific features that should arouse concern about the possibility of serious cerebrovascular causes for headache. These include the following:

Alerting factors

1 Headache which does not conform readily to a benign pattern such as contraction or migraine
2 A change in the pattern of a preexisting headache
3 Headache beginning after age 35
4 Headache occurring in a person with a history of, or phys-

ical signs of, vascular disease such as angina, claudication, congestive failure, valvular disease, hypertension, and bruits

  5 Headache occurring with other symptoms such as diplopia or weakness

  6 The presence of abnormal neurological signs

  7 The presence of meningeal irritation, which in its milder forms is easily overlooked

HEADACHE IN CHILDREN

The term *headache* may be used by a child as a poorly localized description of ear pain, mastoid discomfort, the facial pain of sinusitis, or even eye pain. It may also represent the main area of discomfort of a generalized infection with a high fever or the specific localizer of encephalitis or meningitis.[6]

Psychological causes

As in adults, chronic or recurrent headaches are most likely to be tension headaches (particularly in older children) or migrainous headaches, which may manifest themselves by age 3. Headache can also be the presenting symptom of depression in children.[9] Seldom a prime symptom of brain tumor (cerebellar and brainstem symptoms are much more common), headache in children nevertheless often raises this concern in parents. Headaches may also be used by children to express their reaction to conflict within themselves or with others.

HEADACHE IN THE ELDERLY

Organic causes

Vascular headaches tend to be less common in later life. However, muscle-contraction headaches still occur, although they too occur less frequently. In particular, temporal arteritis, glaucoma, basilar artery insufficiency, cervical arthritis, and chronic brain syndrome may present with headache in geriatric patients. In temporal arteritis, the intense throbbing or burning pain is unilateral and is associated with sudden or gradual visual loss and systemic symptoms of fever, malaise, anorexia, and myalgia. With open-angle glaucoma, the pain may be around the eye orbit or in the forehead or temple. The patient sees "halos" and has a fixed dilated pupil, red eye and steamy cornea, optic cupping, visual field defects, and measurably increased intraocular pressure.

Basilar artery insufficiency may present with a headache and sensory motor disturbance. The headache may be occipital, nuchal, or frontal. Blindness, diplegia, vertigo, dysarthria, dysphagia, hemiparesis, unilateral numbness, and paraplegia may occur.

The vague gradual onset of chronic brain syndrome may include headache, but the headache alone is of little diagnostic help until the personality changes begin to become evident.

EXAMINATION

A minimal examination for a patient with the sole symptom of headache should include temperature, blood pressure, funduscopy, examination for meningeal irritation (photophobia, neck stiffness), palpation of the muscles at the back of the neck for spasm, and a brief assessment of mental and social status. The presence of other symptoms or the finding that any of these tests is abnormal may indicate a need for further examination.

INVESTIGATION

Generally, tension headaches, migraine headaches, and cluster headaches need no investigations unless a simple test can rule out a diagnostic possibility about which a patient is particularly concerned.

Other investigations depend on the history and findings on examination. They may include x-rays of the sinuses, skull x-ray if there is a history of trauma, brain scan if there is a history suggesting tumor or hemorrhage, lumbar puncture (using a small needle) if acute hemorrhage is suspected or if meningitis is likely, sedimentation rate if cranial arteritis is a possibility, tonometry if glaucoma is suspected, and blood sugars if a hypoglycemic cause is considered a possibility.

Limited investigations

APPROACH TO THE PATIENT

It is important to determine why a patient comes with a particular problem on a particular day. Was the pain unbearable? Was the pain interfering with normal functioning? Was the pain a source of anxiety to the patient or to others because of what it might represent?

What does the patient think is the cause? This is worth determining in order to be able to reassure the patient. It also makes it easier for the patient to help the doctor by supplying useful information. Often patients will volunteer that they have been under a lot of tension lately and think that the headache is probably related to stress. A family member may have suffered from "sick headaches" in the past, and the patient may correctly decide that his or her headache is of the same type. Many patients think a headache represents high blood pressure. This is rarely a cause of headache, and it is easy to rule out, thereby reassuring the patient.

Reassurance

Often the patient needs reassurance that there is no danger of a brain tumor or impending stroke or needs an explanation of why the headache is not a "migraine" or a "sinus" headache. Most cases

Acute headache

of "acute" headache presenting de novo are due to acute problems such as acute febrile illness, postconcussion, and acute sinusitis. The exact cause can generally be determined by means of appropriate history taking and a selective examination.

A headache which, even though it may be presenting for the first time to the physician, has been recurring for a considerable period of time is likely to fall into the group we characterize as chronic recurring headaches. For this type of headache it is important from the outset to establish a management program that includes prevention, relief of acute symptoms, physical therapy, appropriate medications, psychological support (including giving support to family members and family members' understanding of the patient's management), and accurate diagnosis.

MANAGEMENT

For each specific kind of headache, particular points deserve emphasis.

Tension headache

In dealing with tension headache, it is important to learn the sources of the patient's anxiety and determine whether conflicts are present. Usually, one can identify repressed hostilities, some dependency problems, or some psychosexual conflicts.

The first approach should be an attempt to change some of the patient's attitudes and perhaps modify the patient's lifestyle. The patient can be encouraged to relax through the use of relaxation exercises or other forms of physical exercise. Analgesics can be used, but narcotics should be avoided for tension headaches. Anxiolytic drugs may help an individual through a stressful period but should be restricted to 2 to 4 weeks without renewal and with built-in follow-up. Factors that aggravate headache (Table 24-3) should be avoided or at least decreased.[10]

Migraine headache

Migraine headaches often have identifiable psychological triggers, which can be avoided or dealt with in much the same manner as the factors causing tension headaches. Medication involves the use of ergotamine with or without antihistamines, with a second line of medication being beta blockers such as propranolol. Antinauseants are often required when nausea is a major problem. Physical treatments, including rest in a dark room, cold compresses, and quiet (if necessary, away from well-meaning friends and family), are an important part of management. Acupuncture and acupressure have been of some help to selected patients. The role of diet is controversial, but one should at least determine any associations of the headache with particular dietary intake, especially with tyramine-containing foods and alcohol. Generally, we would prefer a consultation before prescribing methysergide. For

Table 24-3 Factors That Aggravate Headache

Migraine	Muscular-contraction type
Stress, tension, worry	Stress, tension, worry
Menstruation	Cervical spondylosis
Birth control pills	Neck or head trauma
Hunger and fasting	Neck position in sleep
Bright light	Desk work
Dropping barometric pressure	Driving
High humidity	Gardening
Oversleeping	Working with arms elevated
Lack of sleep	Poor posture
Fumes, odors, cigarette smoke	
Foods, e.g., cheese, nuts, chocolates, smoked meats, cola drinks	

Source: Modified from Murray.[10]

patients in an acute attack for which other therapy has failed, dexamethasone 4 mg given IV over 5 minutes is generally effective. Narcotics should be avoided.

We have observed that a muscular spasm phase often follows the arteriospasm phase of the migraine attack. The treatment of the muscular spasm phase involves the use of ice packs on the neck muscles, massage, and trigger point injection of lidocaine (Xylocaine) and steroid.[11]

Sinus headaches are associated with acute sinus infection or chronic obstruction. The most important part of treatment is drainage, which may be accomplished by means of decongestants (pseudoephedrine) or surgical drainage. In an acute episode, antibiotics are indicated. **Sinus headaches**

Headaches associated with depression usually respond to supportive psychotherapy and antidepressants.

Headaches associated with hypoglycemia may be prevented by means of slight alterations in diet.

Consultations may be helpful in management. One paper[12] points out a decrease in office visits to the practitioner following such consultation for headache.

SUMMARY

For patients with chronic recurring headaches it is extremely important to have a sympathetic, understanding family physician who can communicate and relate comfortably on a continuing basis. To

11 HEADACHE

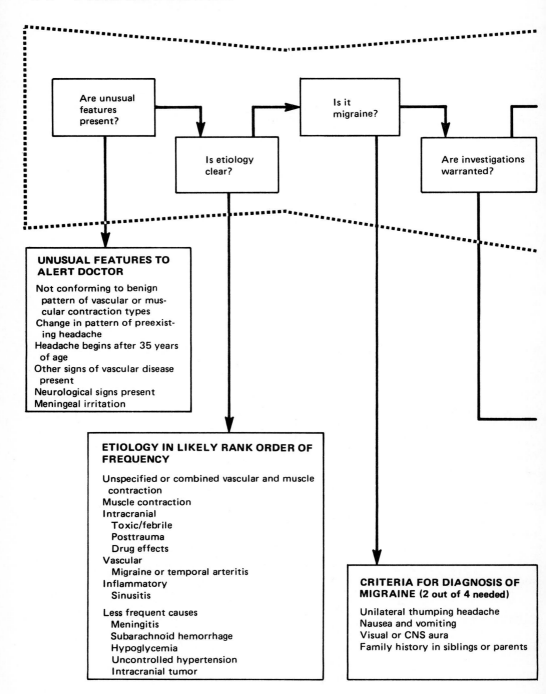

Are unusual features present?

Is etiology clear?

Is it migraine?

Are investigations warranted?

UNUSUAL FEATURES TO ALERT DOCTOR

Not conforming to benign pattern of vascular or muscular contraction types
Change in pattern of preexisting headache
Headache begins after 35 years of age
Other signs of vascular disease present
Neurological signs present
Meningeal irritation

ETIOLOGY IN LIKELY RANK ORDER OF FREQUENCY

Unspecified or combined vascular and muscle contraction
Muscle contraction
Intracranial
   Toxic/febrile
   Posttrauma
   Drug effects
Vascular
   Migraine or temporal arteritis
Inflammatory
   Sinusitis

Less frequent causes
   Meningitis
   Subarachnoid hemorrhage
   Hypoglycemia
   Uncontrolled hypertension
   Intracranial tumor

CRITERIA FOR DIAGNOSIS OF MIGRAINE (2 out of 4 needed)

Unilateral thumping headache
Nausea and vomiting
Visual or CNS aura
Family history in siblings or parents

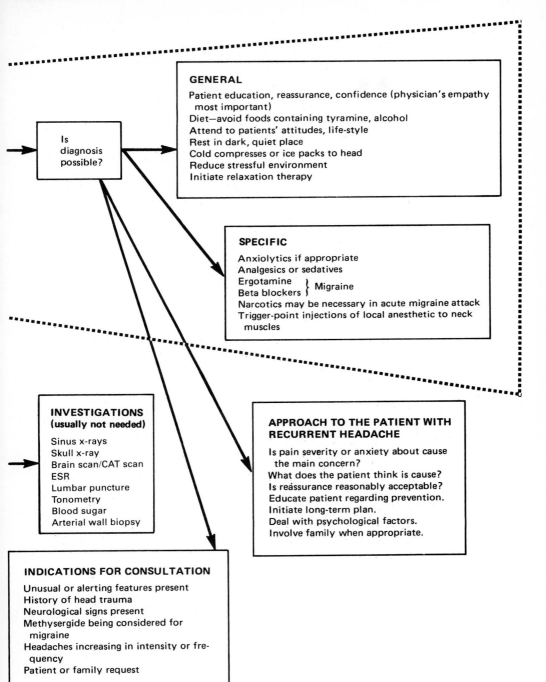

Is diagnosis possible?

GENERAL

Patient education, reassurance, confidence (physician's empathy most important)
Diet—avoid foods containing tyramine, alcohol
Attend to patients' attitudes, life-style
Rest in dark, quiet place
Cold compresses or ice packs to head
Reduce stressful environment
Initiate relaxation therapy

SPECIFIC

Anxiolytics if appropriate
Analgesics or sedatives
Ergotamine ⎫ Migraine
Beta blockers ⎰
Narcotics may be necessary in acute migraine attack
Trigger-point injections of local anesthetic to neck muscles

INVESTIGATIONS
(usually not needed)

Sinus x-rays
Skull x-ray
Brain scan/CAT scan
ESR
Lumbar puncture
Tonometry
Blood sugar
Arterial wall biopsy

APPROACH TO THE PATIENT WITH RECURRENT HEADACHE

Is pain severity or anxiety about cause the main concern?
What does the patient think is cause?
Is reassurance reasonably acceptable?
Educate patient regarding prevention.
Initiate long-term plan.
Deal with psychological factors.
Involve family when appropriate.

INDICATIONS FOR CONSULTATION

Unusual or alerting features present
History of head trauma
Neurological signs present
Methysergide being considered for migraine
Headaches increasing in intensity or frequency
Patient or family request

arrive at a whole-person approach which considers all aspects of management and deemphasizes dependence on medication while at the same time assuring symptomatic relief of pain is a challenging goal for the practitioner of the art. Keeping the patient and family well informed and involved may prevent the upsetting and dramatic scenes that are liable to occur when the frustration of suffering is compounded by a lack of confidence in the correctness of the diagnosis and the appropriateness of the management.

REFERENCES

1 D. W. Marsland, M. Wood, and F. Mayo, *Content of Family Practice: A Statewide Study in Virginia with Its Clinical, Educational, and Research Implications,* J. Geyman (ed.), Appleton-Century-Crofts, New York, 1976.
2 J. S. Milne, "Headaches in General Practice," *Scottish Medical Journal,* **10:** 251–253, 1965.
3 W. E. Waters, "Headache and the Eye," *Lancet,* **ii**(7662):1–4, 1970.
4 A. P. Friedman, *Chronic Recurring Headache: Aspects of Diagnosis and Differentiation,* Sandoz Pharmaceuticals, Basle, Switzerland, November 1973.
5 J. Edmeads, *Headache,* Sandoz, Toronto, Canada, 1980.
6 G. A. Wise, "Headache in Children," *Australian Family Physician,* **6:**813–817, 1977.
7 J. Lubart, "Sinus Headache," *Modern Medicine of Canada,* **25:**19–21, 1970.
8 J. Edmeads, "Headaches and Stroke," *Modern Medicine of Canada,* **33:** 1003–1010, 1978.
9 W. Ling, G. Oftedal, and W. Weinburg, "Depressive Illness in Childhood Presenting as Severe Headache," *American Journal of Diseases of Children,* **120:**122–124, 1970.
10 T. J. Murray, "The Management of Chronic Headaches," *Canadian Family Physician,* **30:**1516–1519, 1984.
11 M. Cohen, "Tension Headaches: A Challenge to the Family Physician," *Canadian Family Physician,* **24:**870–873, 1978.
12 J. L. Grover, P. Butler, and P. A. Millac, "The Effect of a Visit to a Neurological Clinic upon Patients with Tension Headache," *Practitioner,* **224:**195–196, 1980.

Chapter 25

Low Back Pain

B. K. Hennen, M.D.

PRINCIPLE

If people are to be helped to take more responsibility for their own health care, health professionals must emphasize patient education rather than directive advice. At the same time, the ongoing attempt to replace polypharmacy with commonsense prescriptions for nutrition, rest, exercise, physical therapeutics, and even in some cases appropriate job placement requires that physicians understand better the value of such treatment methods. Low back pain is the kind of problem that is helped considerably if patients learn how to take care of their backs and prevent recurrent episodes. As is often the case, the best patient educator is not necessarily the physician. It may be the nurse, the nutritionist, or the physiotherapist.

Teaching patients self-care

DEFINITION

Lumbago, sciatica, ruptured disk, spinal instability, osteoarthritis, degenerative disk disease, prolapsed lumbar disk, acute back spasm, back strain or sprain, and psychogenic backache are among the more common names applied to low back pain in patients who

Table 25-1   Causes of Low Back Pain

1 Viscerogenic
2 Psychogenic
   a Type I: tension
   b Type II: conversion
   c Type III: overlay on underlying organic causes
3 Spondylogenic
   a Trauma
   b Structural defect
   c Lumbar disk
   d Infection
   e Neoplasm
   f Inflammation
   g Metabolic
   h Miscellaneous

Source: MacNab.[4]

present in family practice. The variety of diagnostic labels reflects the difficulty of accurate diagnosis.

PREVALENCE

One of every fifty patients in the family doctor's office will have low back pain as a primary presenting problem. More than two-thirds will be women (except for worker's compensation patients, among whom men predominate), and the peak ages range from the middle thirties to the middle fifties.[1,2] Back pain is the cause of some 60 percent of sickness-related absence from work in the United Kingdom.[3]

ETIOLOGY

Classifications of low back pain causes have been helpful. We offer MacNab's classification modified in accordance with Sergent's consideration of the psychogenic group.[4] (See Table 25-1.)

Viscerogenic

Psychogenic

In the table, low back pain is divided into three main classes: viscerogenic, psychogenic, and spondylogenic. *Viscerogenic* pain refers to pain in the back referred from viscera within the chest, abdomen, or pelvis. There are three types of *psychogenic* pain: type I, *tension,* which occurs in the generally tense patient, who responds to stress by excessive muscle tension ultimately resulting in pain; type II, *conversion,* which refers to a pattern of pain which appears to be a substitute for a strong and undesirable (usually socially unacceptable) emotion, often the result of psychogenic conflicts;[5] and type III, the *overlay* category, which can be associated with any of the physical causes of low back pain and refers to patients' subjective interpretation of their symptoms. The interpretation may be a reflection of many factors, including personality and individual stresses.

Spondylogenic causes of low back pain include physical causes related to the spine and its immediate attachments. In the spondylogenic category, *trauma* includes fractures, fracture dislocations, and soft tissue injuries; *structural defect* includes spondylolysis, spondylolisthesis, scoliosis, facet abnormalities, and spinal stenosis; and *lumbar disk* includes acute herniation and chronic degeneration. The spine, which is subject to continual wear, shows degenerative changes as early as age 30 in postmortem studies and by age 35 in x-rays of patients with new low back pain and no history of previous injury.[6]

With regard to the other spondylogenic categories, *infection* may be pyogenic or granulomatous, *neoplasm* may be benign or malignant (primary or secondary), and *metabolic disease* includes Paget's disease and osteoporosis. The *miscellaneous* category includes diseases such as Scheuermann's disease and coccygodynia.

Spondylogenic

CHARACTERISTICS OF THE PAIN

It is important to determine the onset of the pain. An acute injury may be the final aggravating factor in any existing condition. Pain that is increased by activities such as bending or lifting and is relieved by rest or special posturing is most often associated with disk disease, bony injury, or nonunion of surgically fused vertebrae. The pain of arthritis is often characterized by an early morning ache and stiffness with a relatively quiet midday; however, when accompanied by persistent activity, it can result in tiring and increased pain. Nerve irritation associated with fibrosis or arachnoiditis is increased by activity, is persistent, and is not relieved by rest. It is often described as burning and may also be associated with a tingling feeling.

Differentiating symptoms

If the pain is central in the lower back and there is little or no radiation beyond the upper thigh, the possible diagnoses include persistent midline disk herniation, degenerative or inflamed disk without herniation, and arthritis around the disk or around the joint facets, particularly the sacroiliac joint. Ligamentous tears and avulsions are also possible.

Disk pain is often associated with leg radiation and areas of hypoesthesia. It is usually confirmed by findings of depressed deep tendon reflexes, sensory deficits, and muscle weaknesses localized in the area of the nerve root affected.

The spasm associated with muscle tension usually makes sense in terms of its location and quality and is found in a tense and driving person.

When the only comfortable position is a seated one, one might worry about neoplastic infiltration of the spine.

Conversion "pain" may be associated with a long history of repeated visits to various doctors and more x-rays than would seem necessary. Evidence of psychological conflict can usually be found. The pain may have a bizarre pattern which has no anatomic or physiological rationale. The pain is often categorized by adjectives such as "severe," "awful," "miserable," or "terrible," which do not provide a precise description. The patient may be easily distracted in spite of pain that is supposed to be incapacitating. There is often a history of previous injury at the site of the pain, but in the case of the new presentation there may be no history of a significant trauma that precipitated the current episode and no objective findings on examination.

EXAMINATION

On examination, one must first look for visceral causes such as ureteral colic and renal colic. Examination of the prostate must not be omitted in patients over age 50 (remember to draw blood in order to determine acid phosphatase before palpating the prostate).

Differentiating
physical signs

One should look for deformity and limited range of movement. It is useful to watch the patient undress and climb up on the examining table. It is also useful to continue to observe the patient on the examination table during the interview. Abdominal or gluteal striae often accompany poor muscle tone and obesity. Palpate for muscle spasm, feeling particularly for knots, tenderness, and muscle mass in areas where atrophy may occur, such as in the calves and on the quadriceps. Where muscle spasm is a major factor, trigger points can often be found, especially along the posterior iliac crest.

The tendon reflexes should be tested, as should sensation, by pin prick from the waist down, including the perineal area.

If straight leg raising causes pain on examination, the angle at which it occurs should be noted. One should also note whether the patient can sit upright with the legs extended at other times during the examination. If the patient can do so, seriously doubt the validity of the sign of positive straight leg raising.

One should also examine for psychological status, assessing in particular the patient's previous responses to pain, the presence or absence of internal conflict or conflict with others, and the social situation in the patient's home.

INVESTIGATIONS

A patient reporting low back pain for the first time should be x-rayed, but the x-ray need not be done immediately unless fracture is a possibility or there is evidence of severe compression of nerve roots such as loss of bladder and bowel control. Cancer is much more prevalent in patients over age 50; screening with sedimentation rate, alkaline phosphatase, and serum calcium has found at least one of these three tests to be abnormal in patients with malignant disease.[7] These tests should be done when any patient over age 50 presents with low back pain for the first time or when an apparent recurrence of an old symptom of back pain does not respond to the usual management.

Limit investigations

The presence of congenital vertebral deformities or spondylosis demonstrated radiographically is of doubtful significance in the production of pain.

If active arthritis is likely, a sedimentation rate test and nuclear antibody (ANA) tests are indicated.

MANAGEMENT

Early treatment must address the specific cause of pain, particularly in the case of suspected fracture, nerve root compression, and/or viscerogenic, infective, and neoplastic problems. For other causes of acute low back pain, the initial management can be relatively similar and can proceed consecutively with any investigation needed to make a definitive diagnosis (Table 25-2).

The doctor should reassure the patient about conditions which he or she knows are absent and about which the patient may be concerned. For example, if a malignancy or ruptured disk appears unlikely, the patient should be told as much. However, it is foolish to label a patient with "acute disk" or with any other diagnosis on the initial visit unless the diagnosis is absolutely certain.

The home situation should be assessed on the first visit. It is fruitless, for example, to send a housewife and mother home for rest without ensuring that she will make arrangements for adequate help at home.

Table 25-2   Initial Conservative Management

1   Avoid inaccurate diagnostic labels.
2   Reassurance regarding cancer, "disk," "invalidism."
3   Treatment for causes:
   a   Injection triggers—muscle spasm.
   b   Anti-inflammatory—arthritis.
   c   Psychotherapy.
4   Evaluate home regarding realistic program.
5   Bed rest and advice regarding bathroom privileges, altered activity.
6   Analgesia (watch for constipation).
7   Heal/cold treatment.
8   Consider muscle relaxants, anti-inflammatory agents, sedation.
9   Prophylactic back care.
10 Arrange next visit (set specific time 1 week later).

Specific
instructions

Be specific regarding instructions, expectations for improvement, and follow-up. For example, tell the patient how long bed rest should last, what bathroom privileges are allowed, whether particular aspects of work can be undertaken, and whether sexual activity should be curtailed.

A firm mattress or one supported by a sheet of plywood is best for bed rest. (A mattress on the floor provides the needed support but makes it difficult for the patient to get up to go to the bathroom and is thus a poor suggestion.)

It is important to demonstrate to the patient that the pain can be controlled and will not be a continuous problem. The doctor can make a choice of analgesics based on the patient's previous response to pain and to analgesics but should make sure that they are prescribed in adequate amounts and are taken at appropriate intervals.

Sedation is not needed if the analgesia is adequate. Depending on the particular problem, muscle relaxants or anti-inflammatory agents may be indicated. Again, it is important to use these medications in the proper dosage and with proper regularity.

For acute pain with a great deal of muscle tenderness, cold packs may provide some relief initially. Moist heat, usually after the first 24 hours, is often comforting. If the patient is demonstrating muscle tension and has a palpable and tender knot of tissue, consider injecting the trigger point with local anesthetic with or without a deposteroid. This maneuver is often saved for the second visit and used when the patient has only partially responded to conservative measures.

If the initial episode leads to a modified work program or lost work time for the patient, one should arrange a prophylactic back care program. Whenever a second episode of pain is brought to the doctor's attention, a prophylactic program is warranted. The program should have four major components: (1) instruction regarding posture, (2) flexion exercises, (3) strengthening of abdominal muscles, and (4) weight loss when indicated.

PROPHYLACTIC BACK CARE

The physiotherapist is the ideal person to instruct the patient in back care and exercise. Where physiotherapy is not available, an excellent text on home back care has been written by Livingstone.[8] Patients should be given instructions about posture, particularly regarding lifting, and standing for long periods. Patients should also be told to avoid curling up in bed in such a way that the normal lordosis is lost (a kyphotic posture can cause pressure which will aggravate a threatening disk bulge) and instructed to avoid uneven loads.

    Flexion exercises for the pelvis are important. Have patients lie on the back on a flat surface with the hand in the small of the back and push the back against the hand. The same result can be achieved if the patient leans against a wall in such a way that the lower back is flat against the wall. Strengthening of the abdominal muscles is also accomplished by means of these exercises. These muscles can be tightened 5 to 10 times an hour. Sit-ups should be avoided.

    Yoga back exercises provide particularly useful relaxation for a patient who has a recurrent chronic backache such as occurs after prolonged standing or walking for long periods of time on flat cement surfaces.

    For a patient with no sign of disk involvement, prophylactic back care can begin as soon as pain at rest is absent (with or without analgesia).

    If conversion pain is suspected, Sarno suggests that the physician talk to the patient about a spasm that is aggravated by tension or depression.[5] "Spasm" and "sensitive muscles" are socially acceptable conditions for the patient to have and talk about. Further visits should be suggested to the patient.

Habits

Exercises

When to start

WHEN CONSERVATIVE MANAGEMENT FAILS

When a patient reporting for follow-up has continued pain, the following steps are indicated.

    1 Review compliance. If it has been poor, management should be repeated with stronger emphasis on the reasons for the measures suggested. Including a family member in the plan will

Compliance

Home situation

Reassess
clinically

Consultation

sometimes improve compliance. If compliance has been good, the physician should try to assess what areas of improvement, if any, took place and relate them to particular aspects of management that may be worth emphasizing in a modified treatment program.

2 Reassess the milieu at home. If it is not appropriate or easily changed, the physician might suggest hospitalization to remove the patient from the environment. In some situations, a professional home care program may be a practical alternative. If the home situation seems correctable, the physician may intervene by talking to the spouse, children, or others at home who have a direct effect on the patient's ability to obtain rest, etc. It is also worth finding out if the patient has returned to work. Malingering is rare, but some patients tend not to go back to work because of a fear of reinjury, problems with the boss, or other reasons which, if not brought to light by the physician, may never be dealt with.

3 Reexamine the patient each time as thoroughly as on the initial examination. Records which have been carefully detailed allow assessment of changes, especially in functional movement. When change is slow, the patient may not be aware of improvement.

The options at this point are to repeat the conservative management program, repeat the program for a longer period of time, or seek consultation. *Consultation* with a physiotherapist, neurologist, physiatrist, psychiatrist, orthopedist, or neurosurgeon (Table 25-3) should be sought for specific indications.

Other modes of therapy may be considered. For example, *manipulation* may be appropriate. Contraindications to manipulation include the presence of central nervous system signs, pain that is acutely severe, pain that radiates to the knee or lower, late pregnancy, and referred pain and sciatic distribution that are bilateral.

Acupuncture is another possible therapy. *Relaxation exercises* or *hypnosis* may be helpful to a patient for whom muscle tension is the major problem. *Yoga* can be useful, especially for relaxation.

When a patient requests a consultation, consider whether this

Table 25-3   Indications for Consultation with the Surgeon

1   Severe sciatica
2   Motor weakness
3   Bowel or bladder signs due to cord compression
4   Failure of a conservative regimen with which the patient has been fully compliant
5   Required by an employer, worker's compensation board, etc.
6   Requested by the patient

indicates a failure in the doctor-patient relationship. In such cases the doctor may not have recognized the patient's lack of confidence in the management scheme outlined. We feel the physician should raise the question of consultation before the patient has to ask for it.

A common cause of surgical failure is an initially inappropriate indication for surgery. When this happens, the responsibility for the "error" must rest partly with the referring family physician. Often the failure of his or her conservative management plan was the indication for referral. But if the management plan was not carried out and the family doctor wrongly assumed that it was, he or she might have incorrectly informed the consultant that conservative management had failed. In such cases, the consultant, believing that the family doctor has done everything possible, has a stronger inclination to contemplate surgery as the obvious next step. Here one can only reemphasize that from the beginning, the management plan should have specified goals and detailed expectations about recovery time and the introduction of increased activity and should involve careful and regular follow-up.

Surgical failure

"Once major soft tissue damage has occurred in an intervertebral disk and to its associated ligament of structures, that region will continue to be exposed to constant ever-changing and major stresses, and when such a patient returns to work, there is a strong likelihood of recurrent back trouble."[6] After initial treatment, careful job placement may be a more realistic solution to chronic disability caused by low back pain than surgery or prolonged conservative treatment. One might consider recommending a job change as a logical step in preventing recurrence or continued problems for a patient who has had surgery.

Patients treated in a worker's compensation board hospital and rehabilitation center for 6 weeks had a satisfactory recovery rate from low back pain 2½ times greater than that of patients who were treated for a similar period of time at home.[2] This probably indicates that very specific and careful management, when the doctor has full control and immediate access to others' expertise, does yield better results. To obtain equal results outside the hospital is a challenge to the family physician.

Hospital versus home care

Patients with conversion pain do not appear to do as well as those who have a diagnosis of muscle tension associated with anxiety or depression. However, in a rehabilitation clinic emphasizing psychosocial problems it was found that 70 percent of patients treated were capable of returning to work.[5] Thus a patient with the psychogenic category of back pain is *not* a hopeless case and deserves specific treatment directed toward the cause, which in this case is psychological.

Psychogenic causes are treatable

12 LOW BACK PAIN

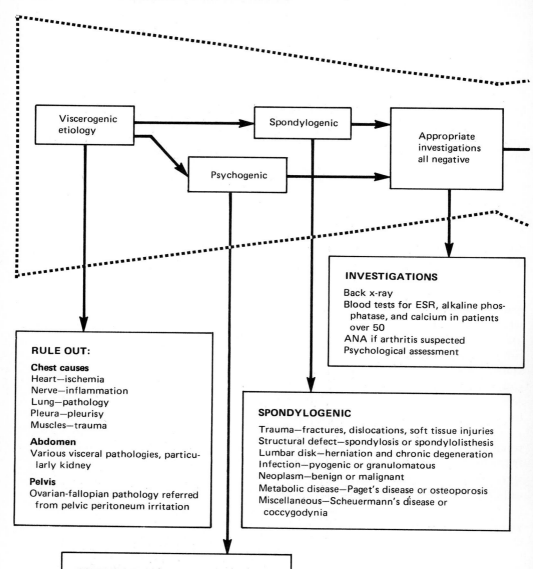

Viscerogenic etiology

Spondylogenic

Psychogenic

Appropriate investigations all negative

RULE OUT:

Chest causes
Heart—ischemia
Nerve—inflammation
Lung—pathology
Pleura—pleurisy
Muscles—trauma

Abdomen
Various visceral pathologies, particularly kidney

Pelvis
Ovarian-fallopian pathology referred from pelvic peritoneum irritation

INVESTIGATIONS
Back x-ray
Blood tests for ESR, alkaline phosphatase, and calcium in patients over 50
ANA if arthritis suspected
Psychological assessment

SPONDYLOGENIC
Trauma—fractures, dislocations, soft tissue injuries
Structural defect—spondylosis or spondylolisthesis
Lumbar disk—herniation and chronic degeneration
Infection—pyogenic or granulomatous
Neoplasm—benign or malignant
Metabolic disease—Paget's disease or osteoporosis
Miscellaneous—Scheuermann's disease or coccygodynia

PSYCHOGENIC (Probably an element in most causes of backache)

Type I: tension
Type II: conversion
Type III: overlay on underlying organic cause

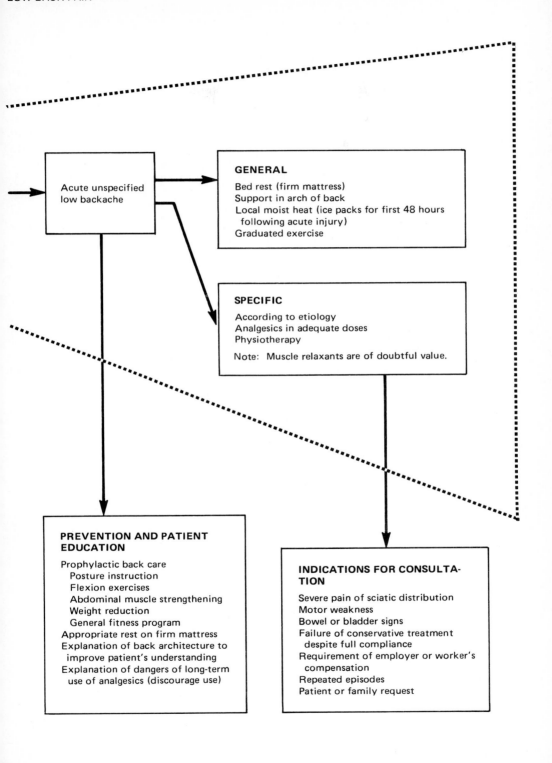

Acute unspecified low backache

GENERAL
Bed rest (firm mattress)
Support in arch of back
Local moist heat (ice packs for first 48 hours
  following acute injury)
Graduated exercise

SPECIFIC
According to etiology
Analgesics in adequate doses
Physiotherapy

Note: Muscle relaxants are of doubtful value.

**PREVENTION AND PATIENT
EDUCATION**
Prophylactic back care
  Posture instruction
  Flexion exercises
  Abdominal muscle strengthening
  Weight reduction
  General fitness program
Appropriate rest on firm mattress
Explanation of back architecture to
  improve patient's understanding
Explanation of dangers of long-term
  use of analgesics (discourage use)

**INDICATIONS FOR CONSULTA-
TION**
Severe pain of sciatic distribution
Motor weakness
Bowel or bladder signs
Failure of conservative treatment
  despite full compliance
Requirement of employer or worker's
  compensation
Repeated episodes
Patient or family request

SUMMARY

The approach to the patient with acute back pain should be aggressive and management should be conducted according to a specific, scheduled plan. Assessment of the cause should be as careful and as accurate as possible, and the management program should suit the etiology as well as the patient's personality and home circumstances. Referrals to consultants should be made on the basis of clear criteria with specific objectives in mind. Medication should be used according to proper dosage and administration guidelines. Records should be detailed and should include ranges in motion and specific neurological findings. Simplistic and premature labeling of the patient's problem should be avoided; the patient should be given the diagnosis only in the degree of specificity that the doctor has determined to his or her satisfaction. Realistic work assignments during rehabilitation will reduce the likelihood of recurrence or chronicity resulting in long-term disability.

REFERENCES

1 D. W. Marsland, M. Wood, and F. Mayo, *Content of Family Practice: A Statewide Study in Virginia with Its Clinical, Educational, and Research Implications,* J. Geyman (ed.), Appleton-Century-Crofts, New York, 1976.
2 A. Kertesz and R. Kormos, "Low Back Pain in the Workman in Canada," *Canadian Medical Association Journal,* **115:**901–903, 1976.
3 M. Polke, "Backache: Diagnosis and Treatment of Mechanical Derangement of the Lumbar Spine," *Update,* **12**(9):955–976, 1976.
4 I. MacNab, *Backache,* Burns and MacEachern, Toronto, 1975.
5 J. E. Sarno, "Psychogenic Backache: The Missing Dimension," *Journal of Family Practice,* **1:**8–12, 1974.
6 K. F. King, "Back Injury," *Australian Family Physician,* **6:**1062–1066, 1977.
7 J. C. Fernbach, F. Langer, and A. E. Gross, "The Significance of Low Back Pain in Older Adults," *Canadian Medical Association Journal,* **115:**898–900, 1976.
8 M. Livingstone, *Your Guide to the Care of the Back—Back Aid,* George Stickley, Philadelphia, 1983.

Chapter 26

Abdominal Pain

D. B. Shires, M.D.

PRINCIPLE

Serious medical problems generally are better managed when diagnosed early. As the primary physician, the family doctor sees most problems before other doctors, often when the developing symptoms are still vague and undifferentiated. The balance between appropriate investigation and premature or unnecessary investigation is often tenuous.

Abdominal pain is the kind of symptom which can represent the ultimate in vagueness. It may be the clue to a life-threatening but treatable condition, or it may be the physical manifestation of a chronically stressful and barely manageable life situation. The care with which the physician approaches the earliest symptom of abdominal pain, even when it is vague and nonspecific, may ultimately ease the difficulties of diagnosis and prevent the occasionally catastrophic complications of late diagnosis.

Early diagnosis

Figure 26-1   Causes of abdominal pain. (*From Marsland et al.*[1])

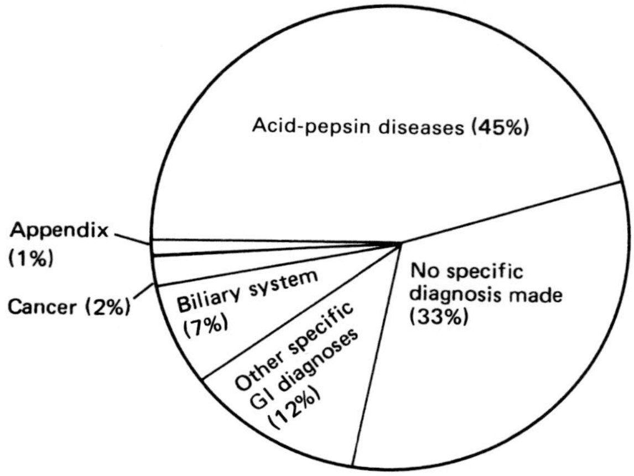

DEFINITION

Patients do not usually complain of "abdominal pain." If the discomfort is in any way related to food, it is often referred to as "indigestion." Complaints of "stomachache," "pain in the stomach," "gas," and "cramps" are often heard. Any of these complaints may be translated by the physician into "abdominal pain."

PREVALENCE AND ETIOLOGY

Causes

In the Virginia study,[1] 17,404 (3 percent) of all patients seen in family doctors' offices had problems related to the gastrointestinal system, in which abdominal pain is usually a symptom. Of these, 33 percent fell into the category of abdominal pain for which no specific diagnosis was made. Acid-pepsin diseases, including gastritis, functional gastric disorders, duodenal ulcer, gastric ulcer, prepyloric ulcer, esophagitis, heartburn, and other nonmalignant diseases of the esophagus, stomach, and duodenum accounted for 45 percent. Only 224 visits were for appendicitis or appendicular pain, and 1260 were for diseases of the biliary system. There were 365 visits by patients with cancer, including carcinoma of the colon (188), carcinoma of the rectum (53), carcinoma of the pancreas (59), carcinoma of the esophagus (42), and carcinoma of the stomach (23) (Figure 26-1).[1]

Diseases of other systems may present with abdominal pain. These include pneumonia; ruptured aortic aneurysm; radicular pain; renal colic and pyelitis; uterine and reproductive problems, in particular pelvic inflammatory disease and ectopic pregnancy

Figure 26-2 Structural and nonstructural causes of abdominal pain in an adult medical clinic. (*From Bain and Spaulding.*[2])

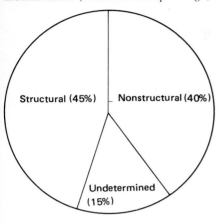

(22 were noted among 7189 visits for pregnancy); abdominal migraine; mesenteric arterial occlusion; and herpes zoster, atypical angina, lymphoma, diabetic ketosis, and other generalized conditions.

Out of 4000 adults presenting in an adult medical clinic, 13 percent had abdominal pain as the main presenting symptom. Of these, 45 percent were thought to have structural diseases (19 percent peptic ulcer, 4 percent gallbladder disease), 40 percent were afflicted with nonstructural diseases (28 percent psychological, 6 percent spastic colon), and 15 percent remained undetermined. Bain and Spaulding concluded that there was good reason to look for psychological disturbances as aggravating factors in abdominal pain, since such a relation was demonstrable in more than half the patients (Figure 26-2).[2]

Recent reviews of presentations of abdominal pain indicate either real changes in disease incidence or improvements in our ability to identify, prevent, or medically treat conditions previously considered primarily surgical. For example, there has been an apparent reduction in the incidence of appendicitis and, at the same time, an apparent increase in the incidence of peptic ulcer disease.

NATURAL HISTORY

The family physician is in the unique position of being able to observe the early symptoms of a developing abdominal crisis. In their early stages, many illnesses are vague, undifferentiated, and often unaccompanied by physical signs. The vast majority of patients

Family physician's role

presenting with abdominal pain to the family physician do not have acute or "surgical" abdomens, but the possibility of acute disease must always be investigated.

Anxiety

Often a patient with a new symptom of abdominal pain is anxious. "What's happening to me?" is a reasonable concern. He or she may also be upset that the day's routine has been disturbed. As a result, the patient may either minimize or overemphasize to the physician those symptoms which seem to be important (usually ones that interfere with function) in an attempt to get quick results. This results in extra pressure on the physician to make the right diagnosis quickly and remedy the situation.[3]

APPROACH TO PATIENTS

Clues before the Interview Begins

Non-verbal clues

The doctor can obtain clues about a patient before sitting down to hear the story of the current illness. How did the patient make contact? Did the patient arrive unexpectedly in the office or was the appointment made a day or two previously or an hour or so previously? Did the patient ask for a house call? All these factors reflect to some degree the patient's concern with and interpretation of the significance of the problem.[4,5]

Characteristics of the Pain

Onset

A clear account of the *onset* of the pain is of prime importance. Knowing the timing of the onset and the circumstances surrounding it often helps to clarify things early on. Inflammatory conditions are more likely to be of gradual and vaguely noted onset, whereas ruptures of ectopic gestation, peptic ulcers, diverticula, and aneurysms tend to have a sudden onset (the patient can recall the exact moment of onset) and are often associated with some activity requiring intraabdominal pressure, e.g., straining at stool or heavy lifting.

Nature

It is helpful to define the *nature* of the pain. Pain that is colicky or spasmodic tends to come from a hollow viscus whose walls are being stretched by gaseous obstruction or by an actual foreign object such as a stone. Pain that comes directly from a solid viscus is more likely to be steady and persistent but also is often less severe than the excruciating pain of colic. Most pains associated with a hollow viscus obstruction have a recognized pattern of radiation

Site

(the ureter to the groin, the gallbladder to the infrascapular area), but often this radiation makes the exact focus of the pain less clear. The pain of a solid viscus, however, tends to be better localized and is more often over the affected organ. Pain involving pathology

Table 26-1 Quality of Abdominal Pain

Affected viscus	Quality of Pain			Pathophysiology
	Nature	Severity	Site	
Hollow	Colicky (spasmodic)	Greater	Poorly localized	Attempting to eliminate cause
Solid	Steady (persistent)	Lesser	Better localized over affected organ	Functional organ disturbance causes constitutional symptoms

Source: Sluglett.[5]

within solid viscus is often associated with a disturbance in general function, and so constitutional symptoms such as malaise are often part of the presentation (Table 26-1).

Quality

Localized pain tends to be associated with the gallbladder, the appendix, the stomach, or the duodenum, whereas pain coming from the colon, small intestine, or pancreas is often more diffuse and less clearly demarcated. Often, the pain itself is the only early physical symptom and there may be no physical findings. Pain described as indigestion, if it occurs 2 to 2½ hours after meals, suggests duodenal ulcer; however, if it is constantly present and is made worse by food, one should become more concerned about the possibility of a malignancy with a chronic gastric ulcer.

Associated symptoms are important. Pain associated with fainting and collapse is most likely to represent perforated ulcer, ruptured ectopic pregnancy, aneurysm dissection, or acute pancreatitis.

Associated symptoms

Vomiting is a common associated symptom. It can be early and severe when associated with the severe pain of colic caused by an obstructed viscus. More frequent and recurrent vomiting which persists may occur later in lower intestinal obstruction. In appendicitis, vomiting rarely occurs before the pain has been present for 3 to 4 hours.

Anorexia is usually associated with vomiting or nausea. Change in bowel habits can be important. In women an accurate menstrual history is essential.

NONSTRUCTURAL CAUSES OF ABDOMINAL PAIN

Bain and Spaulding found that in 40 percent of presenting adults, abdominal pain had nonstructural causes; of these, 28 percent had psychiatric diagnoses and 6 percent had spastic colon. The authors included peptic ulcer (4 percent) as a structural cause.[2] They noted that "psychological disturbances are often fairly easy to identify if

Psychological

care is taken to obtain the personal history and to assess the patient's personality, but the diagnostic terms used to describe psychological disturbances lack precision." Most of the psychiatric disorders found in their study were neurotic rather than psychotic, and many would be more accurately termed problems of living that had exceeded the patients' coping abilities.

Mansfield points out that the neurotic patient without organic disease often complains bitterly of pain caused by even light palpation but lets you continue to palpate or, alternatively, may try to remove your examining hand with his or her own.[4]

GENERAL APPROACH

Presumptive
diagnosis

The practitioner should attempt to clarify the problem when the patient is seen for the first time; attempting a diagnosis at that time often prevents carelessness. Many people who have abdominal pain endure it until the evening and present at a time when physicians are weary and not at their best. Most severe abdominal pains which last as long as 6 hours in patients who have been previously fairly well are caused by conditions of surgical importance.[6] This would seem a reasonable guideline for the family physician to follow in treating patients with abdominal pain, especially pain that is initially vaguely defined and is not accompanied by physical signs. A patient with a new symptom of abdominal pain for which there is no readily apparent diagnosis should probably be seen again by the same physician within 3 or 4 hours of the first assessment. A medication history should also be taken to cover drug-induced events such as tablets sticking in the esophagus (tetracycline and iron), gastritis and ulceration due to ASA and nonsteroidal anti-inflammatory agents, and pseudomembranous colitis due to antibiotics.

Bush[7] has summarized his approach to interviewing the patient with abdominal pain, as shown in Table 26-2.

EXAMINATION

When making a house call, the physician should note whether the patient is in bed, afraid to move, or unwilling to be up and about. These factors may indicate the degree of seriousness which the patient attaches to the symptom.

In the office, the way the patient walks in, sits down in a chair, or climbs up onto the examining table may be significant. Mansfield goes so far as to say, "The patient with a sprightly walk who jumps onto the couch is unlikely to have even an early acute ab-

Table 26-2 Interviewing the Patient with Abdominal Pain: Features to Be Determined

Mode of onset—sudden or gradual?

Character of pain—colicky or continuing?

Natural process—increasing, decreasing, or remaining constant?

Site

Radiation

Aggravating factors

Relieving factors

Effect of sleep

Associated features—vomiting, loss of weight, appetite, bowel habits, micturition, menstrual history, vaginal discharge

Accurate history of any trauma

Source: Bush.[7]

dominal problem."[4] Furthermore, how the patient has tolerated symptoms of discomfort in the past may be a reference point from which to assess the new presenting symptom.

All experienced physicians have preferred examination techniques. Cope[6] relies little on rebound tenderness ("an unnecessary aggravation to an already discomforted patient"), bowel sounds (not very helpful), and abdominal paracentesis (seldom necessary). Wagner, however, makes strong arguments in favor of all three techniques in the emergency room setting.[8] Both authors emphasize the necessity of checking the femoral canals for hidden or unexpected hernias when obstruction seems a possibility.

Differential physical features

The basic signs are temperature, pulse rate, respiratory rate, and blood pressure. Very high initial temperatures are seldom seen in appendicitis, and subnormal temperatures may represent shock. Cope feels that if the respiratory rate reaches twice the norm the likelihood of a thoracic problem being the source of the abdominal pain increases considerably.[6]

Vital signs

Observations should include careful watching of the patient's face during the course of the examination, looking for abdominal distension, observing color (pallor, jaundice), and looking for flaring of alae nasi. Noting whether the patient is restless or lying still helps differentiate between colic and peritonitis. If ileus is a possibility, auscultation of the abdomen without hearing bowel sounds (some say for 5 minutes) will confirm that diagnosis.

A warm hand, gently applied in the areas of the abdomen farthest away from the pain and using the flat parts of the fingertips, should be the initial approach to palpation of the abdomen. Percussion of the liver in the midaxillary line will reveal the loss of normal liver dullness associated with free air under the diaphragm.

Cope emphasized the value of determining the presence of hyperesthesia in the particular anatomic region shared by affected viscera and their related cutaneous dermatome; it occurs in about half of acute inflammatory conditions. Cope also emphasized the value of the iliopsoas and obturator tests to determine irritation of those muscles by peritoneal inflammation.[6] Rectal and pelvic examinations are always indicated, although if one intends to refer the patient to the surgeon forthwith and it is known that the surgeon will perform these examinations, it may be justifiable to defer these procedures.

INVESTIGATION

Basic
investigations

Basic investigations for a patient with a new symptom of abdominal pain should include urinalysis. Hematocrit gives some indication of chronic or subacute blood loss but should not be relied on as an index of the current blood volume in the acute situation. The white count and the differential may be elevated in inflammatory conditions or may be reduced in acute viral illnesses or severe sepsis. Plain x-rays of the chest and abdomen can be done quickly and often provide useful information in the preliminary stages of decision making. Any adult presenting with upper abdominal pain which is not clearly diagnosed should have an electrocardiogram.

SPECIAL GROUPS

There are, of course, special problems in certain groups. For example, one should always consider the possibility of intussusception in childen 6 to 18 months old with periodic episodes of colicky pain.

Abdominal
pain in
children

Recurring abdominal pain in children is said to affect 1 of 10 school-age children. Galler et al. list approximately 70 causes for recurrent abdominal pain in children.[10] Organic causes account for some 5 to 10 percent of cases, with gastrointestinal and urinary diseases contributing equally.[9] In the remaining 90 to 95 percent of cases (usually children aged 5 to 13), the pain is probably psychogenic. Some possible causes include recent death or separation in the family, physical illness in other family members, psychiatric illness in parents (especially depression or alcoholism), unsatisfactory parent-child relationships, poor sleeping arrangements, school problems, and parental preoccupation with the likelihood of illness in the presenting child.

In psychogenic cases, the child almost always reports that the pain is central and occurs at special times such as on school days and after scolding but rarely disturbs sleep. Associated symptoms are vague and often include pain in other body areas with no pathophysiological connection with the abdomen. There may be a history of enuresis or poor sleep habits as well as a family history of similar abdominal pains. It is useful to determine why the child was brought in at this particular time and find out if external pressures (for example, urging of teachers or grandparents) promoted the visit. In such children a careful history concentrating on the stresses in the youngster's life and an equally careful examination not only will reassure the parent and the doctor of the absence of organic disease but also will be therapeutically reassuring to the child and will help direct the child's and parents' thinking toward psychological factors. Investigations should be governed by the history and findings as well as by the response of parents to the assessment.

Old people with acute abdominal conditions tend to react less vigorously and show fewer clinical findings. During their child-bearing years, women are at greater risk for ectopic pregnancy, threatened abortion, and difficult to diagnose abdominal conditions during pregnancy, although they have a low incidence of active peptic ulcer disease during pregnancy. Patients on medication for other reasons, especially on steroids or antibiotics, must be given special attention, since inflammatory conditions are readily masked or altered by such drugs.

Other special groups

MANAGEMENT

In managing abdominal pain, the family practitioner basically has to make one of the following three decisions: (1) hospitalize the patient immediately for further diagnostic maneuvers, consultation, or management, (2) reassess the patient within 2 to 4 hours in order to follow the course of the pain, or (3) discharge the patient with advice and arrange for a follow-up visit.[7]

Decision choices

Admit the Patient to the Hospital and/or Seek Consultation

Having decided that the symptoms and signs of the patient warrant immediate intervention, the physician arranges either that further investigative procedures be done or that a consultant see the patient.

The patient and, where appropriate, the family should be kept informed of the doctor's information as it evolves. Decisions to admit or refer should be made jointly by the patient and the doctor. The choice of hospital and consultant, where choice exists, can be

Patient involvement

put to the patient by the family doctor, who should explain the pros and cons of each alternative.

The patient should be advised to take nothing by mouth and should be told why it is not advisable to relieve the pain with medication before a definitive management decision has been made. Effective explanation can help relieve the patient's anxiety and make it easier to tolerate the pain.

Transport to hospital

Most patients do not need an ambulance for a short trip to the hospital or consultant's office if traffic is not a problem. Patients should not drive themselves.

Consultation process

Most consultants (for emergency abdominal pain the consultant is usually a surgeon, though he or she may be a gastroenterologist, general internist, pediatrician, or gynecologist) prefer to be involved early so that they can follow the progression of the illness. Practical considerations may make it more efficient to arrange for laboratory work and x-rays to be done before the consultant arrives at the hospital. However this is arranged, it is crucial that communication with the consultant be direct and that any divisions of responsibility be clearly understood from the beginning. The referring family physician should remain in continuous contact with the patient; however, when a family practitioner lives in a remote area and is forced to refer the entire responsibility for care to a consultant in the referral hospital, he or she should then communicate with the physician who will direct the care of the patient in the hospital. To refer a patient to a hospital emergency room without directing the assignment of the patient's care to another responsible physician is bad practice and should not be encouraged.

Surgery

If surgery is required, the assistance of a family practitioner who knows the patient can be of value to the surgeon when crucial decisions have to be made quickly. If the family doctor is present during surgery, he or she will know exactly what has been done and what technical problems have arisen; this will help in the early recognition of possible later complications. Also, patients are reassured if the doctor they know and trust is present during surgery and is watching out for them.

Observation

If, rather than surgery or other definitive intervention, continued observation is decided on, the patient should be informed as accurately as possible about facts as they are known, and observation should be started.

Patient kept informed

Explanations to the patient regarding intravenous or altered dietary intake, cautious use of analgesia, and further diagnostic tests (some of which may be repeated ones) should be given clearly and consistently by the attending medical and nursing staff members.

If the problem resolves itself without clear definition and the patient is to be discharged, he or she still requires specific advice.

When we fail to make a diagnosis, we tend to send the patient home without specific advice; this leads to confusion and the often dangerous failure of patients to report recurring or new symptoms.

In summary, it is important to do the following:

1 Communicate directly with others sharing clinical responsibility.
2 Divide up responsibilities clearly.
3 Explain clearly to the patient what is happening.
4 Involve consultants early in the course of the illness.
5 Avoid analgesia when possible before definitive action is determined.
6 As family doctor, stay closely involved, which includes assisting at surgery.
7 Make sure communication among all staff members involved with the patient is consistent.
8 Give specific advice to patients for whom a diagnosis is not established.

Reassess in 2 to 4 Hours

A patient who has abdominal pain which cannot be clearly diagnosed and who has either no abnormal physical findings or vague and nonspecific ones, usually warrants reassessment.

Wait and reassess

The patient should be told what the physician thinks are the possibilities and should be advised to take nothing by mouth, to note carefully any difference in symptoms, and to rest quietly. Explain why analgesia is best avoided. Arrangements can be made to see the patient again in approximately 4 hours in a suitable place. Or it may be agreed that if the symptoms abate noticeably, the patient will inform the doctor and come in for examination the next day.

Admission to hospital for observation

If on reassessment the physician remains uncertain of the diagnosis and the patient has not improved, it is probably wise to admit the patient for observation and, perhaps, more specific investigation, including consultation. Further reassessment (preferably by the same doctor) in 2 to 6 hours is warranted.

If circumstances allow and the patient and family are competent observers, it may be feasible to arrange for further reassessment without admission to the hospital. By this time, however, the repeated visits may be too uncomfortable for the patient or too inefficient for the doctor.

Send Patient Home with Plan for Follow-Up

If the physician makes a specific diagnosis of a nonacute condition, he or she can initiate the appropriate treatment and arrange for follow-up.

13 ABDOMINAL PAIN

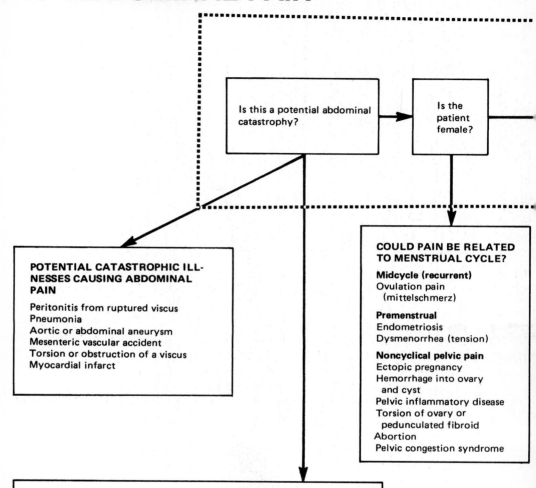

| Is this a potential abdominal catastrophy? | Is the patient female? |

POTENTIAL CATASTROPHIC ILL- NESSES CAUSING ABDOMINAL PAIN

Peritonitis from ruptured viscus
Pneumonia
Aortic or abdominal aneurysm
Mesenteric vascular accident
Torsion or obstruction of a viscus
Myocardial infarct

COULD PAIN BE RELATED TO MENSTRUAL CYCLE?

Midcycle (recurrent)
Ovulation pain
 (mittelschmerz)

Premenstrual
Endometriosis
Dysmenorrhea (tension)

Noncyclical pelvic pain
Ectopic pregnancy
Hemorrhage into ovary
 and cyst
Pelvic inflammatory disease
Torsion of ovary or
 pedunculated fibroid
Abortion
Pelvic congestion syndrome

QUALITY OF ABDOMINAL PAIN (derived from Sluglett[5])				
Affected viscus	Quality of pain			**Pathophysiology**
	Nature	**Severity**	**Site**	
Hollow	Colicky (spasmodic)	Greater	Poorly localized Radiating	Organ attempting to eliminate cause
Solid	Steady (persistent)	Lesser	Better localized over affected organ	Dysfunctional organ causes constitutional symptoms

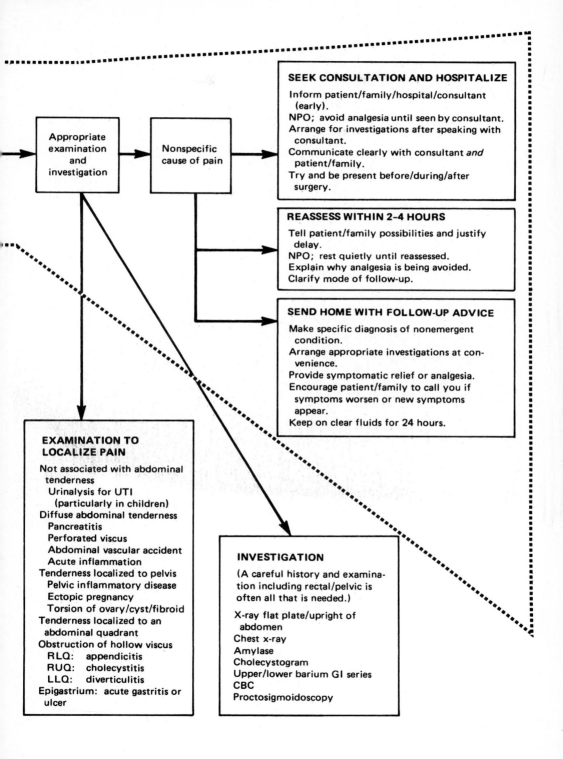

Appropriate examination and investigation → **Nonspecific cause of pain** →

SEEK CONSULTATION AND HOSPITALIZE

Inform patient/family/hospital/consultant (early).
NPO; avoid analgesia until seen by consultant.
Arrange for investigations after speaking with consultant.
Communicate clearly with consultant *and* patient/family.
Try and be present before/during/after surgery.

REASSESS WITHIN 2–4 HOURS

Tell patient/family possibilities and justify delay.
NPO; rest quietly until reassessed.
Explain why analgesia is being avoided.
Clarify mode of follow-up.

SEND HOME WITH FOLLOW-UP ADVICE

Make specific diagnosis of nonemergent condition.
Arrange appropriate investigations at convenience.
Provide symptomatic relief or analgesia.
Encourage patient/family to call you if symptoms worsen or new symptoms appear.
Keep on clear fluids for 24 hours.

EXAMINATION TO LOCALIZE PAIN

Not associated with abdominal tenderness
  Urinalysis for UTI (particularly in children)
Diffuse abdominal tenderness
  Pancreatitis
  Perforated viscus
  Abdominal vascular accident
  Acute inflammation
Tenderness localized to pelvis
  Pelvic inflammatory disease
  Ectopic pregnancy
  Torsion of ovary/cyst/fibroid
Tenderness localized to an abdominal quadrant
Obstruction of hollow viscus
  RLQ: appendicitis
  RUQ: cholecystitis
  LLQ: diverticulitis
Epigastrium: acute gastritis or ulcer

INVESTIGATION

(A careful history and examination including rectal/pelvic is often all that is needed.)

X-ray flat plate/upright of abdomen
Chest x-ray
Amylase
Cholecystogram
Upper/lower barium GI series
CBC
Proctosigmoidoscopy

Home care
follow-up

If the physician is satisfied that the patient does not have an emergency condition but is not completely certain what the problem is, he or she may (1) arrange follow-up the next day for reassessment, (2) arrange for further investigations, or (3) decide to get another opinion. It may be appropriate to provide symptomatic relief during the investigative period. The patient should be encouraged to report new or changing symptoms, with special emphasis on worsening pain, evidence of blood loss, melena, persistent vomiting, and unexpected fever.

It is usually advisable to recommend clear fluids by mouth for 24 hours except in the case of acid-pepsin diseases, in which case food taken frequently in small amounts and avoidance of smoking are part of good management.

SUMMARY

The family doctor who first sees patients with abdominal pain has the particular responsibility to observe carefully and attempt to classify vague symptoms which may or may not be harbingers of serious acute illness. Many problems will not declare themselves as specific diseases, and many will be ultimately diagnosed as acid-pepsin problems. A significant number of patients will have specifically diagnosable gastrointestinal illness. Others will have diseases not related to the gastrointestinal system.

For abdominal pain which may be considered an emergency, the family practitioner must decide with the patient whether to (1) admit the patient to the hospital or refer to a surgeon immediately, (2) reassess the patient within a few hours, or (3) send the patient home with advice.

The relative frequency of emergency conditions presenting with abdominal pain to family practitioners is small. The seriousness of that small number of problems, however, warrants the most careful approach to all patients who complain of abdominal pain.

REFERENCES

1 D. W. Marsland, M. Wood, and F. Mayo, *Content of Family Practice: A Statewide Study in Virginia with Its Clinical, Educational, and Research Implications,* J. Geyman (ed.), Appleton-Century-Crofts, New York, 1976.

2 S. T. Bain and W. B. Spaulding, "The Importance of Coding Presenting Symptoms," *Canadian Medical Association Journal,* **97**(16):953–959, 1967.

3 E. B. Fish, "Early Diagnosis of Abdominal Pain," *Canadian Family Physician,* **22**:134, 1976.

4 F. Mansfield, "The Acute Abdomen in General Practice," *Australian Family Physician,* **5**:1077–1085, 1976.

5 J. Sluglett, "Abdominal Pain in the Adult," *Update,* **7**(11):1477–1478, 1973.

  6 Z. Cope, *Early Diagnosis of the Acute Abdomen,* Oxford University Press, London, 1968.
  7 J. P. Bush, "The Management of Abdominal Pain," *Australian Family Physician FMP Supplement,* **3**(3):2–3, 1976.
  8 D. K. Wagner, "Approach to the Patient with Acute Abdominal Pain," *Current Topics* (Medical College of Pa.), **1**:1, 1978.
  9 J. Appley, *The Child with Abdominal Pain,* Blackwell Scientific Publications, Oxford, 1959.
 10 J. R. Galler, S. Neustein, and W. A. Walker, "Clinical Aspects of Recurrent Abdominal Pain in Children," *Year Book of Pediatrics,* Year Book Publishers, Chicago, 1980, pp. 31–53.

Chapter 27

Chest Pain

D. B. Shires, M.D.

PRINCIPLE

The reasons why a patient reports a given symptom at a particular time depend on the characteristics of the patient as well as on the symptom and other circumstances. Understanding how patients respond to illness can increase the potential for more effective disease prevention, appropriate early management, and rehabilitation.

DEFINITION

For the purpose of this chapter, *chest pain* is defined as discomfort relating to the chest. This definition includes tingling, burning, stabbing, squeezing, and other uncomfortable sensations. The discomfort may be described or identified by a nonverbal response, e.g., clutching one's chest.

PREVALENCE

In adults, chest pain is a common presenting symptom. Depending on the nature of the practice, chest pain is prevalent in 2.3 to 13 percent of patients.[1,2]

ETIOLOGY

Of patients presenting in a family practice with chest pain, 50 percent will have no proven etiology up to 6 months after the initial presentation. The causes found in the remaining 50 percent include: chest wall causes such as traumatic contusions, myositis, and costochondritis; respiratory causes such as bronchitis and pneumonia; vascular causes such as arteriosclerotic heart disease, hypertension, and congestive heart failure; and other conditions such as obesity, depression, anxiety, and viral infection.[3]

Causes

Chest pain is also a frequent presenting symptom for emergent and life-threatening conditions, in particular acute myocardial infarction, pulmonary embolism, dissecting aortic aneurysm, and esophageal rupture. An excellent review of the causes of recurrent chest pain in children has been written by Coleman.[4]

Danger signal

PRESENTING FEATURES

Some characteristic symptoms associated with chest pain are often of great assistance in deciding on the diagnosis and management.

Site

Central chest pain of an acute onset must be taken seriously. Chest pain radiating to the neck, arms, or back is more likely to be cardiac. (All chest pain on exertion must be taken as likely to be cardiac until proved otherwise.)

Nature

Squeezing or pressing chest pain, particularly in individuals with high-risk factors, e.g., men over 30, persons with a family history of heart problems, or persons with obesity, sedentary habits, a stressful existence, or a competitive occupation, should alert the physician to the possibility of myocardial ischemia. Associated symptoms such as sweating; radiation of pain to the neck, jaw, shoulders, or arms; nausea; and dyspnea are important features of myocardial infarction.

Differentiating symptoms

Burning chest pain aggravated by food ingestion and by lying down is likely to be gastrointestinal in origin. Burning pain aggravated by food ingestion but not by lying down may be due to gastritis, cholecystitis, or obstruction. Burning pain in the chest when the stomach is empty, especially if relief occurs on ingestion of food or antacids, strongly suggests peptic ulceration.

Tearing pain is suggestive of aortic dissection or esophageal rupture, especially if preceded by nausea and retching or vomiting. Tearing pain of sudden onset on one side of the chest in a young active adult suggests spontaneous pneumothorax (shoulder pain radiation is often helpful here).

Stabbing chest pain which worsens with deep breathing suggests a pleural cause (a friction rub heard on auscultation is often helpful). Remember that a rub that persists when the patient holds his or her breath is most likely to be pericardial in origin. Pain aggravated by movement suggests a musculoskeletal cause. Sharp stabbing pain also occurs with pulmonary infarction.

Most causes of chest pain are not difficult to evaluate if the pain is clearly defined and if appropriate examination and simple investigation are carried out. Palpation of the chest wall for local tenderness, auscultation, and simple physical examination skills will usually help resolve the dilemma if it is not clear from the history.

MANAGEMENT

Transportation

A patient who has a new symptom of chest pain with any cardiac qualities which has lasted for more than 15 minutes should be regarded as an emergency case requiring immediate medical attention. Whether the patient comes to the doctor or the doctor goes to the patient depends on practical considerations. In some centers, ambulance transportation to the emergency room of the hospital is the usual procedure, but the cardiac rescue team is becoming an increasingly common alternative.[5,6] The initial objectives for a patient with suspected cardiac chest pain are to establish pain relief as fast as possible, reduce anxiety, prevent cardiac arrhythmias, and promptly recognize and manage other complications of myocardial infarction. Every physician should be prepared to travel to a patient if he or she can arrive before the ambulance in order to carry out emergency management. A definitive diagnosis may be reached within 24 to 48 hours, during which period most myocardial infarctions have passed their period of greatest risk.

It has been said that the majority of delays in the management of life-threatening myocardial infarction are caused by the transportation system. Often, however, the patient is responsible for the delay. Table 27-1 lists some of the reasons why patients do or do not put off seeking medical advice for chest pain.[7] This finding has

Table 27-1   Patient Behavior with Chest Pain

Why patients delay	Why patients don't delay
1 Outright denial of existence of pain	1 Concerned relative
2 Interpretation of pain as due to less serious cause (e.g., antacid taken)	2 Concerned friend or colleague
3 Waiting for it to go away	3 Previous personal experience
4 Necessity to finish current task	4 Family experience
5 Belief that normal life after heart attack isn't likely	5 Public education
	6 Medical advice

Source: Hackett and Cassem.[7]

important implications for the planning of anticipatory guidance for patients at high risk or patients with proven heart disease. Such patients should be warned to treat any chest pain with the greatest caution and to alert the physician immediately. More generally, the public should be educated to realize that a normal life is perfectly possible after a heart attack. A review article detailing the cardiac rehabilitation responsibilities of the primary care physician has been written by Wenger.[8]

APPROACH TO THE OFFICE PRESENTATION OF CHEST PAIN

Once it has been determined that the chest pain is not life-threatening, an attempt should be made to find an etiologic cause even though in 50 percent of cases the attempt will be unsuccessful.[3] The approach to recurrent chest pain should be more contemplative, with a special effort made to detect less serious alternatives to chronic coronary heart disease.[9]

Attention should also be paid to fears that patients may have with respect to their chest pain. In one study on adolescents with recurrent chest pain, nearly 70 percent were afraid that the pain was due to heart disease or cancer.[10]

Patient fears

This does not mean that all chest pain without an identifiable physical cause is psychogenic. Such a diagnosis requires evidence of positive factors that may have contributed to the patient's chest pain. The possibility that the patient is suffering from latent depression, anxiety, or emotional distress should be carefully considered.

EMERGENCY TREATMENT
Relieve pain with morphine 10 to 15 mg IV or meperidine 75 to 100 mg IM.

Reduce anxiety by being present, calm, and organized.

14 CHEST PAIN

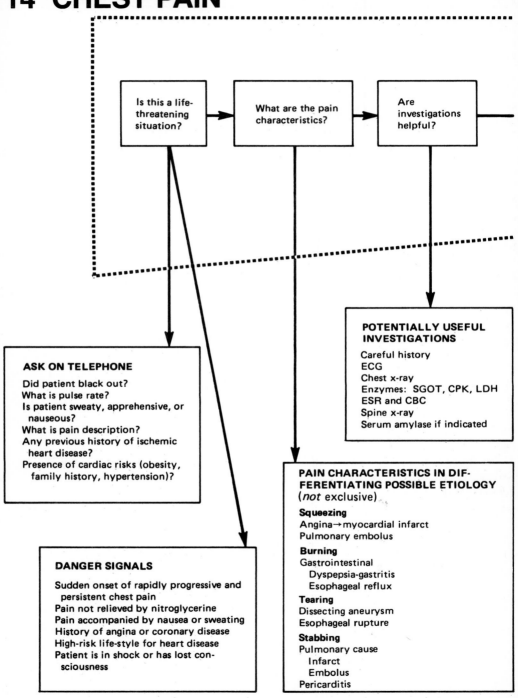

Is this a life-threatening situation?

What are the pain characteristics?

Are investigations helpful?

POTENTIALLY USEFUL INVESTIGATIONS

Careful history
ECG
Chest x-ray
Enzymes: SGOT, CPK, LDH
ESR and CBC
Spine x-ray
Serum amylase if indicated

ASK ON TELEPHONE

Did patient black out?
What is pulse rate?
Is patient sweaty, apprehensive, or
  nauseous?
What is pain description?
Any previous history of ischemic
  heart disease?
Presence of cardiac risks (obesity,
  family history, hypertension)?

**PAIN CHARACTERISTICS IN DIF-
FERENTIATING POSSIBLE ETIOLOGY**
(*not* exclusive)

Squeezing
Angina→myocardial infarct
Pulmonary embolus

Burning
Gastrointestinal
  Dyspepsia-gastritis
  Esophageal reflux

Tearing
Dissecting aneurysm
Esophageal rupture

Stabbing
Pulmonary cause
  Infarct
  Embolus
Pericarditis

DANGER SIGNALS

Sudden onset of rapidly progressive and
  persistent chest pain
Pain not relieved by nitroglycerine
Pain accompanied by nausea or sweating
History of angina or coronary disease
High-risk life-style for heart disease
Patient is in shock or has lost con-
  sciousness

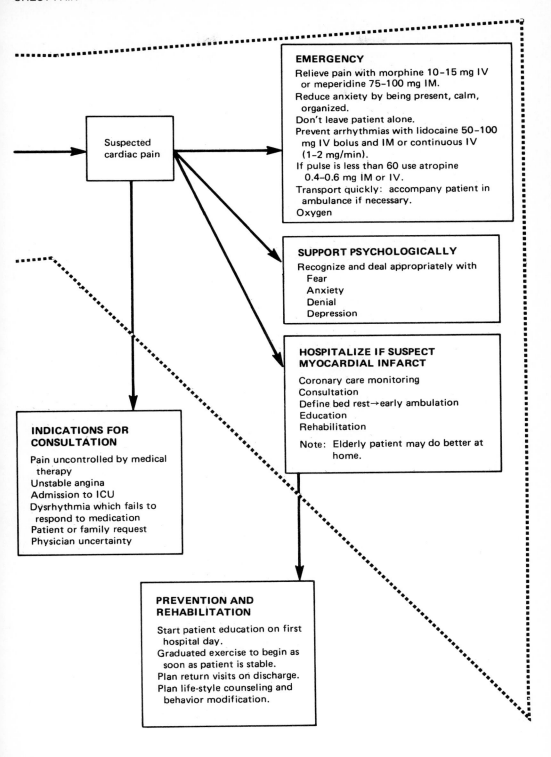

Suspected cardiac pain

EMERGENCY

Relieve pain with morphine 10–15 mg IV or meperidine 75–100 mg IM.

Reduce anxiety by being present, calm, organized.

Don't leave patient alone.

Prevent arrhythmias with lidocaine 50–100 mg IV bolus and IM or continuous IV (1–2 mg/min).

If pulse is less than 60 use atropine 0.4–0.6 mg IM or IV.

Transport quickly: accompany patient in ambulance if necessary.

Oxygen

SUPPORT PSYCHOLOGICALLY

Recognize and deal appropriately with
  Fear
  Anxiety
  Denial
  Depression

HOSPITALIZE IF SUSPECT MYOCARDIAL INFARCT

Coronary care monitoring
Consultation
Define bed rest→early ambulation
Education
Rehabilitation

Note: Elderly patient may do better at home.

INDICATIONS FOR CONSULTATION

Pain uncontrolled by medical therapy
Unstable angina
Admission to ICU
Dysrhythmia which fails to respond to medication
Patient or family request
Physician uncertainty

PREVENTION AND REHABILITATION

Start patient education on first hospital day.
Graduated exercise to begin as soon as patient is stable.
Plan return visits on discharge.
Plan life-style counseling and behavior modification.

Don't leave the patient alone.

Prevent arrhythmias with lidocaine 50 to 100 mg IV bolus and IM or continuous IV (1 to 2 mg per minute). Alternatively, bretylium tosylate can be used in the appropriate dosage.[11]

If pulse is less than 60, use atropine 0.4 to 0.6 mg IM or IV.

Transport quickly: accompany patient in ambulance if necessary.

Give oxygen as required.

REFERENCES

1 K. Hodgkin, *Towards Earlier Diagnosis in Primary Care,* 4th ed., Churchill-Livingstone, Edinburgh, London, New York, 1978.

2 S. T. Bain and W. B. Spaulding, "The Importance of Coding Presenting Symptoms," *Canadian Medical Association Journal,* **97**(16):953–959, 1967.

3 S. Blacklock, "The Symptom of Chest Pain in Family Practice," *Journal of Family Practice,* **4**:429–433, 1977.

4 W. L. Coleman, "Recurrent Chest Pain in Children," *Pediatric Clinics of North America,* **31**(5):1007–1026, 1984.

5 M. M. Kubik, "Mobile Coronary Care Units," *Practitioner,* **216**:303–306, 1976.

6 H. G. Mather, D. C. Morgan, N. G. Pearson, K. L. Read, D. B. Shaw, G. R. Steed, M. G. Thorne, C. J. Lawrence, and I. S. Riley, "Myocardial Infarction: A Comparison between Home and Hospital Care for Patients," *British Medical Journal,* **1**:925, 1976.

7 T. P. Hackett and N. H. Cassem, "The Psychological Reactions of Patients in the Pre- and Post-Hospital Phases of Myocardial Infarction," *Postgraduate Medicine,* **57**:43–46, 1975.

8 N. Wenger, "Rehabilitation of the Patient with Myocardial Infarction," *Primary Care,* **8**(3):491–507, 1981.

9 M. J. Levine, "Difficult Problems in the Diagnosis of Chest Pain," *American Heart Journal,* **100**(1):108–118, 1980.

10 R. M. Pantell, and B. W. Goodman, "Adolescent Chest Pain: A Prospective Study," *Pediatrics,* **71**(6):881–887, 1983.

11 R. E. Hayes et al., "Comparison of Bretylium Tosylate and Lidocaine in Management of Out of Hospital Ventricular Fibrillation: A Randomized Clinical Trial," *American Journal of Cardiology,* **48**:353–357, 1981.

Chapter 28

Confusion in the Elderly

M. K. Laurence, M.S.W., Ph.D
D. A. Gass, M.D.

PRINCIPLE

A confused elderly patient provides the family physician with an opportunity for diagnosis, treatment, and management which probably illustrates the basic tenets of family medicine better than any other example.

Confusion is less a disease than a set of behaviors that usually are caused by a combination of medical and psychosocial problems. Successful diagnosis, treatment, and management depend in large part on the physician's skill in piecing together a variety of clues in order to produce a coherent picture. The process involves some of the most fundamental skills of the family physician: knowledge of the patient, an ability to see the patient as a whole person, knowledge about multiple pathology, psychosocial involvement, use of community resources, and continuity of care. All these elements are basic tenets of family medicine.

INTRODUCTION

Confusion, incontinence, falling, and immobility are common non-specific symptoms of illness in the elderly. Chronic irreversible confusion or dementia is a major disabling condition among a significant percentage of elderly patients.

Importance of diagnostic workup

The reasons for confusion are rarely straightforward. It is therefore necessary to conduct a diagnostic search in order to determine the underlying causes. This search must be broad. It must assess both the patient and the patient's environment and must include the specific investigations needed for a more precise diagnosis. Confusion is not a natural result of the aging process.

DEFINITION

The decreased mental and emotional capacity associated with confusion is characterized by memory loss, agitation and irritability, inappropriate or unsafe behavior, disorientation, and inability to look after oneself. Any or all of these elements may be present in varying degrees of intensity and may reflect either a reversible or an irreversible problem or illness.

ACUTE (REVERSIBLE) CONFUSION

Time course provides diagnostic clues

The time course of the confusion provides the first clue to its cause. Acute confusion or delirium is usually associated with metabolic or drug toxicity or another acute illness such as infection, myocardial infarction, or renal failure.

A careful assessment of the patient's mental status will help differentiate psychiatric problems from organic brain syndromes. A history of early loss of intellectual function followed by loss of memory and the ability to calculate strongly suggests an organic brain syndrome. In contrast, symptoms of depression accompanied by slowness in performing mental tasks suggest a primarily psychiatric problem. Depression is the most common psychiatric illness that is confused with organic brain syndromes. It should be remembered that depression may also represent a reaction to the gradual failure of mental capabilities.

A short portable examination of mental status can be useful in the early assessment of confusion. An outline is provided in Table 28-1. This examination, together with a careful case history of the symptoms, is important in forming a diagnosis.

All cases of organic brain syndrome, chronic or acute, should be the subject of careful medical investigation in order to rule out treatable primary causes. Table 28-2 outlines an appropriate inves-

Table 28-1 Short Assessment of Mental Status

A (Score 1 for each correct response)
    1 What is your name?
    2 What is the name of this place? *or* Where are we now?
    3 What year is this?
    4 What month (or season) is this?
    5 What day of the week is it today?
    6 How old are you?
    7 What is the name of the prime minister or the president of the country?
    8 When did World War I start?

Remember these three items. I will ask you to recall them in a few minutes. (Standard items: bed, chair, window. Have patient repeat before proceeding.)

    9 Count backward from 20 to 1. (For any uncorrected error, score 0.)
   10 Repeat the three items I asked you to remember. (Score ½ for any item remembered or 1 for all three.)

"Normal": 7 or above
Dementia, moderate: 2 to 7
Dementia, severe: < 2

Table 28-2 Laboratory Investigation of Confusion

A General investigations, all cases
    1 Complete blood count
    2 Sedimentation rate
    3 Fasting glucose
    4 Blood urea nitrogen, creatinine
    5 Electrolytes
    6 T_4
    7 Venereal Disease Research Laboratories
    8 Serum B_{12} and folate
    9 Urinalysis
   10 Chest x-ray
   11 Electrocardiogram
B Additional investigations if indicated
    1 Drug levels if indicated by drug history
    2 CT scan of head if indicated by neurological signs or specific history
    3 Lumbar puncture if there is evidence of syphilis or meningeal irritation
    4 Psychological testing if mental status or history suggests affective illness or psychosis

tigation plan for all cases. Other tests should be undertaken in response to the appropriate clinical clues.

Diagnostic Studies

Diagnostic tests should include complete blood count (CBC), a.c. glucose, blood urea nitrogen (BUN), creatinine, electrolytes, thyroid function, Venereal Disease Research Laboratories (VDRL), vitamin B_{12} and folate, chest x-rays, and urinalysis. The presence of lateralized neurological signs, a recent change in the absence of metabolic factors, and the combination of ataxia, incontinence, and confusion are indications for doing a CT scan of the head for intracranial lesions. It must be remembered that cerebral atrophy is not significantly associated with mental dysfunction.

Among patients who have documented and irreversible progressive dementia, 70 percent will have senile dementia of the Alzheimer's type and approximately 30 percent will have multiple infarct dementia related to cerebral ischemia.[1,2] The latter affects men more commonly, has a history of episodic or stepwise deterioration, and is more often accompanied by hypertension, other evidence of cerebrovascular disease, and focal neurological signs.

DRUGS AND CONFUSION

Drugs are major cause of acute confusion

Drugs are one of the major causes of acute confusional syndromes in elderly patients. Elderly patients are more sensitive to the central nervous system side effects of a wide variety of drugs, including the primary psychotropic drugs, cardiovascular drugs (e.g., digitalis), antihypertensives, and analgesics. Avoiding such drugs or starting with a lower than usual dose followed by a gradual increase is the best way to prevent the adverse reaction of confusion. One should be particularly careful to check for the use of over-the-counter drugs or outdated prescriptions.

Paradoxical reactions to common sedatives are not uncommon, perhaps most notably with the benzodiazepines. In this situation, treating confusion and agitation with more psychotropic agents will be counterproductive.

Use of psychotropic drugs

When confusion is accompanied by such agitation that no meaningful communication or management of the patient can be undertaken, it may be appropriate to control the agitation with psychotropic drugs. The use of small doses of haloperidol repeated as necessary will avoid the hypotensive effects of the phenothiazanes. Where the diskinetic reactions sometimes caused by haloperidol must be avoided and the risk of hypotension is not serious, a phenothiazane such as thioridazine may be indicated. Where both of these drugs are contraindicated, a short- to medium-acting benzo-diazepine such as triazolam or lorazepam may be tried. These drugs do not have significant metabolites. Try to quiet agitation through such environmental means as adequate lighting, quiet, and the presence of familiar objects or persons. Psychotropic medications should be limited if possible to a single drug, since the interaction of various drugs complicates the picture.

It should be remembered that bladder retention or constipation can precipitate confusion. Keep in mind that patients with chronic progressive dementia may suffer from acute confusional states which can be relieved through treatment of the primary cause. Such sudden changes in mental status should be pursued independently as separate presentations. The syndrome of benign senile forgetfulness is marked by mild memory deficits, slow development, and relative sparing of intellectual function. Such changes need not affect the patient's daily life significantly. Patients and their families need to be reassured about the benign nature of this disorder.

CHRONIC (IRREVERSIBLE) CONFUSION

Once reversible and treatable causes of confusion have been ruled out, the family physician must consider the likely possibility of chronic confusion. Successful management of this disorder depends on a well-thought-out and organized approach. Otherwise, a confused patient is likely to engender a confused physician.

Management planning

The physician's aims at this point are to retard the progression of the disease as much as possible and to oversee a management plan which will enable the patient to function independently for as long as possible, preferably in the community. To develop a long-term management plan, the physician needs a more thorough assessment of the patient's ability to function.

PROGRESSION OF THE DISEASE

By the time the patient reaches the stage of diagnosis, he or she has been suffering from the disease, and probably has been aware of it, for some time. Usually a critical incident brings the disease to the attention of the family physician. Family members or friends may have found it impossible to cope with changes in the patient's behavior. The patient has probably experienced recent memory loss, inability to pay attention, inappropriate reactions, irritability and emotional outbursts, or inability to complete tasks or follow thought processes. All these factors put stress on the family. Families cope amazingly well until they become frightened or ex-

Stress on family resources

hausted by the need to cover up or compensate for the patient's behavior.

The patient may be depressed by his or her memory loss, which may have to be addressed as such. He or she forgets names, places, where things were put, and where they ought to go. Social masking is common, and the physician should pay attention to this possibility while conducting the examination of mental status. Mental deterioration often carries a social stigma and may be attributed by the ignorant or uncharitable to character flaws, bad heredity, or social inadequacy. The patient and family therefore are motivated to deny the existence of the problem and cover up its symptoms.

As the disease progresses, it begins to involve the patient's physical health. The patient may lose not only the ability to perform activities of daily life but the capacity to control bodily functions. He or she may behave in unsafe ways: leaving the stove on or cigarettes burning, wandering in woods or traffic, driving inattentively, and perhaps dressing inadequately for the weather. Unfortunately, the progress of the disease is neither orderly nor predictable. The physician and family must recognize this and be prepared to vary their modus operandi in accordance with the stage of the disease and its manifestations on any given day.

ASSESSMENT

Examination of Mental Status

Extensive mental status examination

While a short examination of mental status may provide enough information for the initial diagnosis, it is too crude to determine the degree and type of deterioration. A more extensive examination of mental status must be carried out at this point. This examination includes personality assessment and an evaluation of habits, relationships, capacities, judgment, insight, and degree of awareness of and emotional response to deterioration. How does the patient cope with daily life? This is probably one of the most critical functional assessments for determining the degree of compensation or accommodation needed for the ongoing maintenance and management of a patient.

Physical Examination

It is likely that a patient with Alzheimer's disease will also have other medical problems. The history taking and physical examination should assess neurological and mental function and look for hypertension or other medical problems which can affect confusion or complicate management. Confused patients still get sick. At the end of the physical examination and history, a list of problems and current drugs should be drawn up.

Functional Assessment

Assessing the patient's mental and physical condition merely gives a solid basis for a comprehensive functional assessment of the patient. The assessment of physical condition should examine the patient's general capabilities, including special senses (hearing, speech, sight), ability to perform the activities of daily living (washing, dressing, food preparation, eating), bowel and bladder control, and mobility. A complete functional assessment also includes such variables as family resources—personal, emotional, service, financial—and community resources.

Complete functional assessment

PRINCIPLES OF MANAGEMENT

The two principles underlying management are *accommodation* and *compensation*. We may unwittingly and with the best intentions encourage deterioration by failing to keep a proper balance between the two. Stimulation as a means of encouraging continued function often backfires because it fails to take into account changes in the patient's capacities and creates too much stress. However, providing complete care may encourage deterioration by making too few demands on the patient. If we properly assess the patient's level of functioning at a given time, it is possible to compensate for deterioration while continuing to demand that the patient use the resources he or she still has. The kind and degree of accommodation must be adjusted as the disease progresses, and compensations must be adapted to take into account the fluctuations and unpredictability of the disease (Figure 28-1).

Accommodation balanced with compensation

Designing a management program which embraces these principles requires an accurate mental and physical assessment of the patient and knowledge of the resources available in the family and community.

TECHNIQUES OF MANAGEMENT

Stimulation and the use of *reality orientation*, like any other intervention, must be appropriate to the patient's functional level and stage of deterioration. In the earlier stages of the disease, stimulation and reality orientation may help slow the deterioration by forcing the patient to use his or her remaining resources. In the early stages of memory loss, for example, the use of *memory aids* such as lists, labels, and reminders, as well as practicing word association

Stimulation

Figure 28-1   Principles of management: compensation for decreasing function.

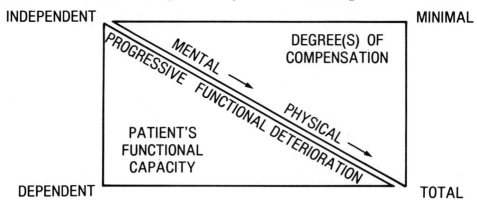

and keeping the patient actively involved in compensatory activity for specific memory loss, is highly desirable.

Reality
orientation

The physician may explain the disease to the patient in the early stages and help the patient both with the emotional reaction and with a planned, organized compensation scheme as well as with specific aids to balance memory loss. In the later stages of the disease and in the period of shifting back and forth between "good days" and "bad days," some stimulation can in fact overload the patient's capacity and precipitate deterioration in function as well as increase agitation and frustration on the part of the patient.

> For example, Mrs. A. has moderately severe mental dysfunction. She wanted to go Christmas shopping but could not cope with the stimulation of a store and the demands it made on her to navigate, negotiate, make decisions, handle money, and deal with other people. Rather than forbidding such an excursion, her husband, with the store's cooperation, took two or three items to her and let her make her choice in the neutral environment of the car. With an accurate assessment of the patient's capabilities and knowledge of the principles of management, the family physician and care givers can clarify such problems and propose creative solutions.

It may be useful to break down a task into parts which the patient is capable of managing or to give single directions or make single requests. Confronting the patient with a closet or drawer full of clothes may be overwhelming, while offering a choice of two garments laid out on the bed may be more manageable. Other activities of daily life may be similarly simplified and adjusted to the patient's functional ability at a given stage of the disease.

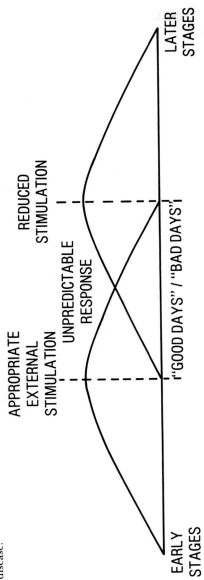

Figure 28-2 Principles of management: accommodation with progression of disease.

15 CONFUSION IN THE ELDERLY

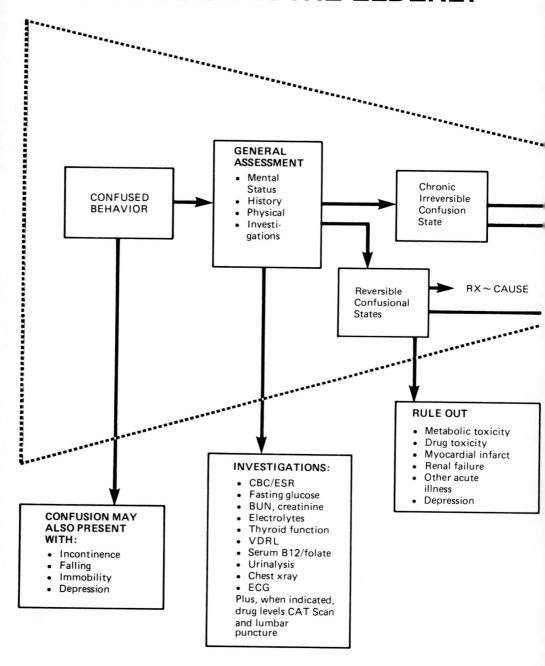

CONFUSED BEHAVIOR

GENERAL ASSESSMENT
- Mental Status
- History
- Physical
- Investigations

Chronic Irreversible Confusion State

Reversible Confusional States

RX ~ CAUSE

RULE OUT
- Metabolic toxicity
- Drug toxicity
- Myocardial infarct
- Renal failure
- Other acute illness
- Depression

CONFUSION MAY ALSO PRESENT WITH:
- Incontinence
- Falling
- Immobility
- Depression

INVESTIGATIONS:
- CBC/ESR
- Fasting glucose
- BUN, creatinine
- Electrolytes
- Thyroid function
- VDRL
- Serum B12/folate
- Urinalysis
- Chest xray
- ECG

Plus, when indicated, drug levels CAT Scan and lumbar puncture

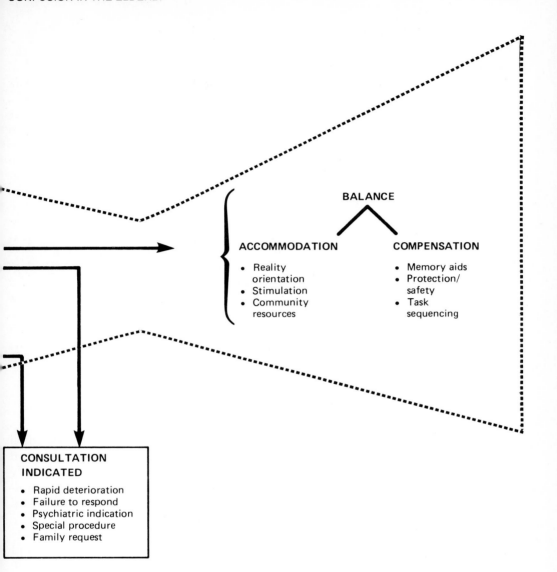

BALANCE

ACCOMMODATION

- Reality
  orientation
- Stimulation
- Community
  resources

COMPENSATION

- Memory aids
- Protection/
  safety
- Task
  sequencing

**CONSULTATION
INDICATED**

- Rapid deterioration
- Failure to respond
- Psychiatric indication
- Special procedure
- Family request

Protection and Safety

Balance risk
with quality of
life

Often the crisis which brings a patient to the doctor and sets the process of diagnosis in motion is unsafe behavior. We feel helpless to control the patient's behavior, and our sense of responsibility and fear for the patient's safety lead us to try to eliminate all risks. One response is to eliminate the patient's access to dangerous items, but this reaction limits the patient's chances of carrying on normal personal and social activities. We tend to try to restrain the patient or get rid of unsafe objects rather than design ways in which the patient can use them safely. Trying to balance risk and the quality of life sometimes calls for creative thinking. For example, if the family worries about the patient leaving the stove burners on, the stove can be disconnected or the circuit breaker can be thrown when supervision is unavailable. This will allow the patient to stay home when the family is out.

Restraints

The use of restraints is a double-edged sword. They often aggravate the patient, causing increased agitation. We must be careful to assess the use of restraints; the operative principle is that it is better to manipulate the environment than the patient. Bed rails may cause more falls than they prevent. Lower beds are easier to get into and out of, especially with a properly placed fixed chair; if the patient falls from a low bed, the distance fallen and the impact are reduced.

THE ROLE OF THE FAMILY PHYSICIAN

From the moment of presentation through diagnosis and initial management and often until the patient dies, the family physician is in a position of leadership.[3] He or she must provide anticipatory guidance, whole-person care, medical expertise, emotional counseling, psychological and behavioral management and therapy, and access to community and social service organizations.[4]

Ongoing
management
plans

Initially, the family physician can help the patient and family by providing them with a sense that the disease is a legitimate and serious one, not a reflection on their worth. The physician can use his or her long-term knowledge of the patient and family and their circumstances to help develop an ongoing management plan. Perhaps the most difficult aspect of irreversible confusion is its unpredictability and the fluctuations which occur as the disease progresses. The physician may help by working out a range of options so that the care givers can alter their approach to the patient in accordance with the patient's state. A patient who has been "doing well" for some time may abruptly "get much worse"; if the patient's family members have been prepared for this possibility and have a variety of management plans from which to choose, they will be better able to cope. Understanding and preparation can go a long way toward easing the frustrations, fear, and stress which accompany the progress of a disease.

The family physician can help the patient's care givers keep their perspective and solve problems as they arise. It is easy for everyone—not just the patient—to be overwhelmed and confused. Just as, for example, dressing must be broken down into individual parts if the patient is to cope, so must management of the confused patient be approached step by step.

Community resources—home health care, day care, intermittent admission to appropriate institutions, professional or lay counseling, and organizations such as the Alzheimer's Society and Widow-to-Widow—are invaluable in providing support and relief to physician and family.

Community resources

If and when institutionalization is the appropriate intervention, the family physician can help the family choose an institution and arrange admission and then support the family through the process of separation, guilt, and grief. When the patient dies, the physician always has a patient in need of help in the person of the survivor, who after the long siege is faced with loss, grief, and the need to mourn.[5]

REFERENCES

1 R. Katzman, "The Prevalence and Malignancy of Alzheimer's Disease," *Archives of Neurology*, **33:**217, 1976.
2 F. R. Freeman, "Evaluation of Patients with Intellectual Deterioration," *Archives of Neurology*, **37:**658, 1976.
3 M. K. Laurence, "Dealing with Confusion in the Elderly," *Canadian Family Physician*, **27:**1565–1568, 1981.
4 C. Eisdorfer and D. Cohen, "Management of the Patient and Family Coping with Dementing Illness," *Journal of Family Practice*, **12**(5):831–837, 1981.
5 M. K. Laurence and R. Weikart, "Grief, Loss, Mourning: What to Do," *Canadian Family Physician*, **30:**669–674, 1984.

Chapter 29

Breast Cancer

D. I. Rice, M.D.

PRINCIPLE

Cancer ranks second only to heart disease as the most common cause of death among adults in most countries in the western world.

Carcinoma of the breast has been selected for inclusion in this section on common health problems not with a view to providing a complete treatise on this complex disease but because it provides an opportunity to demonstrate the unique role that the family physician can play in the comprehensive management of a relatively common and always serious illness.

Overall role of family physician

In the management of breast cancer, the role of the family physician includes patient education, the identification of patients at risk, early detection and diagnosis, appropriate selection of consultants, supportive care to the patient and family with emphasis on psychological support, information and guidance concerning therapeutic options, follow-up care including continued surveillance for recurrence, and, because of the sometimes fatal nature of the disease, management of terminally ill patients.

DEFINITION

Like cancer in general, breast cancer is not one disease but many, depending on the breast tissue involved. The great majority of invasive cancers arise from the epithelium of the ducts and have no particular distinctive characteristics. So-called noninvasive carcinomas and lobular carcinomas are far more frequent than might be thought and may remain silent for years or decades.[1] Because untreated breast cancer is inevitably fatal, at an early date it must be identified and distinguished from more common but less serious diseases of the breast, including fibrocystic disease, fibrous mastopathy, mammary dysplasia, chronic cystic mastitis, and cystic hyperplasia. It should also be remembered that breast cancer can mimic every benign condition of the breast.

Breast cancer has many types

PREVALENCE

While cancer in general is not a common problem in the average family practice, cancer of the breast is among the most common forms of cancer seen by the family physician. It is currently the leading cause of cancer deaths in women (cancer of the bronchus may surpass it before 1990) and the leading cause of all deaths among women aged 35 to 54 years.[2] According to current estimates, 1 of 11 women in North America will develop cancer of the breast at some time during her life, with more than two-thirds of all breast cancers occurring among women aged 50 years or older.

Breast cancer is common

ETIOLOGY

Despite significant advances in detection and treatment, breast cancer remains in many respects an enigma, with its etiology uncertain. Many myths and misconceptions about this illness continue to exist, including the possible relation of bumps and bruises to the development of breast cancer. Fortunately, few people still believe that breast cancer is contagious. Both myths should be dismissed as misleading and incorrect.

Etiology remains uncertain

PATIENT EDUCATION

Until more reliable information and scientific evidence becomes available, there will be no known way to prevent the disease. The control of breast cancer must therefore begin with a combined public and patient education program. Through opinion surveys conducted by both the American and Canadian cancer societies and designed to determine the knowledge and attitude of the public toward breast cancer, a good deal of information has been made available to be mobilized for use in an education program.

The focus of patient education

Patient education should focus on the asymptomatic woman as well as on the patient who has already developed breast symptoms. It should include information regarding the known risk factors for developing breast cancer, the importance of early detection through breast self-examination (BSE) and regular physical examination, the normal cyclic changes in the breast that occur before menarche or during the normal menstrual cycle, and most important, the reassurance that follows a mature knowledge and understanding of the symptoms of breast cancer and the various successful treatment and rehabilitation opportunities that are now available.

Depends on accurate diagnosis

A woman who visits her family physician with breast symptoms should be reassured that her complaint does not necessarily indicate that cancer is present. This should be followed by a thorough explanation of the appropriate tests and procedures that will be used to confirm or rule out a diagnosis of cancer. Once these procedures have been completed, the patient should receive a clear and frank explanation of the results.

In instances where breast cancer is suspected or confirmed, patient education will focus on information about the disease itself, particularly on initial or follow-up therapy. The patient may also require specific instructions on postoperative exercises, the selection and use of prostheses, the technique of breast self-examination, and the availability, benefits, and potential risks of reconstructive breast surgery.

Communication with other professionals essential

The family physician must know what the patient has been told by the surgeon, the radiation therapist, and the medical oncologists and other health professionals who have helped in the patient's care and must be prepared to provide appropriate reinforcement of these instructions whenever possible.

Involve the family

Patient education also involves counseling and the provision of psychological support to all members of the patient's family. Cancer is a complicated, highly emotional disease. Most people require time to identify their concerns and formulate questions, and the availability of the family physician to deal with these questions contributes to the development of a support system that better enables the patient to cope with her disease.

Community agencies offer much help

In addition, the voluntary cancer agencies in most countries, as represented by national cancer leagues and societies, play a prominent role in cancer education directed toward the individual cancer patient and toward society in general through public education programs. The Reach for Recovery program, which initially was developed by the American Cancer Society and subsequently was adopted by the International Union Against Cancer (IUCC) for promotion to other cancer leagues and societies, is designed specifically to help patients with breast cancer live more comfortably with the disease. Family physicians who assume responsibility for the care of cancer patients should be familiar with the services provided to cancer patients through these important voluntary agencies.

RISK FACTORS

All women are susceptible to cancer of the breast, but certain women are at greater risk than others. As previously noted, two-thirds of all breast cancer occurs in women aged 50 years or older. To establish the degree of risk, it is essential to complete a detailed personal and family history on all patients presenting with breast complaints. A history of breast cancer in a mother or sister doubles the risk for developing the disease. A previous history of breast cancer in the patient triples the risk of developing cancer of the opposite breast. Patients with early menarche, those who are nulliparous, and those with a first pregnancy after age 30 years may also be at higher risk. Cancer of the breast in other female relatives (a grandmother or aunt) may increase the risk, although the degree of risk remains unknown.[3]

Known risks

There is evidence to suggest that diet may be a factor in the development of breast cancer. Rats fed a high-fat diet showed an increased incidence of breast cancer, and some comparative studies suggest that overweight women, particularly after menopause, and women whose diet includes an excess of fats, especially animal fats, may have a higher incidence of breast cancer.[2]

Suggested risks

The use of certain medications is associated with a variety of changes in the breast, including lactorrhea. While evidence is lacking to confirm a specific cause-and-effect relation, particular attention should be paid to patients using such drugs as oral contraceptives, estrogens and progestins, thiazide diuretics, phenytoin (Dilantin), levodopa (L-dopa), phenothiazines, and methyldopa.[3]

Some medications are suspect

EARLY DETECTION AND DIAGNOSIS

A shorter delay between the appearance of symptoms and the diagnosis of breast cancer may lead to a reduction in premature mortality.[4] Data from the Breast Cancer Detection Demonstration Projects of the American Cancer Society and the National Cancer Institute (United States) indicate that early detection of breast cancer at an "asymptomatic" stage followed by appropriate therapy may result in a significantly higher rate of survival, e.g., an average 5-year survival rate of 87 percent, with some centers reporting

Evidence supports value of early recognition

rates as high as 95 percent.[5] This represents the best survival rate for any type of localized cancer.

However, when cancer has spread beyond the primary site, survival rates drop to 56 percent. Expressed in another way, 30 percent more lives are lost, and clearly a great deal more suffering results from the disease.

The increased emphasis on early detection of breast cancer means that the majority of patients are now being seen with early disease which may be appropriately treated with less extensive surgical procedures. Awareness by both the family physician and the female patient of the importance of breast self-examination in the early detection of breast cancer cannot be overemphasized.

Lumps and other signs

The initial sign of breast cancer is commonly the presence of a lump in the breast. Usually the lump is detected by the patient herself accidentally or during routine breast self-examination. Breast cancer may sometimes be detected by other signs and symptoms, such as nipple discharge, dimpling of the breast and/or skin retraction, axillary nodes, nipple retraction, and localized inflammation. Less frequently, a mass may be discovered during the course of a routine physical examination by the physician or during screening programs such as mammography of an asymptomatic patient at risk for breast cancer.

A team approach

For most patients with carcinoma of the breast, a definitive diagnosis and initial therapy will be the responsibility of someone other than the family physician. In many instances a team of health professionals including a surgeon, a radiologist, and a medical oncologist will be involved. Nonetheless, the family physician will continue to play a central role in the management of the disease. This role will consist primarily of providing the patient with adequate and accurate information regarding diagnosis and treatment and with appropriate psychological support. To properly assume this role, the family physician must have a complete understanding of the pathophysiology of breast cancer, the currently accepted options for therapy, and the available procedures for monitoring the patient's response to therapy.

Initial tests and consultants

When a tentative diagnosis of breast cancer follows a careful personal and family history combined with a complete physical examination with particular attention to inspection and palpation of both breasts, the patient will be referred to a surgeon for consultation and confirmation of the diagnosis, usually by means of a biopsy of the suspicious lesion. The stage of referral will be influenced by the availability of additional diagnostic procedures such as mammography, cytological examination of nipple secretions (if indicated), and laboratory tests such as alkaline phosphatase, routine blood examination, chest x-ray, and Papanicolaou's test. Regardless of who assumes the responsibility for these additional diagnostic procedures, the physician's aim must be to reduce the delay between the time when the patient first seeks medical attention and the time when initial therapy begins.

THE CONSULTATIVE PROCESS

Increasing public awareness of different options for the local treatment of malignant disease and of the palliative nature of much cancer treatment (as well as knowledge that the intent of cancer treatment is frequently palliative rather than curative) is having a growing effect on cancer management.[6] The controversy that surrounds the definitive treatment of carcinoma of the breast has been heightened by the knowledge that there is no conclusive scientific evidence to prove that one method of treatment will ensure the best long-term results for all patients.

In selecting consultants, it is important for the family physician to select a surgeon who is objective, familiar with the current state of the art concerning the treatment of breast cancer, and prepared to involve other available experts in the selection of appropriate therapy for the patient.

Choosing consultants

The family physician, acting as patient advocate, has a responsibility to explain to the patient, and if necessary to selected members of the family, the results of the clinical examination, laboratory tests, and other diagnostic procedures. In particular, the physician must provide a supportive explanation of the need for surgical consultation. Once the consultation has been completed, it is important for the family physician to obtain complete information concerning the recommended therapy and to explain the relative risks of optional therapy to the patient.

Providing accurate information

In addition to information about current approaches to therapy, the patient may wish to have information concerning reconstructive breast surgery. The family physician must be aware of the possible risks associated with such procedures and must assess these risks in relation to the cosmetic benefits to a particular patient.

THERAPEUTIC OPTIONS

It is not within the purview of this discussion to describe in any detail the controversial and complex issue of the current treatment of breast cancer. Given the family physician's responsibility for counseling the patient and her family in regard to therapeutic matters, it is essential that the physician be familiar with these options as described in well-controlled validated studies reported in the current literature.

Know about the therapeutic options

Accurate staging leads to optimal selection of therapy

With the increased emphasis on early detection of breast cancer, the majority of patients today are seen with early disease and may be appropriately treated with less extensive surgical procedures. In select instances, radiation therapy may be employed as the primary treatment. These more moderate approaches produce the same survival rate as more drastic procedures, depending on the stage of the disease, and cause less disruption in the patient's life.[3]

The selection of therapy is determined by the stage at which the disease is first diagnosed. In general, the outcome of improved staging has been to reduce the number of radical surgical operations, since frequently these procedures cannot be justified if there is any chance of local treatment achieving a cure.

The stages of breast cancer are shown in Table 29-1.

The forms of therapy available include surgery, radiation therapy, chemotherapy, and sex hormone manipulation (Table 29-2). These therapies may be used alone or in combination depending on the stage of the disease. The standard form of therapy for patients with stage I and stage II breast cancer is a modified radical mastectomy.[7] Recently, interest has evolved in partial mastectomy and radiation therapy as the primary treatment for breast cancer. However, the benefits of radiation therapy as an adjunct have not been established, and such therapy is not generally recommended.[3]

Among patients in whom axillary nodes are found to contain tumors (stage II), early systemic chemotherapy is usually prescribed for 12 to 18 months. This therapy has been shown to prolong the disease-free interval in premenopausal patients, but its value in postmenopausal patients is still under study. While the effects of early systemic chemotherapy on long-term survival have not been determined, most medical oncologists favor the use of early chemotherapy in all patients with positive axillary lymph nodes.

Therapy for patients with stage III breast cancer will be selective and modified in accordance with the location and size of the tumor, edema of the skin, or fixed axillary nodes. Either preoperative radiation therapy or chemotherapy may be employed. The entire tumor may be resected. In most instances, there will be a period of at least 12 to 18 months of postoperative chemotherapy and, in some instances, postoperative radiation therapy.

Most patients with stage IV breast cancer are candidates for a form of systemic therapy using either chemical agents or hormonal manipulation if the tumor is estrogen receptor–positive. This will follow surgery of the breast and axilla and local radiation therapy. When the tumor is progressive after hormonal therapy, multiagent chemotherapy is usually employed. Hormonal manipulation may consist of oophorectomy or an antiestrogen in premenopausal

Table 29-1   Clinical Stages of Breast Cancer

Stage I	Small tumors (less than 2 cm) with negative nodes
Stage II	Tumor up to 5 cm with positive ipsilateral axillary nodes or tumor 2 to 5 cm with negative axillary nodes
Stage III	More advanced local disease including tumor greater than 5 cm and large axillary nodes
Stage IV	Far advanced local disease such as inflammatory cancer, recurrent cancer following a cancer-free interval after initial therapy, or cancer overtly disseminated beyond the ipsilateral axilla when first diagnosed

Table 29-2   Therapeutic Options

Stage I/II	Modified radical mastectomy Partial mastectomy plus radiation
Stage II	The above options plus systemic chemotherapy
Stage III	Preoperative radiation therapy Chemotherapy Radical mastectomy Postoperative radiation and/or chemotherapy
Stage IV	Mastectomy and/or local radiation Chemotherapy (multiagent) Hormonal therapy (medical and/or surgical)

cases or an antiestrogen or an estrogenic steroid in postmenopausal cases.

Increasing media coverage of all aspects of breast cancer, particularly in regard to women's choices of the extent of surgery used in treatment, appears to be having a positive effect on people's attitudes toward breast cancer. This should contribute to an improvement in early detection, an improved prognosis, and an improvement in quality of life for breast cancer patients.

SURVEILLANCE

The follow-up of a patient who has been treated for breast cancer can usually be provided by the team of surgeon, radiotherapist, medical oncologist, and family physician. The particular responsibility of the family physician is to provide continuing surveillance for recurrence, monitor the patient's psychological status, and help provide the intervention that may be required to ensure optimum rehabilitation of the patient physically, emotionally, and socially.

Local recurrence and metastatic spread are more likely to occur

Coordinating follow-up

Timing of follow-up visits

within the first 3 years after primary therapy. Follow-up visits should therefore be arranged at 3-month intervals for the first 18 months after the initiation of therapy and at 3-month to 6-month intervals for the following 18-month period. There appears to be no consensus regarding long-term follow-up; this should be determined on an individual basis with the knowledge that there is no evidence to suggest a permanent cure for cancer of the breast but considerable evidence to support prolonged control of the disease.

The follow-up visit

At each follow-up visit, the family physician should ask about symptoms that suggest deterioration in general health, recurrence of lumps or nodes, pain in the chest or back, weight loss, cough, or difficulty in breathing. On physical examination, particular attention should be directed to symptoms identified during the history taking, with laboratory tests and other procedures if indicated. On each visit, the breast should be examined with special attention to the surgical scar and adjacent skin and regional lymph nodes.

Annual review

On an annual basis, surveillance should include a Papanicolaou's smear, complete blood picture, serum alkaline phosphatase, chest x-ray, mammogram of the opposite breast, and bone scan as indicated by symptoms or physical findings.

TERMINAL ILLNESS

The cause of death in many women with a diagnosis of breast cancer will be unrelated to the primary diagnosis, while in other patients death will be the direct result of complications from the disease itself.

In his chapter on "Death and Dying," Brian Hennen has described in detail (chapter 30) the responsibilities of the family physician in caring for terminally ill or dying patients. All these tenets have application to the management of patients who are terminally ill as a result of breast cancer. Unlike death that results from trauma, acute myocardial infarction, and other causes where the contributing factors have been abrupt and unexpected, the lead time in patients dying of breast cancer is in most instances gradual and prolonged.

Anticipating the likelihood of death

Since the outcome of breast cancer, as in more serious forms of cancer, is so frequently fatal, the preparation of the patient for ultimate death from the disease begins once the diagnosis of malignancy has been confirmed. While this preparation is in most instances subconscious on the part of both physician and patient, it becomes an integral part of the communication process between physician and patient, essential to the proper management of a patient with cancer.

The responsibility of the family physician for continuity of patient care provides an opportunity to establish a relationship with the patient and the patient's family that is built on mutual trust, respect, and confidence—the basic ingredients of an effective communication process. This doctor-patient relationship contributes to the acceptance by the patient of cancer as a serious and life-threatening illness; from the outset, it better enables a patient with a diagnosis of breast cancer to prepare for the eventual outcome of the disease: death.

While it is not possible to determine exactly when a patient enters the terminal phase of illness, at some point the end appears to come more clearly in sight both for the patient and for those involved in the patient's care. The patient's mental awareness of the approaching end is not always conscious but rather is described as the preconscious premonitions of impending death.

Doctor Adriaan Verwoerdt, professor of psychiatry at Duke University Medical Center, Durham, North Carolina, at a national conference on Human Values and Cancer sponsored by the American Cancer Society in June 1976, addressed the subject of communicating with the fatally ill. He described four major goals of communications that are important during the terminal phase of illness. The major goals are

Communication goals in managing terminal illness

"(1) to prevent a sense of hopelessness, helplessness, and loneliness; (2) to preserve dignity, both in the patient's own eyes and in the eyes of others; (3) to prevent the massive psychopathology that results from terminal ego breakdown, and (4) to help the family with their grief, feelings of guilt etc. and to assist the patient in facing the loss of his life, working through this loss, toward the final acceptance of death—and thereby the acceptance of his life".[8]

In realizing these goals, a major challenge for family physicians is to be able to deal with their own sense of helplessness, inadequacy, and frustration that results primarily from the limitations placed on the health professions and the scientific community in effectively dealing with the complexities of cancer as well as from the inability of many physicians to personally cope with the emotional and spiritual aspects of death and dying.

Doctors have to deal with frustration

For many patients, the fear of desertion is greater than the fear of death. Too many physicians insist that in not sharing with patients the full extent of their illness they are somehow being more humane, when in fact the physician is engaging in a conspiracy of silence in order to defend himself against his or her own fears and anxieties.

What do patients actually fear?

The family physician who accepts responsibility for the care of a terminally ill cancer patient can hope for no greater commendation than that expressed by Bernard Martin in his book *If God Does Not Die*:

> The cancer patient who has a physician who can prescribe therapy either specific or non-specific, curative or palliative, choosing appropriately among them, and one who will care for the patient whether there is a medical success or failure is indeed fortunate. The physician who knows enough to accept his role as both scientist and humanist, parent and friend, will eventually become comfortable enough to successfully care for his patient even to death.[9]

REFERENCES

1 *Clinical Oncology: A Manual for Students and Doctors*, edited by the Committee on Professional Education of the International Union Against Cancer, Springer-Verlag, Berlin, Heidelberg, New York, 1973.

2 *Facts on Breast Cancer*, Canadian Cancer Society, Toronto, 1982.

3 *Carcinoma of the Breast: Reference Guide #1*, American Board of Family Practice, 1983.

4 S. Nichols and W. E. Waters, "The Effect of a Health Education Intervention about Breast Cancer amongst General Practitioners on Speed of Referral and Outpatient Workload," *Community Medicine*, **6:**115–118, 1984.

5 L. H. Baker, "Breast Cancer Detection Demonstration Project: Five Year Summary Report," *CA* **32**(4):194–235, 1982.

6 M. H. M. Tattersall, "Cancer Management in the 1980s," *Medical Journal of Australia*, **41:**10–15, 1981–1982.

7 "Special Report: Treatment of Primary Breast Cancer," *New England Journal of Medicine*, **301:**340, 1979.

8 A. Verwoerdt, "Some Aspects of Communication with the Fatally Ill," *Proceedings of the American Cancer Society's National Conference on Human Values and Cancer*, The American Cancer Society, New York, 1973.

9 B. Martin, *If God Does Not Die*, John Knox Press, Atlanta, GA, 1966.

Chapter 30

Death and Dying

B. K. Hennen, M.D.

PRINCIPLE

Identifying and relieving the patient's fears throughout the course of an illness helps to clarify the appropriate focus of management.

INTRODUCTION

This chapter deals with the patient for whom the decision has been made to stop treatment that aims at curing or arresting a life-threatening disease and to turn entirely to palliative symptom control and care in the anticipation of death. According to Sampson, dying begins "when no specific therapy can or should be given, when drug and radiation resistance have developed, when palliative surgery is unreasonable, when intravenous therapy should no longer be given, and when further admissions to Intensive Care Units would only result in a few days of prolongation."[1]

It is easier to focus on palliation if the decision to stop trying to cure has been made. However, family physicians often provide care for patients whose diseases are being managed by others, for example, specialists in oncology or surgery. Even while curative treatment is being attempted (perhaps with a small but statistically possible chance of success), the family physician can ensure that necessary palliation is adequately provided.

PAIN

Symptom control is extremely important. Pain, nausea, sleeplessness, depression, and fatigue are commom symptoms and are often interrelated.

Accurate pain history

The Canadian Expert Advisory Committee on the Management of Severe Chronic Pain in Cancer Patients cited three main reasons for poor pain control: (1) lack of factual knowledge about analgesics and existing techniques for controlling pain, (2) inappropriate attitudes, fears, and behaviors in the health care team (including the family) and the patient, and (3) lack of access to the appropriate resources.[2]

They stress the importance of assessing the pain accurately and trying to identify its cause. Is it due to the cancer itself, to the treatment, or to factors unrelated to cancer therapy? Examples of pain directly caused by cancer include bone infiltration with or without muscle spasm, nerve compression, bed sores, and herpetic neuralgia. Pain related to treatment includes postoperative pain, phantom limb pain, postradiation inflammation, postradiation myelopathy, and postchemotherapy neuropathy. Pain unrelated to the cancer or therapy would include arthritis, cardiovascular pain, headaches due to migraine or tension, and musculoskeletal pains due to other causes.

Analgesic use

In regard to the administration of medication, they stress the importance of the proper dose, regularity of administration, the patient's attitude toward the use of the medication, the way the medication is being administered (orally, intravenously, etc.), and the side effects of the medication.

Their approach to analgesics is basically a simple one, with ASA, codeine, and morphine being the mainstays of pain control. It is useful to be familiar with one or two alternatives to each of these agents. One should consider switching to the next more potent level of analgesic only if the analgesic is being given regularly around the clock, the frequency of application is appropriate, the dose has been increased to its highest acceptable range, and the pain remains.

Analgesic side effects

For morphine-induced nausea or vomiting, they recommend prochlorperazine or haloperidol if the symptoms are due to stimulation of the chemoreceptor trigger zone in the medulla, metoclopramide if the symptoms are due to gastric stasis, or dimenhydrinate if the symptoms are due to vestibular stimulation. Most medication, including morphine, can be given orally, and this is preferable. Morphine and some of its alternatives can be given in rectal form, intramuscularly, subcutaneously, intravenously, or even epidurally.

Other modes of treatment may control pain, including surgical decompression, radiotherapy, nerve blocks, transcutaneous electrical nerve stimulation (TENS), acupuncture, steroid injection, massage, hot packs or cold packs, elastic stockings, elevation of limbs, splints and slings, and relaxation exercises.

Other pain treatments

FEAR

It is important to deal with the patient's fears. Patients who realize that they are soon to die fear different things. Some fear dying in pain. Some fear being incontinent. Others are most disturbed by a loss of control over the management of their everyday lives. Some fear the mode of death; for example, dying short of breath (smothering) is a source of fear for some people. Dying alone is also a major concern. There is also the anticipatory grieving of the loss of loved ones by the person who is about to die. As one person put it, "I am not afraid of death, I am afraid of not living anymore." Other fears include the unknowns of cancer treatment, hair loss, disfigurement, bleeding, drug addiction, vomiting, going crazy, and family bankruptcy.

Patients' understanding

It may be useful to distinguish between premature and timely death and determine which the patient feels he or she is facing. A premature death is one which any person experiences who faces the likelihood of actual death before feeling that he or she has completed the business of this world. For want of a better expression, a timely death is one in which the dying person feels that his or her "time has come" and is ready for it. It is important to determine whether the patient's family members feel that their sick member is experiencing a premature or a timely death.

People respond to illness in individual ways. It is easy to make incorrect assumptions about how a problem is perceived by one person after having just helped another person deal with the same problem. For example, having determined that a patient's insomnia was due to fear of dying alone, a doctor might mistakenly attribute another patient's insomnia to the same cause, when pain was keeping the second patient awake.

It is sensible to go with the odds, that is, to anticipate that certain problems are more likely to be due to certain causes, as long as we check out our suspicions with the patient in each instance.

Raising the question whether care is best planned primarily for home or hospital, Sampson suggests three major steps.

Home or hospital?

First, bring up the subject with the patient directly by asking opening questions: "Have you thought about what lies ahead?" "Have you been making any personal plans?" If the patient appears not to understand, be more direct and ask where he or she wants to spend his last days.

Second, clear the decision with the family, making it plain what the patient's wishes are if he or she has not informed them. Explain that you will attempt to support them and reassure them that the hospital can always be used if things do not work out.

Third, enlist the help of community-based resources such as visiting nurses and home care organizations.

HOME CARE

The wishes and motivation and the emotional capacity of the patient and the patient's relatives are obviously vital. The physical circumstances of the home are important, for example, the avoidability of stairs, the availability of commodes, and the need for a hospital bed in the home.

Home care is not always best

Circumstances which make home care difficult include intractable pain, persistent nausea and vomiting (particularly if dehydration and electrolyte imbalance ensue), choking spells and/or breathlessness, and incontinence of either bladder or bowel. Severe hemorrhage or fecal incontinence may make hospitalization on a short-term basis desirable.

Inability to cope on the part of family members may be expressed as anger and should be anticipated. Worries that "she hasn't eaten anything in days" require practical reassurance. Intravenous therapy should not be necessary for terminally ill patients if family anxieties can be quieted.

Symptom control is essential, especially in regard to pain and bowel and bladder dysfunction (catheters can relieve the necessity for painful movement of aching limbs).

Home care is team care

The planning of home care for a dying patient has to be developed in a team atmosphere. The Expert Advisory Committee included on the cancer pain team the patient, family members, physicians, nurses, social worker, pharmacist, chaplain, physiotherapist, occupational therapist, nutritionist, psychologist, and volunteers. Those members of the team to whom the patient and the key care givers can relate best should be given the prime communication responsibilities for direct contact. Others should provide their necessary skills and not push themselves on the patient or the care givers. An office nurse can contribute through frequent telephone contact and may benefit from participation in at least an occasional home visit.

The events surrounding death can be enriching and rewarding when the dying person can be helped and the family can contribute to that help.

How family members can contribute is exemplified in a situation where a fairly noncommunicative husband was pacing outside in the garden during my visit to his dying wife. I suggested that for her to move to the bathroom, which was only several feet away, was quite uncomfortable and that it might be a good idea for him to fashion some kind of commode for her. The next day he had fashioned an extremely practical and feather-light commode chair out of a commode appliance from the local drugstore and a webbed aluminum garden chair. Having contributed his best to the care of his wife, he was then more able to feel a part of the caring team. Another example involved a professional man dying at home of cancer. His family had not been particularly close in a physical or "touchy-feely" way. His sons and daughters, however, read sensitive and warm poetry to him by the hour. Within the family, this was their way of sharing their deepest feelings for one another.

The avoidance of last-minute admissions to hospital emergency rooms and unnecessary resuscitation attempts can usually be assured by providing accurate information about the terminal state to the family. Prevention of feelings of panic and helplessness is important.

Advising family what to expect

Other hints regarding home care include knowing the particular personal resources within the entire family and the resources of the community. The keeping of a record of care at the patient's bedside in the home is an essential part of communication among the various health care professionals, support personnel, and family members.

In summary, an approach to the dying patient should include the following elements.

1 When you suspect a serious problem and even before you confirm it, be honest with the patient as investigations progress.

2 Make an assessment of the patient's personality from a psychological and social point of view. Include an assessment of the patient's philosophy and attitudes.

3 Make an assessment of the patient's family.

4 Confirm the diagnosis of the disease.

5 Take the attitude of intending to tell the patient the truth. Look carefully for opportunities to do so, trying to determine the patient's optimal state of readiness to accept the news.

6 As a general rule for an adult and responsible patient, try to communicate the truth about the diagnosis.

7 Having discussed the likelihood of death with the patient, gain his or her endorsement to communicate the necessary facts to the family and those health professionals who may be involved in management.

8 Be prepared to be doubted, to be asked for another opinion, and to be asked for further tests and confirmation.

9 Be prepared to reassure the patient of your continuing interest and involvement even in the face of anger or rejection.

10 Always offer hope and aim your activities toward improved quality of life in whatever dimensions are appropriate.

11 Be prepared to protect the patient from wasting his or her remaining health looking for "quack" cures.

12 Remember that you and the patient need not carry the whole burden alone. Make use of the family and the many appropriate health professionals available.

13 There is never nothing to be done.

At the time of death, it is important for the patient's family to know what to do. Do they call the doctor or the doctor's deputy? Is there a funeral director to be called? Has there been discussion about an autopsy or body donation?

The doctor may also be called on to help close family members with their acute grief. A common request is to give sedation. This may be inappropriate, especially if unaccompanied by a personal contact that fosters the free expression of grief.

FOLLOW-UP

Some follow-up contact with the family physician is well advised. A visit or phone call a week or so after the death is appropriate. By then support from the immediate family and friends may have dissipated. Quarterly visits during the year following a death can be helpful, and subsequently arranging some contact on the anniversary of the death is worthwhile. If the family feels that the death was premature, more extensive follow-up may be necessary.

REFERENCES

1 Sampson, W. I., "Dying at Home," Journal of the American Medical Association, November 28, 1977, Vol. 238, No. 22.
2 Expert Advisory Committee on the Management of Severe Chronic Pain in Cancer Patients, "Cancer Pain," Minister of Supply and Services Canada, 1984.

Part Three

Facilitating Health Maintenance

Chapter 31

Ecology of Health in Communities

D. B. Shires, M.D.

Health is a dynamic entity. Health maintenance—that is, freedom from disease or the threat of disease—requires consideration of some of the interacting forces that affect an individual's ability to resist disease-causing agents. Physicians generally think in terms of the medical aspects of illness in the individual. As a result, they often neglect the broader issues, such as the effects of ecological and environmental factors on health.

While it is difficult to draw up an inclusive list, an initial assessment of broader health factors, both positive and negative, can facilitate an understanding of the health status not only of individuals but also of the community. As the continuous provider of primary care, the family physician must accept the major responsibility for utilizing these factors to promote good health.

    What are the ecological variables that enhance health? We shall review some of them and suggest ways in which the physician and the health team can use their knowledge of ecological factors to increase the quality of care.

    Most important are the indigenous remedial and health education programs available within a community. In many third world societies, western-style health services, even at the emer-

Family physician responsibility

Ecofactors

Societal attitudes

Third world

gency remedial level, are conspicuously absent. Nevertheless, a variety of traditional healers such as herbalists, bone setters, and priests practice a form of indigenous "traditional" primary care. In western society, if health care services are to be used effectively at all levels of society, the family physician must understand social attitudes toward the concept of health. In some societies, being sick means being unable to get out of bed. In others, the slightest nasal drip sends individuals running to expensive health services. Both attitudes may result in poor health: the first because services are not used when remedial intervention is necessary, and the second because services are used unnecessarily, thus depriving those in greater need.

Another complicating factor is that even when free health education and medical services are available to them, many people disregard obvious signs of ill health and/or fail to comply with seemingly simple therapeutic regimens. All these factors must be considered in the ecological "balance of health."

NUTRITION

Starvation and obesity

Poor nutrition is probably the greatest contributor to ill health in the world today. In third world countries the problem is an undersupply of food or maldistribution of food, whereas in the western world an oversupply of the wrong types of food is one of the main causes of poor nutrition. (See chapter 35, "Nutrition.") It is sad to reflect that after thousands of years of so-called civilization, a large part of the world is slowly starving to death while in much of the remainder, nutritional overindulgence (obesity) is a serious health problem.

Both excessive and inadequate nutrition have major effects on morbidity and mortality. Certainly the consequences of starvation as seen, for example, in the marasmic infants of central Africa and Asia and in the rising incidence of kwashiorkor and various vitamin deficiency diseases, are well documented. It is astonishing and not as well publicized that even in Canada and the United States—countries with an annual food surplus—a significant percentage of the population is malnourished.[1]

LIFESTYLE

Positive lifestyles

The habits of life that may play havoc with an individual's future health are well known to most people: smoking, uncontrolled food intake, poor choice of food items, and lack of exercise. A *positive* lifestyle conjures up the image of glowing bodily health and is considered desirable. Health buffs who jog, reject smoking (for themselves or those in their immediate vicinity), select natural foods, use seat belts, drive defensively, and reject alcohol and other drugs are regarded as eccentric in many societies. However, this sort of eccentricity is becoming more common.

New understanding of the effect of lifestyle on health is finally starting to have some impact on the population.

Positive lifestyles in terms of health can lead to greater productivity if enough people participate and may result in generally improved health in a community. Failure to use seat belts and to drive defensively as well as failure to acquire adequate anticipatory health care such as the Pap smear and immunization are common lifestyle habits. However, lifestyles can be altered for groups and individuals by means of health education, reading, peer group discussion, audiovisual materials, and mass media. The goal is to reduce morbidity from chronic illness, which is the ultimate result of "negative" lifestyles.

Negative lifestyles

HIGH-RISK OCCUPATIONS

Some people have occupations that are associated with a high risk of morbidity and mortality; among them are miners (particularly in dusty locations such as asbestos mines) and air traffic controllers, among whom stress diseases are prevalent. In some industries workers are protected by strict work regulations, worker's compensation laws, and the use of protective clothing, while in others (e.g., in third world countries) they are not.

Occupational hazards

Constant activity and vigilance are needed to ensure that individuals at risk are adequately protected. Programs such as those which provide protective helmets and safety laws for construction workers or goggles for welders to protect their retinae from high-intensity light are essential. Family physicians should make themselves aware of occupational health problems in their communities.

ENVIRONMENT

Housing and working conditions have been a focus of social workers' concern for decades. A poor physical and social environment has a highly deleterious effect on individual and community health. Bad housing leads to an increase in respiratory disease; rodents and insects, contamination of drinking water, and overpopulation have caused epidemics and disasters throughout history. Cities with rapidly expanding populations such as Lagos, Mexico City, and Manila are experiencing such problems today.

High-risk neighborhoods

As the effects of pollutants and careless social habits become known, industrialized societies, which traditionally have been re-

Ecology

garded as conservative, are beginning to take action. New industry, new construction, and new housing developments are carefully evaluated in terms of potential disruption of psychosocial and physical health in the community. Ecological action means actively resisting the geophysical and political forces that prevent a community from enjoying maximum good health.

GENETICS

Inheritance

Genetic mutation has only recently begun to be understood. Approximately 40 percent of admissions to children's hospitals are for conditions rooted in the child's genetic background.[2] The challenge is to identify individuals possessing the genetic makeup of these diseases so that problems can be discovered early (by means of amniocentesis and other techniques) and appropriate action can be taken. These interventions are, of course, ethically contentious.

Some diseases—for example, diabetes, obesity, alcoholism, migraine, convulsive disorders, and smooth muscle disorders—are affected by genetic factors. Awareness of familial disease patterns can form the basis for preventive education.

GEOGRAPHY

Allergies

The geographic formation of certain areas causes inversion of temperatures or wind conditions, which, combined with the indigenous flora and fauna, will produce symptoms related to allergenic and vasospastic diseases. The high-mortality smogs of Los Angeles and London are good examples.

MENTAL OUTLOOK

Patient attitudes/moods

The negative mental outlook of many people with chronic ill health may be a result of mischance, unknown and complicated factors, or an emotional state commonly known as "the dumps." There is no question that people with a negative body image show a pattern of frequent visits to the doctor. If these individuals could be made more aware of the deleterious effect of mood, their state of health and that of their families might be considerably improved.

MISCHANCE

Accidents

Mischance is one factor the family physician cannot influence. Accidents, whether they involve motor vehicles or quirks of nature, are a variable that explains why the group statistics used in predictive medicine are not entirely accurate. Preventive measures can be of great use but are not infallible. Motor vehicle injuries can be reduced but not eliminated if drivers avoid the consumption of alcohol and mood-altering drugs and if they and all passengers routinely use seat belts. Preventing accidental childhood poisoning by removing detergents and harmful chemicals from the bottom shelf and putting them out of the toddler's reach is another example.

FINANCES

Inability to pay for health services may prevent an individual from following good health practices. Paradoxically, too much money may also lead to poor health practices. For example, individuals who are well-off financially may seek health resources on the basis of their own diagnoses, referring themselves at personal expense to a tertiary care specialist. If the knowledge and understanding of the patient and the physician are adequate, the self-referral approach may work. However, we have found that it results too often in a sequence of needless cross-referrals which end when the physically and financially exhausted patient returns to the family physician or generalist to put it all together.

Costs

Abuse of health services

The negative impact of either too little or too much money on health is most apparent in North American society, where overuse of health resources is sometimes found in the same cities in which the infant mortality rates exceed those of much poorer countries. Some cultures provide health care regardless of the individual's ability to pay, such as the People's Republic of China and Tanzania, where health care is provided to the people through rural health programs. Similar programs exist in North America in the provision of health care to indigenous groups, for example, the Inuit and Indians in Canada and the United States.

EDUCATION

An understanding of health and its continuous maintenance is necessary if we are to avoid the deleterious effects of poor health habits, whether they are physical or result from lifestyle (e.g., smoking, eating to excess, and consuming too much alcohol). In some parts of the world people must learn to avoid streams infected with *Bilharzia*. People everywhere should be made aware of the process of toxin-producing bacterial contamination and its effect on frozen and canned foods. Understanding is the first step in obtaining pa-

Patient education

tient acceptance and willingness to adopt good health habits. (See chapter 40 on Patient Education.)

FAMILY

Family life

A good home and a stable family situation are thought to be important contributors to health. It is well known that some diseases are managed better in the familiar home situation than in a strange institution such as a major city hospital. This is particularly true with elderly patients. It is essential that the principles of primary care and community medicine, where they help to strengthen family life, be used by the family medicine team in planning appropriate patient management.

Seniors

Strong family support, particularly for geriatric and pediatric patients, is a most valuable asset of home care. It has been shown that physical ailments for which intensive care seemed indicated could be managed equally effectively in the home.[3] However, home care can fail unless families are carefully screened before being encouraged to provide care. Where appropriate, home care can be supplemented by the use of institutional care. A good example is long-term care for senior citizens (particularly those who have strong family ties), in which the direction is provided by a personalized program set up by a health institution and involves alternating home care with hospital care.

BALANCE OF HEALTH

Balance

The balance of health is a fragile matter that can be easily tipped in either direction. (See Table 31-1.) The health team must seek ways to ensure a positive direction and attempt to reduce the negative factors in the community.

Table 31-1 The balance of health-promoting and health-depleting factors.

Negative
Poverty
Societal Attitudes
Negative Lifestyles
Genetic Disorders
Poor Environment
Poor Nutrition
Geography
High-Risk Occupation
Poor Home/Family Life

Negative Mental Outlook
Mischance

Positive
Availability of Health Services
Positive Lifestyles
Active Health Protection Program
High Motivation
Strong Community Resources
Strong Family Support
Positive Mental Outlook
Good Fortune

Health status can be defined only in relative terms; it is subject to constant change and is always in a state of positive (health) or negative (disease) balance. Health maintenance is the continuity of a positive balance.

Procedures for maintaining health can be carried out in the office while the physician is seeing a patient for another reason. (See chapter 32, "A Rationale for Early Disease Detection.") It is true that busy family practitioners may have little time, financial incentive, or training for health maintenance procedures. But if this situation were changed by means of education, appropriate financial reward, and office reorganization, there would be no need for alternative health maintenance facilities.

SUMMARY

The family physician's role is to assist the patient in tipping the balance of health toward the positive side. Physicians, especially family physicians, must expand their horizons to take account of the societal factors that affect their patients' health. Effective management requires consideration of the effect of ecology and environment.

REFERENCES

1 Canada, Department of Health & Welfare: *Nutrition—A National Priority,* a report from Nutrition Canada, Ottawa, 1973.
2 C. R. Scriver, J. L. Neal, R. Sheinur, and A. Clow, "The Frequency of Genetic Disease and Congenital Malformations among Patients in a Pediatric Hospital," *Canadian Medical Association Journal,* **108:**1111–1115, 1973.
3 J. D. Hill, J. R. Hampton, and J. R. A. Mitchell, "A Randomized Trial of Home-versus-Hospital Management for Patients with Suspected Myocardial Infarction," *Lancet,* **i:**837–841, 1978.

Chapter 32

A Rationale for Early Disease Detection

D. B. Shires, M.D.

Advanced technologies (including computer technology), new laboratory instruments, well-controlled epidemiologic studies, and a recognition of the concept of health risk identification have led to renewed interest in early disease detection. Some concepts that are basic to our philosophy of health maintenance can help health providers introduce techniques of early disease detection and maintenance of health into their daily practice.

The principal objectives of health maintenance are as follows:

To alert and educate individuals about their roles and responsibilities in maintaining their own health

To detect disease at an early stage and alter its progression

To provide entry into the health care system

To improve health care, especially among socially disadvantaged groups

To gain understanding of disease trends both in populations and in individuals

To make the best use of proven (cost-benefit) techniques

THE VALUE OF CASE FINDING

If an average practitioner decides to use some sort of case-finding protocol in office practice, what kind of yield can he or she expect? Table 32-1 presents an approximation of the number of patients with high-risk factors (such as hypertension, obesity, and alcoholism) and preventable problems (such as some motor vehicle accidents, infectious childhood diseases, and diabetes) that can be expected to occur in the population seen in an average office practice.[1] Since 75 percent of patients with such problems contact the doctor within 1 year and 95 percent do so within 2 years,[2] it is reasonable to suppose that these cases could be detected (case finding) by family physicians in the course of their daily practice.

What to expect

Effective Case Finding in Practice

The literature on screening and case finding reviews the results of a number of double-blind control studies and population surveys; material is also available from federal health protection agencies on the ways in which good health is linked to lifestyle habits. The results of these studies show that there is widespread confusion in the minds of doctors who are interested in both predisease screening and improving the quality of care offered to their patients. Some direction must be provided to practitioners so that they can assess current thinking on what constitutes good clinical practice. Table 32-2 shows disorders for which screening has been shown to be effective, conditions for which further proof of the value of screening is awaited, and conditions for which screening has been shown to be of little value.

Controversy in screening

Effective screening procedure

Table 32-1   Potential Yield from Physician's Office Screening Program

High-risk factors	No. of cases per year	Possible preventable disease	No. of cases per year
Hypertension	150	Childhood infectious diseases	50
Obesity	150	Diabetes	15
Alcoholism	75	Cerebrovascular accidents (CVA)	5
Adjustment reactions (adolescence, menopause, retirement)	50	Myocardial infarcts (MI)	5
		Motor vehicle accidents (MVA)	10
Communication problems (sexual problems)	30	Obstructive lung disease (COLD)	20
		Suicide and attempts	15
High-risk pregnancy	5	Accidental poisoning	5
Trauma	15	Chronic renal disease	5
Anemia	10		

Table 32-2   Effective and Ineffective Screening

Disorders for which screening has been shown to be effective	Procedures that should be maintained awaiting further proof	Procedures that have been shown to have little value
Phenylketonuria	Periodic health examination	Routine chest x-ray
Rhesus incompatibility	High-risk identification (Bodycheck)	Multiphasic biochemical screens
Gestational—bacteriuria, diabetes	Pap smears in high-risk group	Annual physical
High-prevalence TB		Routine sigmoidoscope
Neural tube deformities (α-fetoproteins)	Emotional assessment	Yearly electrocardiogram
Down's—amniocentesis, women over age 37	Perceptual testing in preschoolers	
Diastolic BP over 105	Breast self-examination in all women	
Childhood immunization	Health education	
Trauma—sports equipment, seat belts	Tonometry	
Breast cancer screening by mammography in women over age 50	Counseling parents about accidental child poisoning	
	Hemoglobin at age 1 and in menstruating women	

Source: Canadian Task Force.[3]

PREVENTION IN OFFICE PRACTICE

The family physician needs to know the difference between case finding, screening, and surveys in order to evaluate the literature on the value of preventive strategies. The three terms are defined as follows:

Case finding

Screening

Surveys

Case finding: administering a test, examination, or questionnaire to a patient who is in the physician's office for another reason, e.g., taking the blood pressure of someone who is in your office for a minor respiratory illness.

Screening: establishing a service that invites apparently well (asymptomatic) people to come in for a checkup, e.g., well-women's clinics.

Surveys: programs set up to measure certain parameters of a group defined by geographic, ethnic, age, or other characteristics, e.g., a survey of rubella antibody titers in 11-year-old children.

The cost-effectiveness of screening and surveys is questionable except in the case of research studies conducted to answer specific questions. In fact, there is a possibility that screening can be harmful, either because the treatment given to the asymptomatic patient may be worse than the potential disease or because negative results may give the patient a false sense of security.

Case finding, however, may provide three advantages—cost-effectiveness, clinical usefulness, and patient satisfaction—particularly if Table 2 and the life protocol schema discussed in this book are used as a guide.

SUMMARY

There is considerable controversy about the value of screening in patients with chronic disease. Nevertheless, the identification of precursors, environmental factors, and high-risk situations and the evaluation of lifestyles may help defer the relentless downward progress of an already established disabling disease.

REFERENCES

1 J. N. Barber and F. A. Roddy, *General Practice Medicine*, Churchill-Livingstone, Edinburgh, 1974.
2 *National Health Services Statistical Report*, HM Printers, London, 1975.
3 Canadian Task Force, "The Periodic Health Examination," *Canadian Medical Association Journal*, **31:**1–45, 1979.

Chapter 33

A Prospective Approach to Health Maintenance

D. B. Shires, M.D.

With the knowledge that screening for disease is less productive than initially hoped, efforts have been made over the past 10 years to identify those at risk in particular populations and apply selective screening tests to them. The compilation and computation of risks has resulted in health risk appraisal programs such as Bodycheck, which is described in this chapter. A mechanism for its rationale and implementation is also suggested.

Health maintenance encompasses screening for abnormalities, early detection of disorders that can be alleviated, and prevention of ill health. One problem the family physician faces is how to approach preventive practice.

We suggest the approach of *prospective medicine*,[1] in which risk factors are identified for an individual, a family, or a community. The factors are then grouped together so that a personalized program for health maintenance can be set up before certain abnormalities develop. We think this approach is the most promising one for the future. By refining this technique and combining it with morbidity statistics and fitness risk factors, we can develop a risk appraisal tool suited to the family practitioner: health risk appraisal (HRA).

THE HISTORY OF HEALTH RISK APPRAISAL

The concept of health risk appraisal was initiated by Robbins and Hall in Indianapolis during the early 1960s.[1] Since then, it has been adapted and sometimes modified by a number of groups. The data collected for an individual include lifestyle characteristics, physical measurements, and family history. The results are given to the individual, usually in the form of a computer printout, and provide an individualized analysis of the risks of disease within the next 10 years. Suggestions are then made as to how the risk of various diseases may be reduced.

Bodycheck, which is one version of this approach, uses a patient-oriented protocol based on the work of Harold Colburn[2] of the Health Protection Agency in Ottawa, Canada. Colburn's group took the 1971 Canadian mortality statistics and applied them to the risk factors established for the Canadian population, which were modified from risk factors established for the United States. The group then developed a computer program to identify the risk for an individual patient by peer group, age, and sex.

The concept of the prospective approach is depicted in Figure 33-1, where it is shown how the identification of risks precedes the usual screening procedures that depend on the presence or absence of signs, symptoms, or test abnormalities.

Rationale

Bodycheck

PRIMARY PREVENTION

Most of the research on screening has demonstrated that the presence of signs or symptoms indicates a late stage of disease, a point

Figure 33-1   The concept of predisease risk appraisal.

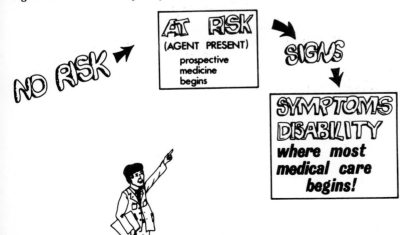

Figure 33-2   Accumulative risk of individual factors in motor vehicle accidents.

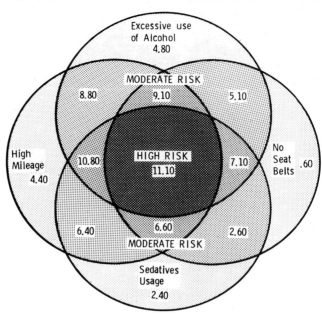

<table>
</table>

at which it is questionable whether the outcome of the specified disease can be materially affected.

Risk detection

By identifying high-risk factors at a much earlier stage, physicians may be able to eliminate or decrease the incidence of some diseases which cause great loss of potentially productive years. A classic example is, of course, cardiovascular disease, which is largely a phenomenon of middle age. Here the identified risk factors are hypertension, obesity, diabetes, sedentary habits, family history, smoking, and lack of exercise, most of which are remediable. The accumulated risks for motor vehicle accidents are illustrated in Figure 33-2.

Advantages of the Prospective Approach

Advantages of lifestyle

The prospective approach has many advantages. Patients develop increased awareness of their own contributions to possible diseases and the deleterious effects of poor daily habits. The personalization of risks and the ranking of the leading causes of death tend to make individuals aware that disease and death do not choose their victims but rather are chosen to a large extent by the individuals themselves. In the prospective approach, health risks are not presented as separate from disease but as interrelated factors that eventually cause disease. The threat of potential illness becomes more real. Individuals are ranked into 5-year age groups and are made aware of the leading causes of death in their group so that health maintenance becomes more personalized. Individuals are free to choose whether they will undertake a program that may minimize the risks of disease.

It is our belief that techniques such as Bodycheck are of special benefit to younger people, whose minds are more flexible. Furthermore, it may be easier to cultivate good lifestyle habits in persons whose bodies have not already been exposed to conditions of health risk for many years. Even though the mortality statistics used in the calculations are crude, representing death statistics and not necessarily morbidity, the concept of the prospective approach to health maintenance has promise and deserves careful consideration for practice.

Target is younger age group

Disadvantages of the Prospective Approach

There are also disadvantages to the prospective approach, including the following.

1 Anxiety may be created in an individual who already has a strong family history of fatal disease or other irreducible factors. (One approach to dealing with such a person is to accentuate good lifestyle habits positively and reinforce the maintenance of health.)

2 There is little hard evidence that the reduction or elimination of high-risk factors will necessarily reduce the risk of a specific disease entity.

3 Groups labeled as high-risk may be discriminated against by insurance companies or employers, just as persons labeled by screening procedures are.

4 Assessments made on the basis of total population risk factors in the United States in the late 1960s may not be appropriate for other populations. There is obviously an urgent need to develop specific risk factors for specific populations. The statistics used in the assessments are crude population and group statistics and therefore must be subject to broad interpretation. Unless this concept is clearly understood, misinterpretations and inappropriate programs to reduce risks may be undertaken.

5 The computer printouts confuse some individuals and therefore may reduce compliance.

The selection of patients will vary with the type of practice. People in the under-35 age group are more receptive to lifestyle change, but their prime risk is motor vehicle accidents, which lessens the importance of using the technique for other preventable chronic diseases. For people under 35, one might use the data for the 45 age group in order to demonstrate the possible future results of their risk-taking behavior.

Strategies for improving compliance

Figure 33-3 Bodycheck input forms.

BODYCHECK
(Health Hazard Appraisal)
Fenwick Place
5599 Fenwick Street
Halifax, Nova Scotia
B3H 1R2

NAME:
HEALTH I.D. NUMBER
HEALTH PROFESSIONAL _____ R.N.
M.D.
Address: _____
City: _____

PLEASE RECORD THE MOST APPROPRIATE RESPONSE BY WRITING THE CODE NUMBER IN THE COLUMN ON THE RIGHT HAND SIDE OF THE PAGE.

TO BE COMPLETED BY ALL PATIENTS ————————— RECORD ALL ANSWERS IN THIS COLUMN —————

SEX	(1) male	(2) female
AGE	(in years)	
HEIGHT (without shoes)	(centimeters) or (feet & inches)	cm
WEIGHT (naked)	(kilograms) or (pounds)	kg / lb

ALCOHOL HABITS (average number of drinks per week including beer, wine, aperitifs and hard liquor)
(1) 41 or more   (2) 25-40   (3) 7-24
(4) 3-6   (5) 1-2   (6) stopped
(7) never drank

SERIOUS DEPRESSION (i.e. disabling)   (1) often   (2) seldom or never

SMOKER
(mark the number for current habits or heaviest amount smoked in last 5 years)
(If cigarettes and pipes/cigars, mark only code for cigarettes)

QUIT SMOKING LESS THAN 10 YRS. AGO (mark the number for heaviest amount smoked in year before quitting)

CIGARETTES-PACKS PER DAY
1) 2 plus
2) 1-2
3) ½-1
4) ½ or less

PIPES/CIGARS-NUMBER/DAY
5) 5 plus or any inhaled
6) 4 or less not inhaled

NON-SMOKER OR QUIT SMOKING FOR MORE THAN 10 YEARS
mark 7. do not smoke

STOPPED SMOKING   mark number of years stopped
OR mark "O"
{ If still smoking
{ If non smoker
{ If stopped more than 10 years

MILES DRIVEN PER YEAR AS DRIVER AND/OR AUTOMOBILE PASSENGER (in thousands of miles)

SEAT BELT USE % of time in automobile
(1) seldom or never   (3) 25-75%
(2) 10-24%   (4) almost always

EXERCISE (including work and leisure activities)
(1) No deliberate activity to improve my physical fitness
(2) Occasional moderate activity (walking, jogging, calisthenics, cycling, tennis, recreational sports, swimming etc.) but not on a regular basis
(3) Regular moderate activity (some as above) but averaging 2-3 sessions per week
(4) Very Frequent regular activity (same as above) but averaging 4-5 sessions per week.

HEART ATTACK
Natural Parents Died of Heart Attack before age 60
(1) both parents
(2) one parent

Natural Parents Died under age 60 (of other causes) or still Alive Below age 60
(3)

None of these
(4)

FAMILY HISTORY OF SUICIDE (mother, father, sister, brother)   (1) yes   (2) no

FAMILY HISTORY OF DIABETES (mother, father, sister, brother, child)   (1) yes   (2) no

DO YOU HAVE DIABETES?   (1) yes-no treatment   (2) yes-under treatment   (3) no

RECTAL DISORDERS (history of disease other than hemorrhoids)
Growth   (1) yes   (2) no
Bleeding   (1) yes   (2) no

HAS YOUR PHYSICIAN EVER SAID YOU HAVE chronic bronchitis and/or emphysema?   (1) yes   (2) no

Figure 33-3   Continued

BODYCHECK

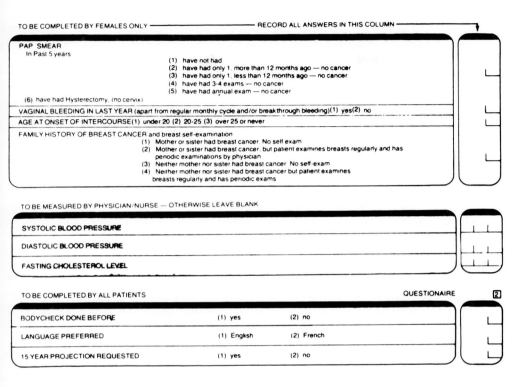

TO BE COMPLETED BY FEMALES ONLY ——————————— RECORD ALL ANSWERS IN THIS COLUMN ——

PAP SMEAR
In Past 5 years
 (1) have not had
 (2) have had only 1, more than 12 months ago — no cancer
 (3) have had only 1, less than 12 months ago — no cancer
 (4) have had 3-4 exams — no cancer
 (5) have had annual exam — no cancer
(6) have had Hysterectomy, (no cervix)

VAGINAL BLEEDING IN LAST YEAR (apart from regular monthly cycle and/or breakthrough bleeding)(1) yes(2) no

AGE AT ONSET OF INTERCOURSE(1) under 20 (2) 20-25 (3) over 25 or never

FAMILY HISTORY OF BREAST CANCER and breast self-examination
 (1) Mother or sister had breast cancer. No self exam
 (2) Mother or sister had breast cancer, but patient examines breasts regularly and has
   periodic examinations by physician
 (3) Neither mother nor sister had breast cancer. No self-exam
 (4) Neither mother nor sister had breast cancer but patient examines
   breasts regularly and has periodic exams

TO BE MEASURED BY PHYSICIAN/NURSE — OTHERWISE LEAVE BLANK

SYSTOLIC BLOOD PRESSURE

DIASTOLIC BLOOD PRESSURE

FASTING CHOLESTEROL LEVEL

TO BE COMPLETED BY ALL PATIENTS   QUESTIONAIRE 2

BODYCHECK DONE BEFORE   (1) yes   (2) no

LANGUAGE PREFERRED   (1) English (2) French

15 YEAR PROJECTION REQUESTED (1) yes   (2) no

MECHANICS OF BODYCHECK

The completed input forms used in Bodycheck or HRA (see Figure 33-3) are mailed from the physician's office and are then processed by computer. As with many laboratory tests, the results are returned to the physician in time for the patient's next appointment. Thus, the doctor will have the results of the risk appraisal available to review with the patient during the periodic selective health screening examination.

Sequence of analysis

The forms require data from both the patient and a health professional, and it may be reasonable to suggest that these forms be completed at the same time so that comparisons can be made. It should be noted that the data do not necessarily have to be collected by a physician; a well-trained nurse, receptionist, or health educator can perform this task.

Explanation of results

The data returned to the doctor's office include the following.

Figure 33-4 Bodycheck—graphic display of individual risks.

```
                              HEALTH AND WELFARE CANADA - SMOKING & HEALTH
SUBMITTED BY- JUNIOR RISKO           - - - B O D Y C H E C K - - -(MARS VERSION 2.0)            FILE NO-    1
DATE-  78/05/17.****DR. A. P. PRAISED
*****

                    (((((( 1 5   Y E A R   P R O J E C T I O N ))))))

            THE RISK REGISTRY DATA HAVE BEEN ANALYSED AND THE RESULTS ARE SUMMARIZED BELOW
            AS THEY RELATE TO THE 12 MOST FREQUENT CAUSES OF DEATH FOR MALES AGED 55.

            THE AVERAGE RISK IS THE NUMBER OF CHANCES A PERSON OF YOUR AGE AND SEX HAS OF
            DYING IN WITHIN THE NEXT 10 YEARS OF SPECIFIC CAUSES,PER EVERY 100,000 CNDNS.

            THE APPRAISED RISK IS THE NUMBER OF CHANCES   Y O U   HAVE OF DYING WITHIN THE
            NEXT 10 YEARS IF YOU CONTINUE TO FOLLOW THE SAME LIFESTYLE.

            THE ACHIEVABLE AGE IS THE REDUCED NUMBER OF CHANCES OF DYING IN THE NEXT 10
            YEARS IF ??   Y O U   C H A N G E   YOUR LIFESTYLE AS SUGGESTED.

            ACTUAL AGE 55          APPRAISED AGE 61.4        ACHIEVABLE 53.4
```

CAUSE OF DEATH	CHANCES OF DYING PER 100,000			APPRAISAL GRAPH
	AVERAGE RISK	APPRAISED RISK	ACHEIVABLE RISK	

```
                                                    0      1      2      3      4      5      6
                                                    +..........+..........+..........+..........+..........+..........+
                                                    +          +
HEART ATTACK                6811      15052     4303  +-------WWWEEEEEEEEEEESSSS
                                                    +-------WWWEEEEEEEEEEESSSS
                                                    +-------WWWEEEEEEEEEEESSSS
                                                    +-------WWWEEEEEEEEEEESSSS
                                                    +-------WWWEEEEEEEEEEESSSS
                                                    +-------WWWEEEEEEEEEEESSSS
                                                    +-------WWWEEEEEEEEEEESSSS
                                                    +-------WWWEEEEEEEEEEESSSS
                                                    +-------WWWEEEEEEEEEEESSSS
                                                    +-------WWWEEEEEEEEEEESSSS
                                                    +-------WWWEEEEEEEEEEESSSS
                                                    +-------WWWLEEEEEEEEEESSSS
                                                    +-------WWWEEEEEEEEEEESSSS
                                                    +-------WWWEEEEEEEEEEESSSS
                                                    +-------WWWEEEEEEEEEEESSSS
                                                    +-------WWWEEEEEEEEEEESSSS
                                                    +-------WWWEEEEEEEEEEESSSS
                                                    +-------WWWEEEEEEEEEEESSSS
                                                    +-------WWWEEEEEEEEEEESSSS
                                                    +-------WWWEEEEEEEEEEESSSS
                                                    +          +
LUNG CANCER                 1484      2671      2136  +---------------SSSS
                                                    +---------------SSSS
                                                    +---------------SSSS
                                                    +---------------SSSS
                                                    +          +
STROKE                      931       993       806  +---------SS
                                                    +---------SS
                                                    +---------SS
                                                    +          +
INTESTINAL CANCER INCL. RECTUM   533   399       349  +--------- +
CHRONIC BRONCHITIS AND EMPHYSEMA  521   937       656  +-------------SSSSSS
CIRRHOSIS OF LIVER          390       780       390  +----------AAAAAAAAAA
DISEASES OF ARTERIES ARTER. CAPS  355   378       307  +----------SS
MOTOR VEHICLE ACCIDENTS     330       989       593  +-----------------AAAAAAAAAABB
SUICIDE                     305       305       305  +----------
DIABETES                    267       299       153  +-------WWWWWW
                                                    +          +
                                                    +..........+..........+..........+..........+..........+..........+
```

```
LEGEND..A =  ALCOHOL         B = SEATBELT        H =  BP-SYST         M =  BP-DIAS         C =  SELF-EXM
        D =  DIABETES        W =  WEIGHT         E =  EXERCISE        S =  SMOKING         Y =  PAPSMEAR
        C =  SELF-EXM
```

1 A bar graph that can be used to discuss reducible and non-reducible risk factors with the patient. This graph may be detached from the remaining part of the computer printout and handed to the patient during the selective screening examination. (See Figure 33-4.)

2 Statistical tables depicting the mortality information based on specific tables for the patient's age and sex as well as compliance ratios, etc. This should be detached from the rest of the computer printout and stored with the patient's chart. (See Figure 33-5.)

3 A computer-generated letter. This may be kept by the physician, who will then have the option of either signing the letter and mailing it or asking the receptionist to type it on the doctor's own stationery. The letter may help reinforce the advice given by the physician when the patient receives it in the mail several days later. (See Figure 33-6.)

A suggested schedule for implementing a Bodycheck-type program is as follows.

Four weeks prior to the annual selective screening physical examination, the nurse does the following:

Suggest schedule

Weighs the patient
Measures blood pressure
Collects blood for cholesterol check
Records information on the Bodycheck form

Two weeks prior to the annual physical examination, the remaining information on the Bodycheck form is completed by the patient and mailed to the computer center.

At the annual physical examination, the doctor or nurse does the following:

Reviews the Bodycheck printouts
Detaches the statistical table and files it with the patient's chart
Tears off the bar graph output and writes comments, which are then handed to the patient
Signs the computer-generated letter, which may then be mailed to the patient or given to the receptionist to type on the physician's stationery

Many techniques are used in risk reduction programs, and several documented patient-oriented materials, for example, Risko[3] (Michigan Heart Foundation), are available from Canadian and American manufacturers. The choice of program will vary according to the type of practice and the resources available in the community. However, many of the programs are simple enough to be administered by a single individual, family group, or community.

Other office risk assessments

Figure 33-5   Computer-generated mortality risk table.

* * * DETAIL * * *   FILE NO- 1

CAUSE OF DEATH	CONTRIB. CHARACTER.	APPRAISAL			COMPLIANCE		
		AS SUBMITTED	ACTUAL COMPO. RISK	RISK	AS COMPLIED	APPLIED COMPO. RISK	RISK
HEART ATTACK	BL.PRESS	135/ 90	.7/1.0		135/ 90	.7/1.0	
	CHOLESTR	220-279	1.0		220-279	1.0	
	DIABETES	NOT DIABETIC	1.0		NOT DIABETIC	1.0	
	WEIGHT	195	1.1		163	.9	
	EXERCISE	NO DELIBERATE ACT.	2.5		EXERCISE PROGRAM	1.0	
	SMOKING	STILL SMOKES 20+	1.5		STOPPED SMOKING	.7	
	FH/HEART	NO	.9	3.00	NO	.9	.55
MOTOR VEHICLE ACCIDENTS	ALCOHOL	7-24/WEEK	2.0		3-6/WEEK	1.0	
	MIL/YEAR	20000	2.0		20000	2.0	
	SEATBELT	10-24 %	1.0	3.00	ALMOST ALWAYS	.8	1.80
SUICIDE	DEPRESS	SELDOM OR NEVER	1.0		SELDOM OR NEVER	1.0	
	FH/SUICD	NO	1.0	1.00	NO	1.0	1.00
LUNG CANCER	SMOKING	STILL SMOKES 20+	1.5	1.50	STOPPED SMOKING	1.2	1.20
CIRRHOSIS OF LIVER	ALCOHOL	7-24/WEEK	2.0	2.00	3-6/WEEK	1.0	1.00
STROKE	BL.PRESS	135/ 90	.7/1.0		135/ 90	.7/1.0	
	CHOLESTR	220-279	1.0		220-279	1.0	
	DIABETES	NOT DIABETIC	1.0		NOT DIABETIC	1.0	
	SMOKING	STILL SMOKES 20+	1.2	1.17	STOPPED SMOKING	1.0	.97
INTESTINAL CANCER INCL. RECTUM	POLYP	HAS HAD	2.5		HAS HAD	2.5	
	RCTBLOOD	NO BLOOD IN STOOL	1.0	.75	NO BLOOD IN STOOL	1.0	.75

* RISK FACTORS ADAPTED FROM [HOW TO PRACTICE PROSPECTIVE MEDICINE(, DRS. ROBBINS AND HALL, METHODIST HOSPITAL OF INDIANA.

** LUNG CANCER RISK DECREASES STEADILY AND REACHES NON SMOKER LEVEL 10 YEARS AFTER STOPPING.

FOR HEIGHT 71 INCHES,195 LBS. IS APPROXIMATELY 24 % OVERWEIGHT - - - DESIRABLE WEIGHT IS 157 LBS.

- - - COMPLIANCE - - -

EXERCISE FROM-	NO DELIBERATE ACT. TO-	EXERCISE PROGRAM
SMOKING FROM-	STILL SMOKES 20+ TO-	STOPPED SMOKING
ALCOHOL FROM-	7-24/WEEK TO-	3-6/WEEK
WEIGHT FROM-	195 LBS. TO-	163LBS.
SEATBELT FROM-	10-24 % TO-	ALMOST ALWAYS

THE ACHIEVABLE CHANCES OF DYING ARE BASED UPON THE ASSUMPTION THAT FACTOR(S) ARE MODIFIED AS FOLLOWS-

Figure 33-6 Computer-generated physician's letter.

```
DEAR JUNIOR RISKO

     I HAVE REVIEWED YOUR BODYCHECK REPORT AND WANT TO SUMMARIZE
YOUR HEALTH RISK AGAIN.YOUR APPRAISED AGE IS NOT AS LOW AS THE
REPORT SHOWS YOU CAN GET IT.THIS MEANS YOU HAVE A GREATER RISK OF
DYING IN THE NEXT 10 YEARS THAN IS NECESSARY.

     THE FOLLOWING ARE THE MOST PROBABLE CAUSES OF DEATH WHICH
YOU CAN AFFECT BY CHANGES IN YOUR LIFESTYLE.


          1.HEART ATTACK

          2.MOTOR VEHICLE ACCIDENTS

          3.LUNG CANCER

          4.CIRRHOSIS OF LIVER

          5.STROKE


     IF YOU IMPROVE YOUR LIFE PATTERN,YOU COULD LOWER YOUR
HEALTH RISKS.MY RECOMMENDATIONS FOR YOU ARE,IN ORDER OF RELATIVE
IMPORTANCE.

     EXERCISE FROM-    NO DELIBERATE ACT. TO-    EXERCISE PROGRAM
     SMOKING FROM-     STILL SMOKES 20+ TO-      STOPPED SMOKING
     ALCOHOL FROM-     7-24/WEEK TO-             3-6/WEEK
     WEIGHT FROM-      195 LBS. TO-              163LBS.
     SEATBELT FROM-    10-24 % TO-               ALMOST ALWAYS

     I SUGGEST THAT YOU WORK ON THE FIRST RECOMMENDATION AND AS
MANY OTHER CHANGES AS YOU FEEL YOU ARE ABLE TO HANDLE AT ONCE.


     PLEASE REMEMBER THAT THIS IS A STATISTICAL ANALYSIS OF YOUR
HEALTH RISKS AND SHOULD ONLY BE USED TO POINT OUT AREAS OF CON-
CERN.I SINCERELY HOPE YOU HAVE LEARNED SOMETHING ABOUT YOUR LIFE-
STYLE FROM THIS PERSONALIZED REPORT.IF YOU HAVE ANY FURTHER QUES-
TIONS ABOUT YOUR HEALTH RISKS OR GENERAL HEALTH,FEEL FREE TO CON-
TACT ME.

               YOURS SINCERELY,

                    DR. A. P. PRAISED
```

Future potential

What is lacking in all current risk-assessment programs is an assessment of morbidity rather than mortality and the ability to detect high-risk emotional problems such as adjustment reactions and potential or actual problems of communication.

SUMMARY

Health risk appraisal programs such as Bodycheck are gaining increasing acceptance. Bodycheck is relatively simple to institute in the physician's office and can be accomplished with already available office help. It is supported by current concepts of preventive medicine that advocate lifestyle and risk assessment and is in tune with the thinking of the federal governments in both the United States and Canada, which consider lifestyle as a major element affecting health.

REFERENCES

1 L. C. Robbins and C. Hall, *How to Practice Prospective Medicine,* Slaymaker Enterprises, Indianapolis, Ind., 1970.
2 H. N. Colburn and P. M. Baker, "Health Hazard Appraisal—a Possible Tool in Health Protection and Promotion," *Canadian Journal of Public Health,* **64:** 490–492, 1970.
3 Risko: See D. Woods, "Two Epidemiologists Discuss Myths and Realities and Health Maintenance," *Canadian Medical Association Journal,* **109:**1146–1155, 1973.

Chapter 34

Life Protocols: A Schema for Health Maintenance

D. B. Shires, M.D.

The need for protection from proven health hazards such as infectious disease, lifestyle hazards, and occupational hazards requires that family practitioners use a prescribed framework to plan health maintenance for their patients. This chapter deals with the problem on a chronological basis and outlines a series of age sets for which appropriate health maintenance procedures are suggested.

This chapter presents a rationale for a health maintenance program and suggests protocols for groups from before birth to old age. (See Tables 34-1 and 34-2.) These protocols are in no way meant to be cast in concrete; they are merely guidelines that may be considered by a physician who is contemplating the establishment of a health maintenance program.[1,4]

PREBIRTH

Some of the most dramatic achievements of modern medicine have been wrought in the womb. The almost complete eradication of Rhesus isoimmunization by sophisticated antibody detection methods and by the use of Rhesus antibody (RhoGAM) has been a major

Rh disease

Table 34-1 Life Protocol for Health Maintenance: A Schema for Noncrisis Visits—Prebirth, Preschoolers, and School-Agers

Age or interval	Test or procedure
Prebirth	
Fetus	Family and maternal history for potential high-risk delivery, e.g. rubella, Rhesus isoimmunization
Less than 15 weeks' gestation	Amniocentesis for chromosomal analysis, sex typing, blood grouping biochemical tests (where indicated) Ultrasound if indicated
Prenatal (monthly)	Family-life education Regular measurements of prenatal development using standard flowchart Urinalysis
Preschoolers (0 to 5 years)	
Newborn	Full physical examination including rectal, hips, physical measurments; hemoglobin after 48 hours; phenylketonuria; silver nitrate to eyes; vitamin K injection; T_4 test Encourage infant bonding
6 weeks	Repeat physical examination including cardiac and physical measurements; counsel as to feeding, paternal and maternal health Encourage motor vehicle child seat restraints
3 months	Reinforce counseling to parents; begin Denver Grid behavioral assessment; start diphtheria, pertussis, tetanus, oral polio (DPT) Eye examination for strabismus
4 months	Second DPT plus polio
6 months	Third DPT plus polio; physical measurements and Denver assessment
10 months	TB test (with PPD) ~ risk; lead level ~ risk
12 months	Repeat measurements and Denver assessment; hemoglobin ~ risk; measles, mumps, rubella (MMR); antipoison counseling; nutritional guidance
18 months	DPT plus polio booster, repeat booster, physical measurements, and Denver assessment
2 years	Physical examination; counseling to parents regarding normality; encouragement of seat belt use; dental care
5 years	Perceptual screening, behavioral assessment, physical measurements, DPT plus polio booster, blood pressure, dental care, urinalysis Eye examination for strabismus

Table 34-1   Continued

Age or interval	Test or procedure
School-agers (6 to 16 years)	
8 years	Physical measurements, check immunizations, screen for learning problems, measure blood pressure
12 years	Physical measurements, health education, lifestyle risk assessment, nutrition, sexuality, puberty and adolescence, rubella antibody titer in females, annual dental examination

Table 34-2   Life Protocol for Health Maintenance: A Schema for Noncrisis Visits—Young Adults, the Middle-Aged, and Seniors

Interval	Test
Young adults (17 to 38 years)	
6 months, annual, or biannual	Pap smear and pelvic examination in females; breast examination in females; testicular examination in males; family and sexual education; premarital counseling; dental examination
Annual	Hemoglobin in females; health risk assessment and life-style counseling; blood pressure; reinforce oral hygiene
5 years	Behavioral assessments; tetanus and polio
10 years	Tetanus and oral polio
The middle-aged (38 to 55 years)	
6 months, annual, or biannual	Hemoglobin; breast examination; Pap smear and pelvic examination in females; testicular examination in males
Annual	Counseling; preretirement, menopause in females, identity crisis in male; health risk assessment; selective physical examination including blood pressure, tonometry, and rectal examination; dental examination
10 years	Tetanus and oral polio
Seniors (56 years and over)	
Annual	Pap smear and pelvic examination, breast examination in females; physical including nutrition and podiatry, social and health maintenance; retirement planning; counseling and anticipatory guidance; influenza shots; dental care; blood pressure
2 years	Examine for hypothyroidism in postmenopausal women
10 years	Tetanus and oral polio

High-risk
pregnancy

Amniocentesis

Family-life
education

triumph of obstetrics and neonatology. The identification of high-risk pregnancy has resulted in increased fetal survival. Rubella vaccine given to non-pregnant women can eradicate the possibility of a deformed child in a rubella-exposed, susceptible mother. Amniocentesis and developments in microchemistry, chromatography, and cytogenetics allow us to detect many abnormalities in the developing fetus which may lead to intervention.

Equally important are those aspects of family-life education that deal with the family's understanding of the impact of parenthood. Although we generally recognize sibling rivalry, we tend to underestimate father rivalry and other emotional problems that take place in the family. These questions should all be raised well before delivery in order to prevent or control such problems.

PRESCHOOLERS (0 to 5 years)

PKU

6 weeks

3 months

Immunizations

The newborn examination is well described in obstetric, neonatologic, and pediatric textbooks, and we shall not elaborate on it except to stress the importance of a thorough examination. It has also been shown that screening for phenylketonuria (PKU) is a valid cost-benefit procedure that deserves routine inclusion. Although its validity is not well established, the postbirth hemoglobin test is useful in the newborn period if it is done after the hemodilution phase has been accomplished.

Conducting a 6-week examination to establish baseline physical measurements and to detect murmurs not apparent in the neonatal period is a wise practice; the prudent family physician will use this opportunity to assess not only the child but also the coping mechanisms of the mother and family. Infant bonding should be assessed.

When a child is 3 months old, one should begin the immunization schedule and also undertake a behavioral and physical assessment using the Denver Grid and other growth and development protocols. Again, the opportunity to assess the whole family should not be overlooked. The second and third triple vaccine or quad boosters should be given at 4 and 6 months of age. At 10 months, a screening test for tuberculosis should be done. The current suggestion is a Mantoux test using purified protein derivative (PPD) as an antigen in place of old tuberculin (OT). At 12 months, the physical measurements using the Denver Grid and behavioral assessment should be repeated and a hemoglobin should be done (preferably using an electronic counting method, a hematocrit, or both) for those at high risk because of prematurity, poor socioeconomic circumstances, or intrauterine-perinatal problems. At about 14 months, the measles, mumps, rubella (MMR) vaccine should be given. Before the child reaches the crawling stage, accidental poison prevention should be discussed with the parents, who should then be given a simple emergency poison handbook and the telephone number of a poison control center or even an emergency kit with a universal antidote and an emetic. One year of age is also the time to investigate any risks of impending or actual child abuse and take corrective action. Parents should be cautioned about the high risk of bicycle accidents in the under-5 age group. The use of motor vehicle child seat restraints should be encouraged.

Poisoning prevention

Child abuse

Trauma

    When the child reaches 18 months, the physician should reinforce any counseling action already taken, although in most cases this will not be necessary. At this time a triple vaccine or quad booster should be given, and physical measurements and the Denver Grid assessment should be repeated.

    The age of 2 years is a difficult stage in a child's behavioral development, and parents, particularly first-time parents, need reassurance that the child's development is normal. A gentle physical examination of a well child at this time will provide both physician and child with an opportunity to get to know each other and should lead to an easier relationship later.

Reassurance

    Around 4 years of age is a good time for the first dental visit.

    At 5 years (preschool), perceptual development (hearing and seeing) and intellectual abilities should be assessed for the purpose of detecting potential learning disabilities. Another triple or quad booster should be given; in addition, the blood pressure should be taken, using a pediatric cuff, and recorded on the chart. Urinalysis to detect asymptomatic bacteriuria is helpful at this time. Eye examination for strabismus should be done at 2 to 4 months and again before the child starts school.

Dental care
Perceptual disorders

SCHOOL-AGERS (6 to 16 years)

The child's emotional and learning capabilities should be reevaluated after 2 to 3 years at school, at about age 8. The annual or "camp" physical should be discouraged, but particular attention should be paid to any child who is considered at risk. Blood pressure should be recorded.

At-risk assessments

    Twelve years of age is an excellent time to reassess physical development and reestablish a good interpersonal relationship with the adolescent. Good rapport is needed to provide health education in the areas of lifestyle risk assessment, nutrition, sexuality, puberty, and adolescence; indicate your openness to further discussions should these be necessary.

Adolescent anticipatory guidance

    At this time, girls will require a rubella antibody titer. If it is below an acceptable level (1:16), the advisability of rubella immunization should be discussed. At this age, it may not be too early to

Rubella

raise questions of sexuality, contraception, and so forth for children of both sexes.

An annual dental examination in early adolescence should be encouraged.

YOUNG ADULTS (17 to 38 years)

Preventive
health
counseling

Bodycheck

Pelvic exam

Periodic health
exam

Young adult females are among the most frequent visitors to the family physician's office, and this group is probably the most susceptible to health maintenance counseling. Recent evidence provided by the Canadian Task Force on Gynecological Cancer[2] suggests that a pelvic examination and Pap smear should be performed every 6 months in a high-risk woman and every 2 to 3 years in a low-risk woman. Breast self-examination on a monthly basis should be taught and should be practiced at every visit to the physician. However, the idea that the pelvic examination provides an excellent opportunity to discuss intimate problems with young female adults seems to us invalid. If such problems have not been discussed before, bringing them up during the examination will only embarrass the patient and may even dissuade her from any kind of communication. Testicular examination should be done in men.

Premarital counseling provides an excellent opportunity to get to know both partners, deal with health questions, and build a lasting bond with the new family.

The periodic health examination, if it is considered appropriate, should include a blood pressure reading, a hemoglobin test in women, and a lifestyle assessment as well as dental advice. A biannual visit to the dentist should be encouraged.

Giving a polio-tetanus booster every 10 years is good practice.

THE MIDDLE-AGED (39 to 55 years)

Family and
individual crisis
anticipation

As in the young adult female, the pelvic and Pap examination should be done periodically in middle-aged women according to risk assessment. In this age group, one should begin to look selectively for warning signals of the identity crisis of the early forties in men and menopausal problems in women. Plans for retirement should be discussed, and appropriate counseling should be sought. The periodic physical should include blood pressure, tonometry, and rectal examination, particularly in men over 40. Men should also have a testicular examination.

Dental care should not be forgotten.

Again, giving a booster of tetanus and polio every 10 years is a wise precaution.

SENIORS (56 years and over)

Unless other evidence is present, it is probably unnecessary to persist with the Pap smear for women over 60. A regular protocol of breast self-examination is far more important, and an abnormality at this age must be carefully evaluated. Influenza shots and dental care should be provided as required. Postmenopausal women in particular should be examined for hypothyroidism.

Additional causes of concern for this age group are foot problems and nutrition. Some studies have shown that at least 50 percent of people over age 60 have correctable foot problems.[3] The tetanus and polio booster should still be continued.

Social and general health counseling is vital, and anticipatory guidance to avoid the crisis of retirement is important. Probably the most valuable health maintenance the physician can provide to patients in this age group is interest in and concern for their well-being; a friendly visit with the doctor is as good as any tonic.

Encourage regular visits

REFERENCES

1 L. Breslow and A. R. Somers, "The Lifetime Health-Monitoring Program: A Practical Approach to Preventive Medicine," *New England Journal of Medicine,* **296:**601–611, 1977.
2 J. Walton, "Cervical Cancer Screening Programs" (DNH & W of Canada Report), *Canadian Medical Association Journal,* **114:**1003, 1976.
3 G. F. Adams, *Essentials of Geriatric Medicine,* Oxford University Press, Oxford, United Kingdom, 1977.
4 College of Family Physicians of Canada, Toronto, Ontario, Canada, "Health Maintenance Guide," 1983.

Chapter 35

Nutrition in Family Practice

S. E. Dyer, B.Sc., P.Dt.

Many current health problems in North America are a reflection of a lifestyle characterized by sedentary living, overeating, and poor dietary habits. Since modern transportation, storage, and technology have made a wide variety of foods available year-round, people are faced with having to make wise food choices to foster good health. They are influenced by high-pressure advertising, a vast amount of confusing and conflicting advice in popular books and magazines, and their own schedules, which leave little time for meal preparation and eating at home, leading to a greater reliance on snacks, fast foods, and convenience foods. This style of eating may contribute to an increased risk of developing chronic diseases such as atherosclerosis, diabetes, and some forms of cancer. In recent years, the role of nutrition as a means of promoting health and delaying and/or preventing the onset of chronic disease has begun to be appreciated.

To realize fully the potential role of nutrition in family practice, the family physician must have a good understanding of normal nutrition throughout the life cycle, be able to anticipate and identify the need for nutritional intervention, provide basic preventive dietary counseling, and where more complex nutritional problems exist, refer patients to professional dietitians or nutritionists.

CASE STUDY

Mrs. Young is a white 70-year-old widow who has continued to maintain the family home since her husband died 3 years ago. Although her two children are busy raising their own families in another community, they still manage to visit once a month. Mrs. Young fell and fractured a hip as she was bringing groceries into the house. A hip replacement was considered necessary. At the hospital, Mrs. Young was diagnosed as having osteoporosis. The medical history revealed a total hysterectomy at age 43 and two bouts of nephrolithiasis. Questioning revealed the following relevant facts: not physically active; calcium intake averaging 400 mg a day, mainly from milk in beverages and on cereal; six to eight cups of coffee a day; one-half pack of cigarettes a day; always weight- and diet-conscious.

1 How long will she be hospitalized? Who will look after her house? Who will pay for the hospitalization? Will she require nursing care when she goes home?

2 How long will she be immobilized? Will immobilization cause further medical problems (e.g., increased risk of thrombosis, pulmonary disease, loss of lean body mass)?

3 What are her chances of making a full recovery medically or financially? Can she maintain her home? Her independence?

Questions the family physician must answer

NUTRITION RECOMMENDATIONS

As a basis for providing information on nutrition to patients, physicians should be familiar with federal nutrition recommendations.[1,2] These recommendations have been designed to maintain and improve the health of the general population and to reduce the risks associated with poor health and illness. They are not a replacement for special diets that may be required in the treatment of a particular disease or condition (see Table 35-1).

Canada's Food Guide[3] and *Food for Fitness*[4] are plans which enable individuals to meet their nutrient needs by following a simple daily food pattern based on four food groups. Table 35-2 provides a

Food guides

Table 35-1 Nutrition Recommendations

1 Consume a nutritionally adequate diet as outlined in the food guides.

2 Reduce fat in the diet to 35 percent of total energy intake. At the same time, include a source of polyunsaturated fat.

3 Consume a diet that emphasizes whole grains, fruits, and vegetables and minimizes alcohol, salt, and refined sugars.

4 Prevent and control obesity by reducing excessive consumption of food and increasing physical activity.

Table 35-2   Daily Food Guide

Food group	Key nutrients	Family needs, no. of servings — All members	Pregnancy needs, no. of servings — 13–15 years	16–35 years	Examples of one serving
Milk and milk products	Calcium, protein, vitamins A, D, B_6, B_{12}, riboflavin	Child, 2–3 Adolescent, 3–4 Adult, 2	5	4	250 ml (1 cup) milk 175 ml (¾ cup) yogurt 45 g (1½ oz) cheese
Fruits and vegetables	Vitamins A and C, folic acid	4–5	5	5	125 ml (½ cup) fruits or vegetables 125 ml (½ cup) juice
Meat and meat alternatives	Protein, iron, thiamine, niacin, riboflavin, B_6, B_{12}, folic acid	2	2	2	60–90 g (2–3 oz) cooked meat, fish or poultry 60 ml (4 tablespoons) peanut butter 250 ml (1 cup) cooked dried peas, beans, or lentils 125 ml (½ cup) nuts or seeds 60 g (2 oz) cheddar cheese 2 eggs
Breads and cereals	Iron, thiamin, niacin, riboflavin, B_6	3–5	5	5	1 slice of bread 125 ml (½ cup) cooked cereal 175 ml (¾ cup) ready-to-eat cereal 125 ml to 175 ml (½ to ¾ cup) cooked rice or pasta

summary of the food guides. They are designed for healthy individuals of all ages except infants. The central themes of the food guides include the following.

Variety: A widely varied diet increases the probability of receiving all essential nutrients.
Moderation: Cut down, not out.
Energy balance: Balance intake with expenditure.

The food guides provide about 4000 to 6000 kJ (1000 to 1400 kcal) per day, which makes them a good basic guide for weight reduction. The key to the food guides lies in the recommended numbers and sizes of daily servings from each food group. The guides provide a range in the number and size of servings that allows for variations in personal nutrient, energy, and lifestyle needs. People with greater energy requirements can meet their needs by increasing the number and size of servings or by adding other foods. The food guides are quite useful as an educational tool, and by comparing an individual's food intake with that recommended in the food guide, they also provide a rapid screening device for assessment of diet.

Canada's Food Guide and *Food for Fitness* are based respectively on the *Recommended Nutrient Intakes for Canadians,* or RNI (1983),[5] and the *Recommended Dietary Allowances,* or RDA (revised in 1980).[6] These standards describe the recommended intake of nutrients and the average energy requirements necessary for maintaining health in already healthy individuals; they are not designed to cover therapeutic needs. Individual variability is taken into account. Because the RNI and the RDA meet the needs of practically all persons, they exceed the minimum requirements of most individuals. An intake below the standard does not mean that an individual has failed to meet his or her requirement, but the further the intake falls below the standard, the greater the probability that this will be the case.

Deviations from the recommended intake are significant only in terms of an individual's total health status, which must also include evaluation of biochemical, clinical, and anthropometric measurements. With this in mind, the following section examines nutritional concerns at various stages throughout the life cycle.

Basic requirements

NUTRITION CONCERNS DURING PREGNANCY

Requirements for almost all nutrients, in particular for protein, calcium, phosphorus, iron, and folic acid, increase during pregnancy. The increase in energy requirements is not large by comparison: an additional 400 kJ (100 kcal) in the first trimester and 1200 kJ (300 kcal) in the second and third trimesters. Therefore, the nutrient density (i.e., nutrient quality) of the diet must be stressed.

Prenatals identified as being at high risk on the basis of current nutritional status and diet history should be referred to a professional dietitian for nutritional counseling. (See chapter 16 on "High-Risk Pregnancies.")

The *recommended weight gain* during pregnancy is a range of 9 to 16 kg (20 to 35 lb) with an average gain of 11 kg (25 lb) for a woman of normal weight at conception, 9 kg (20 lb) for an over-

Recommended weight gain

weight woman, 14.5 kg (30 lb) for an underweight woman, and not less than 14.5 kg (30 lb) for a pregnant adolescent.[7] Even more important than the total weight gain is the pattern of weight gain. A gain of 1 to 2 kg (2.2 to 4.4 lb) is appropriate for the first trimester, with an increase of 0.3 to 0.4 kg (0.9 lb) per week thereafter to term. Weight loss should *not* be attempted during pregnancy. Overweight prenatals should not be placed on a diet of less than 7500 kJ (1800 kcal) and should consume sufficient energy to achieve an appropriate weight gain.

Dietary supplements

Nutrient supplements should be prescribed only after assessment of nutritional status and evaluation of diet shows that they are necessary. Some women may benefit from additional iron and folic acid because of the magnitude of the increased requirement, low body stores, and difficulty obtaining these nutrients from foods. If a pregnant woman is unable or unwilling to make changes in her food habits, a supplement containing 50 to 150 percent of the RNI and/or RDA should be recommended. The appropriate dosage for iron is 30 to 60 mg of elemental iron in the ferrous form per day; for folic acid, it is 200 to 400 mg a day.

Calcium

Alternative sources of calcium must be recommended to a prenatal who dislikes milk, e.g., yogurt, cheese, ice cream, milk in cooking and baking, milk powder added in cooking or baking, canned fish with bones, tofu, and broccoli. If the patient cannot eat dairy products, she will need a supplement for calcium and vitamin D as well as an extra 4 ounces of protein from the meat and "alternates" food group.

Sodium

Sodium should not be unduly restricted. An intake as found in healthy foods and moderate use in cooking and at the table will provide the appropriate amounts. Salt should be iodized; diuretics should not be used.

Alcohol and caffeine

Alcohol should be cut out if at all possible. *Caffeine* should be limited to 600 mg per day (four cups of drip coffee).

Food-Related Concerns of Pregnancy

Symptom	Suggestion
Nausea, vomiting	Eat crackers or dry toast before rising Eat small, frequent meals instead of three large meals Avoid irritating foods (coffee or spicy or fatty foods) Eat meals and snacks without fluids; drink fluids at other times
Heartburn	Avoid spicy, fried, or fatty foods, caffeine, and alcohol Eat small meals; take fluids between, not with, meals Remain upright for 1 to 2 hours after eating
Constipation	Increase intake of high-fiber foods, e.g., bran, whole-grain breads and cereals, fresh fruits and vegetables, dried fruit

Constipation   Increase fluid intake
(continued)   Increase physical activity
                              Stool softeners are preferred to laxatives

Nutrition Concerns during Lactation

The family physician can encourage breast feeding in several ways.
Counseling should be provided to prenatal patients and their
spouses well before delivery in order to provide time for a decision
to be made. This will also allow time for breasts to be prepared for
nursing. Many reasons can be offered to justify breast feeding: The
nutrient compositon of breast milk is ideally suited to needs of an
infant; there is less chance of allergies; breast milk has immunologic properties; breast feeding reduces the chance of overfeeding;
breast milk is at the right temperature, free of bacterial contamination; breast feeding is convenient and inexpensive, with no formula to make and no bottles to sterilize; infant-mother bonding
develops naturally; breast feeding helps the uterus return to normal size and may help the patient lose weight.[8]

Encouraging
breast feeding

In the hospital, breast feeding can be supported by encouraging feeding as soon as possible after birth, ensuring that adequate
instruction is provided, referring mother and infant to a community health nurse when they are discharged from the hospital, and
arranging for an early follow-up appointment to allow problems to
be detected early.

The lactating woman must continue to eat as well as she did
during pregnancy. An adequate calcium intake is important to ensure that calcium will not be withdrawn from the mother's endogenous resources. The additional energy required to support lactation is estimated to be about 3000 kJ (710 kcal) a day. For a lactation
period of 100 days, 840 to 1300 kJ (200 to 300 kcal) per day will
come from fat reserves laid down during pregnancy and an additional 1900 kJ (450 kcal) per day will be supplied by diet. Daily
energy requirements will be greater for a mother who nurses
longer than 3 months, especially if her weight falls below normal
for her height. Because of the need for sufficient energy to produce milk, breast feeding is not a time for weight reduction, as the
volume of milk may be adversely affected. Adequate rest and sufficient fluid (eight glasses daily) tend to increase the volume of
milk.

Mother's
dietary needs

Caffeine, cigarettes, and alcohol should be avoided or limited.
Some women may benefit from iron supplementation to replenish
iron stores after their depletion during pregnancy.

Infant Feeding

Questions about feeding infants generally center on the type of
milk to use; what, how, and when solids are to be introduced; and

Keep up-dated

what vitamin supplements to use. Family physicians not only must be able to offer reliable and up-to-date information on feeding but, perhaps more important can also use this opportunity to promote good nutrition for the whole family.

Milk Feedings   Ideally, full-term newborns should be breast-fed for the first 6 months. For infants with a family history of allergy, breast feeding constitutes an important preventive measure. If the mother cannot or will not breast-feed or discontinues nursing before the end of the first 6 months, the infant should be given a commercially prepared infant formula. Whole cow's milk is not recommended in the first 6 months, and skim and 2 percent milk should not be used in the first year.

Breast feeding may be continued beyond 6 months of age or may be replaced with one of the following: (1) commercially prepared infant formula, (2) whole cow's milk when the infant is consuming the equivalent of two bottles of baby food a day—6 to 9 months at the earliest (the combination of solid food and whole milk provides the appropriate ratio of protein, fat, and carbohydrate), and (3) diluted whole evaporated milk (one part water to one part milk).

Milk allergies   It is possible for exclusively breast-fed infants to develop sensitivity to foods in the mother's diet. The range of symptoms is similar to symptoms experienced by formula-fed infants who are allergic to cow's milk. Cow's milk, eggs, and citrus fruits appear to be the major offenders. The mother should continue to breast-feed while eliminating the offending foods from her diet. The extent to which this is carried out depends on the baby's symptoms and the foods involved. The mother may be able to eat the food once every 4 days. In this way she can continue to eat a varied diet, and the baby will remain symptom-free.

Parents should be cautioned against giving a child a nursing bottle containing milk or sweetened liquid as a bedtime pacifier. This may result in a dental condition known as nursing bottle syndrome. The erupting teeth are bathed in sugar all night, leading to tooth decay, usually of the upper front teeth when they come through the gums. Both baby teeth and permanent teeth can be affected.[9]

Vitamin and Mineral Supplements   A breast-fed infant requires 10 μg (400 IU) of vitamin D per day while being completely breast-fed. As breast-feeding is reduced, the vitamin D will be supplied by formula or fresh milk. Iron in breast milk has increased bioavailability, and so an iron supplement is not needed until about 6 months, when an iron-fortified infant cereal will provide it.

Iron   Iron supplements are necessary at about 3 to 4 months in healthy full-term bottle-fed infants. Iron supplements may be provided as iron drops in a daily dose of 1 mg per kilogram of body weight or in an iron-fortified commercial infant formula. Introduction of iron-fortified infant cereal and, later on, meat makes iron supplementation unnecessary. A reasonable intake of 1 ounce (11 tablespoons) of infant cereal daily provides 8.4 mg of iron. The RNI for iron in 6- to 12-month-old children is 7 mg per day.

Commercial formulas generally have vitamins and minerals added, and so further supplementation is not required. However, the label should be checked. Fluoride supplementation for breast-fed infants is controversial. In Canada, ready-to-feed formula is made with fluoridated water, and so a fluoride supplement is not needed. If concentrated liquid formula, powdered formula, or evaporated milk formula is used, fluoride should be given only if the local water supply is not fluoridated. The appropriate dosage is 0.25 mg per day until age 1 year.

Vitamins and minerals

Introduction of Solids   The timing of the introduction of solid food should be determined by the needs of the growing infant, not by chronological age. Height and weight gain should be plotted on appropriate growth charts, and food should be given when weight gain decelerates. In general, solids are not needed before age 4 months and should not be delayed beyond age 6 months. A child of 6 to 7 months is beginning to make chewing motions and is developmentally ready to learn to chew lumpy foods. Delaying such foods beyond 6 to 8 months may result in later feeding difficulties.

Practical tips

There are several practical tips for introducing solids.

1   A reasonable order of introduction for solid food is cereal, vegetables, fruits, meat, dairy products, bread products, cooked egg yolk, whole egg.

2   Infant cereals are appropriate as first food because they are iron-supplemented, are of the right consistency, are easily digested, and keep the right ratio of protein:carbohydrate:fat.

3   Use a small rounded spoon, placing food on the tongue.

4   Use single-ingredient foods, e.g., single grain, meat, or vegetable.

5   Introduce one new food at a time to allow detection of food sensitivities; allow 1 week between new additions. Rice and barley cereals are the least allergenic.

6   Begin with one teaspoonful and gradually increase the amount as the need increases. Infants eat according to their energy needs, not by volume of food. Forcing the child to consume a predetermined amount of food may result in excessive consumption of kilocalories.

7   Do not add salt, sugar, or fat to baby food.

By the end of the first year, infants should be consuming a variety of foods from the basic food groups.

TODDLERS AND PRESCHOOLERS

Establishing
good food
habits

The toddler and preschool years are a time for parents to establish patterns of good nutrition, normal weight, and an active lifestyle in children. Experience and example are the two major influences on a child's eating habits. The family physician can emphasize to parents their special responsibility to set a positive example by their own eating habits and to provide their children with a wide variety of food from the four groups.

The role of the family physician at this time is to provide anticipatory guidance. Parents are often not prepared for the erratic eating behavior that occurs in children during the preschool years. The rate of growth slows, and growth becomes irregular. This slowdown is reflected in decreased appetite and food consumption, dawdling over food, and strong likes and dislikes. If parents are prepared for this, they will be in a much better position to handle the situation and prevent feeding problems. During this time, the child still needs all the necessary nutrients; the best way of assuring this is through the use of a daily food guide. Emphasis must be placed on foods of high nutrient density.

Several practical points should be stressed to parents by the family physician in order to foster the development of good eating habits in the child.

1   Respect the child's appetite by serving small portions. For meats, fruits, and vegetables, servings are approximately one tablespoon per year of age, e.g., to a child of 2 years, offer a serving of 2 tablespoons.

2   The child may not be able to eat enough at one meal to get through to the next; snacks high in sugar and fat can interfere with the child's appetite for more nutritious food and can contribute to dental caries. Therefore, offer nutritious snacks which count toward the day's total nutrient intake.

3   Offer snacks 1½ hours to 2 hours before the next meal so that they do not affect the child's appetite.

4   Try new foods in small amounts; serve with a favorite food. Children like finger foods, soft foods, and foods at lukewarm temperatures.

5   Keep mealtimes happy and relaxed; allow the child 10 to 15 minutes to relax beforehand.

Practical
pointers

6   Allow the child enough time to eat, with no distractions, e.g., television.

7   If possible, the family should eat together.

8 Have regular mealtimes; lack of structure in eating patterns provides no opportunity for the child to develop hunger.

9 Be prepared for the child to be messy; allow time for the development of eating skills.

10 Remove emotional overtones from food; food should not be used as a reward or punishment.

11 Avoid arguments over the meal. A child quickly learns that refusing to eat wins rewards or attention. Children develop dislikes of foods that are associated with unpleasant experiences. If a child has not finished eating after 30 to 45 minutes, allow the child to get down from the table. Avoid bribery, coaxing, or force.

Some other concerns with this age group include the following.

1 *Milk anemia*: Occurs in children who drink milk to the exclusion of other foods. The mother is pleased that her child is drinking milk and does not realize that the child is missing certain nutrients, e.g., iron. *Management*: Keep milk back till the end of the meal; fill the child's glass only then. Use an iron supplement if necessary.

2 *Child does not like vegetables*: Try raw vegetables instead of cooked; let the child have a hand in preparation; offer small amounts. The preferences of parents and older siblings are quickly apparent to the child, who is apt to copy.

3 *Child does not like meat*: Check food habits. The child may be consuming adequate protein through eggs, peanut butter, chicken, cheese, etc., but is unable to chew more fibrous meats (roasts or chops). Explain sources of protein in the diet and the amount needed.

Specific problems

4 *Should the child be given vitamin and mineral supplements?* Always ask the parents what and how much food the child eats each day. Check how this compares with the food guide. If the child has poor appetite and low food intake over an extended period, a supplement that meets the daily nutrient requirement may be temporarily necessary. Always emphasize that what the child does eat should be as nutritious as possible. A poor appetite and low intake of food over a long time can reflect a zinc deficiency; the serum zinc level should be checked.

Parents should also be given guidance about safety in feeding small children. To prevent choking, children under 48 months should be fed sitting upright with the knees bent, with adult supervision while eating. Children should not be allowed to run around while munching finger foods. For children under age 3, those foods which are difficult to control in the mouth, chew, and swallow should be avoided, e.g., nuts (especially peanuts), raw carrots, hot dogs, whole grapes, gumdrops, and jelly beans. Food

Avoiding choking

should be modified to reduce the risk of choking, e.g., hot dogs cut lengthwise and then crosswise, carrots cooked, grapes quartered, pits removed from fruits such as plums. Because peanut butter can form a semisolid sticky bolus that cannot be removed from the vocal cords, it should never be served in bulk but only as a spread on bread or toast. Raw carrots, often used as a teething food, should not be fed to the child until the primary molars are fully functional.

5 TO 12 YEARS

Fostering good
nutrition

The main objective of nutrition during the school-age years is to continue to foster the development of healthy eating habits. Many more influences affect the child's eating habits, e.g., school, teachers, peers, vending machines, corner stores, and television. The child is becoming more independent and eating more meals away from home. The child must be encouraged to "think" nutrition when he or she eats.

The family physician should check the following.

Does the child eat a balanced breakfast? It should include three of the four food groups.

Does the child eat lunch? It should include all four food groups.

Does the child eat snacks at recess? After school? Are they low in sugar for dental health? Parents may need to be reminded to supply good snack fixings.

The family physician should be on the alert for the development of obesity and underweight. Height and weight should continue to be monitored.

TEENAGERS

Rapid growth
phase

The nutritional concerns that arise with this age group stem from the fact that this is the second period of rapid growth during the life cycle. Energy and nutrient requirements are highest when the velocity of growth is most rapid, and this depends on physiological, not chronological, age. The multiple changes that occur—rapid physical growth, sexual maturation, changes in body shape and appearance—cause most adolescents to be very concerned with and sensitive about their bodies. They may develop a distorted and unrealistic view of the body image if it does not fit accepted standards. This may lead to inappropriate food choices and compromised growth.

Nutritional concerns during adolescence include the following:

Lifestyle effects
Obesity
Anorexia nervosa
Pregnancy
Effects of participation in sports

Lifestyle Effects

A teenager's busy schedule can result in poor food selection, irregular hours of eating, missed meals, and increased frequency of snacks.

Management Emphasize making snacks count to compensate for missed meals. Snacks should be good sources of calcium and iron, two nutrients that are especially important during growth. Advice should be offered on how to eat out; e.g., order a hamburger or cheeseburger, skip the French fries, and choose a carton of milk instead of pop or a milkshake. Fast foods are generally high in fat, salt, and calories. Encourage breakfast and lunch, as teenagers often skip these meals.

Obesity

Obesity is probably the most common nutritional problem among adolescents in developed countries. Physical inactivity may be more important than consuming excessive calories, since an adolescent may be too embarassed by his or her size to exercise. Girls in particular are susceptible to fad diets, which may provide an inadequate level of the nutrients needed for normal growth.

Management Management should include counseling the whole family, behavior and lifestyle modification, increased physical activity, and referral to a professional dietitian or nutritionist for nutrition education that will correct misinformation about diet. Set realistic goals for weight, activity, and food-related behavior. For teenagers experiencing growth spurts, weight should be maintained or slowly increased over time, allowing for changes in the ratio of lean body mass to fat. After growth spurts have finished, the plan may include actual weight reduction.

Anorexia Nervosa

Anorexia nervosa is an eating disorder with underlying serious developmental and psychological disturbances. It occurs almost exclusively in girls and requires early intervention. Initial symptoms include amenorrhea, weight loss, compulsive physical activity, preoccupation with food, bulimia, and purging. Anorexics have a distorted body image and continuously strive to achieve a lower body weight.

Management Management should include restoration of normal nutrition by tube feeding in advanced cases if necessary, psychological help, and nutritional counseling from a professional dietitian.

Pregnancy in Teenagers

The nutritional needs of pregnancy are superimposed on the woman's own extra needs for growth and development. Irregular eating habits (e.g., missed breakfast) and poor food choices may cause her to consume suboptimal amounts of essential nutrients.

Management Refer to a professional dietitian for diet assessment and counseling.

Athletics and Sports

Teenage athletes are susceptible to much misinformation regarding the role of diet in promoting increased performance. Several points should be stressed in this area.

Specific advice

1 The athlete has an increased need for water and electrolytes and needs sufficient calories to cover normal growth requirements and physical activity.
2 Energy requirements can best be met by increasing food intake across the board without altering the balance of macronutrients in the diet.
3 A well-balanced diet with sufficient calories to meet energy requirements will supply adequate protein.
4 The most common deficiency in teenage athletes is water loss from sweating; an athlete should drink water periodically throughout exercise.
5 Generally, eating extra food and normal salting practices will replace salt.
6 Watch for iron deficiency, especially in female athletes, because of poor diet and high requirements.

ADULTS

The adult years are an important time for education and medical care in order to preserve health and prevent or delay the onset of chronic disease. Lifestyle and one's habits of exercise, drinking, smoking, and food choices do make a difference in regard to health in both the short term and the long term.

Weight control

Probably the greatest nutritional problem during the adult years is control of body weight. Because the basal metabolic rate declines about 2 percent per decade and because activity often declines with age, people gradually gain weight during the adult years if their eating habits remain constant. Being fat is associated with an increased risk of hypertension, increased blood lipids, and type II diabetes mellitus, all of which may lead to an increased risk of heart attack and stroke. Obesity is also associated with osteoarthritis, gallbladder disease, surgical risks, and certain types of cancer.[10]

Management of obesity includes evaluating current food habits and making necessary changes, evaluating eating habits and using behavior modification techniques, assessment of physical activity through fitness testing and changes in exercise habits, and long-term follow-up.

Several methods may be used to help determine an ideal body weight. These methods include the following.

1 Metropolitan Life's height and weight table (1983). A weight which is 20 percent above a desirable body weight indicates obesity.

2 Use of skin fold calipers. A desirable percentage of body fat for males is 15 to 18 percent, and for females it is 20 to 25 percent. A body composition of more than 20 percent body fat for males or 30 percent for females represents obesity.

Ideal body weight

3 Weight status may be determined by the following rule of thumb. For females, allow 45 kg (100 lb) for the first 150 cm (5 ft) of height and add 2.2 kg (5 lb) for each 2.5 cm (1 in) of height thereafter. Add 10 percent of the total for a large frame; subtract 10 percent of the total for a small frame. For males, follow the same procedure but allow 50 kg (110 lb) for the first 150 cm (5 ft).

A weight goal should be established jointly by the doctor and the patient. Some people may choose an unrealistically low weight that is both unsuitable and unhealthy to achieve and maintain.

Weight goal

Because of the proliferation of fad diets, commercial weight reduction ventures, and misinformation about weight loss, the following guidelines are offered as a way of evaluating the safety and potential effectiveness of a diet program. Each statement should be checked yes if the diet in question is to be recommended.

Does the diet do the following?

1 Recommend choosing foods each day according to an established food guide?

2 Include a variety of foods normally eaten and enjoyed?

3 Include a variety of foods from all four food groups (no one food or group is emphasized)?

Questions to be asked when considering a diet

4 Rely on food, not supplements or meal replacements, for essential nutrients?

5 Provide for gradual weight loss (0.5 to 1 kg per week)?

6 Allow nutritious snacks?

7 Emphasize portion control?

8 Recommend increasing physical activity?

9 Suggest consulting a doctor and a nutritionist?

10 Recommend regular meals, at least three per day, with food regularly spaced over the day?

11 Include behavior modification to encourage and reinforce positive changes in eating habits?

12 Increase knowledge of the nutrient content of foods and their role in the promotion of health?

13 Provide long-term follow-up to assist in the maintenance of new eating habits and activity patterns?

Alcohol

In addition, people need to be aware of the contribution of alcohol to energy intake. One bottle of regular beer contains 150 kcal, while one jigger of hard liquor has 120 kcal, with mix counting as extra. People who choose "fast food" meals often need to be careful to avoid excess fat.

Regular physical activity is an important component of weight control management. Exercise affects such management in the following ways.

Exercise

1 Exercise contributes to energy deficit directly by increasing energy expenditure.

2 The energy-expending efforts of exercise are cumulative; they may be substantial over time.

3 A combination of diet and exercise results in a loss of fat *and* an increase in lean muscle mass. This is desirable, as lean muscle mass is more metabolically active than fat. Diet alone causes loss of lean body mass as well as fat.

4 Regular exercise can offset to some degree the adaptive reduction in metabolic rate that occurs with dieting. This exercise-induced increase in BMR may extend beyond the exercise period.

5 Exercise increases cardiorespiratory fitness.

6 Exercise helps ease tension and decrease stress.

Sending the patient for a fitness test will provide baseline data against which progress can be measured. This can be a motivating factor. In addition, an exercise program that is safe and appropriate for the individual's fitness level will be recommended. Make sure that only qualified people conduct the fitness testing, e.g, a certified or registered fitness appraiser.

Heart Disease

The best general nutrition advice to offer to patients in order to reduce the risk of heart disease is the nutrition recommendations for Canadians or the American Heart Association's prudent diet.[11] In addition to a well-balanced, varied diet, weight control, and exercise, fat intake should be reduced from 40 percent to 35 percent of the total energy intake. At the same time, a good source of the essential fatty acid linoleic acid should be included in the diet.

There are several ways to control the amount and type of dietary fat.

1 Choose lean cuts of meat; eat smaller portions; trim visible fat; discard fat rendered out during cooking; cut down on gravy.

2 Use low-fat meat alternatives, e.g., poultry, fish, legumes; cut down on high-fat processed meats.

3 Avoid fried foods; broil or bake foods.

4 Avoid high-fat dairy products such as cream, cream cheese, ice cream, and whole milk.

5 Use 2 percent or skim milk and low-fat cheese, cottage cheese, and yogurt.

6 Limit the intake of high-energy, high-fat desserts or snack foods (e.g., potato chips).

7 Good sources of linoleic acid include sunflower, corn, safflower, and soy oils and margarines with a label which declares the relative content of saturated and unsaturated fatty acids. However, even these added fats should be eaten in moderation.

Specific recommendations

As fat calories are reduced, carbohydrates should be increased to supply the body's energy needs. Complex carbohydrates supplied by whole-grain cereals, vegetables, fruits, dried legumes, nuts, and seeds are preferable to refined forms since they contain essential nutrients as well as a variety of different types of fiber. Some types of fiber have been found to lower cholesterol and low-density lipoprotein (LDL) and to contribute to better control of blood glucose levels.

The nutrition recommendations also advise cutting down on salt. Levels of salt consumption vary widely from 5 to 8 g per day, with the average intake being 10 to 12 g. The RDA is 3 to 8 g per day. This involves cutting down on very salty foods (e.g., processed meats, canned soups, salty snack foods, and salty condiments) and using salt sparingly in cooking and at the table.

Salt restraint

Based on current research, similar recommendations of maintaining a desirable body weight, eating less fat, increasing fiber, eating a variety of fruits and vegetables, using alcohol in moderation, and cutting down on salted, smoked, and pickled foods may have a protective effect against the development of cancer.

Counseling for the prevention of *osteoporosis* should begin in the teenage years and continue throughout the adult years. Although the cause of osteoporosis is more complicated than simple calcium deficiency, there is considerable evidence that adequate dietary calcium is important in both the prevention and the treatment of this disease.[12] As a result of less than desirable intake of calcium during the years of peak development of bone mass,

Osteoporosis

women may never reach maximum bone mass. The situation is made worse after menopause, when decreased estrogen production is associated with a reduced ability to absorb calcium.

Dairy foods are the best nutritional source of calcium, and calcium from these sources is well absorbed. In addition, many dairy products are enriched in vitamin D, which enhances calcium absorption. High consumption of soft drinks may reduce consumption of dairy products. Also, in an effort to lose weight, women may limit their intake of dairy products. Current recommendations are 700 mg of calcium for women from 16 to 49 years and 800 mg for women over 50. Many women consume less than this. Recent calcium balance studies have shown that perimenopausal women require a calcium intake of 1000 to 1200 mg per day to produce calcium balance, whereas postmenopausal women need 1400 to 1500 mg per day.

Women of all ages should be encouraged to consume more dairy products. Low-fat dairy products should be chosen when energy intake is a matter of concern. If a woman is unable (e.g., through lactose intolerance) or unwilling to increase calcium intake through diet, a calcium supplement should be considered. An estimate of actual calcium intake should be made to help determine an appropriate level of supplementation. Alcohol, caffeine, and smoking are also thought to adversely affect bone mass and should be used in moderation. Regular physical activity or weight-bearing exercise such as walking has been found to be effective in slowing the rate of calcium loss even in elderly and osteoporotic individuals and should be a part of any program of prevention or treatment for people undergoing age-related bone loss.

THE ELDERLY

Nutrition in the elderly presents special challenges. The multitude of factors that have influenced an individual throughout his or her life must be considered and appreciated. The nutritional status and health of each individual will vary. For physicians to provide nutritional care for the elderly, they must be able to identify those who are at risk nutritionally and are in danger of deteriorating health because of poor nutrition. The following guide classifies the elderly in increasing order of risk.[13]

Nutritional risk groups

1 Seniors who are physically, mentally, and socially active are most apt to consume a nutritionally adequate diet.

2 Men with spouses will benefit from a wife's cooking and shopping skills.

3 Recently widowed men may lack skill in planning, buying, and preparing meals.

4 Because of chronic disabilities, medications, less freedom of choice, and problems in communication, the institutionalized are at greater risk.

5 Those who are housebound, isolated, physically or mentally handicapped, or unable to shop or prepare food are at greatest risk.

Drug Use

Nutrient needs do not decrease with age. Although there is less metabolically active tissue, nutrient utilization and appetite decrease at the same time. Therefore, the choice of food is still important. Nutritional adequacy is determined by nutrient intake and utilization, which may be affected by drug use. The elderly use more drugs than other age groups and may be on multiple-drug therapies at any given time. In addition, aging itself may potentiate drug metabolism. Drugs used for different purposes may have an additive effect in producing nutrient depletion. Drug ingestion may diminish appetite or produce nausea or vomiting or may affect the absorption or excretion of nutrients, leading to drug-induced malnutrition. However, some drugs may produce hyperphagia and cause obesity. Several examples follow.

Laxatives: Mineral oil prevents absorption of fat-soluble vitamins.

Antacids: Those containing aluminum or magnesium can result in phosphate depletion.

Analgesics: Aspirin can cause gastrointestinal blood loss and iron deficiency. Salicylates also compete for sites on serum protein that transport folate and thus may cause folic acid deficiency.

Diuretics: These agents may cause calcium, potassium, zinc, and magnesium depletion.

Digitalis: This drug may produce anorexia and contribute to protein-calorie malnutrition.

Coumarin: Anticoagulants can cause vitamin K deficiency.

Elderly persons who have several chronic disorders, take multiple medications, use over-the-counter drugs, and eat poorly must be considered at increased risk for drug-induced malnutrition.

Drug-induced malnutrition

Vitamin Supplements

The elderly frequently take vitamin and/or mineral supplements. Their use should always be checked. They are often taken for inappropriate reasons: to prevent colds, for energy, or for general health. Supplements are of proven value *only* where a deficiency exists. This requires a clinical and biochemical assessment of the nutritional status as well as a checking of food habits. Improving

Table 35-3   The Life Cycle

Stage	Concern	What to Look For
Pregnancy	Optimal total weight gain	Appropriate energy intake
	Optimal rate of gain	High-quality diet to meet the increased needs of pregnancy
	Calcium, folate, iron, and protein	
	Prevention of fetal alcohol syndrome	Check alcohol intake
Lactation	Inadequate breast milk	Rest, fluids, balanced diet, correct positioning of baby to breast
	Calcium intake	No reducing diets
Infancy	Inappropriate growth	Poor nursing habits Infant sleeping through feedings Poor maternal diet Improper dilution of formula
	Allergies	Quantity and type of solids Introduction of single foods one at a time
	Iron deficiency anemia	Use of iron-fortified infant cereals
Toddlers and preschoolers	Erratic eating habits	Overreaction on part of parents to child's small appetite Type of snacks, when given
	Iron deficiency anemia	Overconsumption of milk
School-age children	Inappropriate growth	Type of snacks, meal pattern, food habits of parents, exercise patterns
	Dental caries	Consumption of sweets, snacks
Adolescence	Obesity	Misinformation, fad diets
	Underweight, anorexia	Identify early
	Pregnancy	Diet must meet own needs for growth and development *plus* requirement for fetal growth
	Sports	Water is key nutrient to be replaced
Adults	Insidious development of obesity	Regular physical exercise Balanced diet, moderation in eating habits Alcohol intake
	Delay or prevent development of chronic disease	Check calcium intake, stress exercise Decrease fat intake Smoking habits

Table 35-3   Continued

Stage	Concern	What to Look For
Elderly	Malnutrition	Food-drug interactions Abuse of over-the-counter drugs, e.g., laxatives Special diets, too restrictive Food faddism, quackery Alcohol intake Poverty Poor diet, decreased food intake

the quality and quantity of diet is the preferred means of improving nutrition. Supplements may create imbalances among nutrients or lead to toxicity. They are expensive and create a sense of false security in both patient and physician.

The elderly are susceptible to dietary fads which claim to improve health, relieve symptoms, or slow aging. As a primary source of information for the elderly, the family physician must discourage patients from these practices, which are potentially harmful, waste money, and may cause an elderly person to delay seeking medical treatment.

Diet modifications

The elderly have many chronic diseases, some of which may require modifications of diet as part of treatment, e.g., chewing problems, constipation, cardiovascular diseases, overweight, diabetes, osteoporosis, osteoarthritis, malnutrition, and cancer. Special diets are a major cause of malnutrition among the elderly.

Modifications to a regular diet should be considered only when a significant improvement in health can be expected as a result of intervention. Diets may be too difficult to follow if they omit foods to which seniors are emotionally attached. There is also a risk of misinterpretation as to the severity and duration of restriction. Elderly patients should be referred to a professional dietitian for nutrition counseling in order to ensure that their nutrient needs are met, especially when their diets must be modified.

Meals on wheels

Poverty is a major cause of malnutrition among the elderly. Use should be made of community resources such as Meals on Wheels and Wheels to Meals.

A nutritional assessment should be performed when an elderly patient is first admitted to a nursing home. The patient's nutritional status and needs should be reviewed periodically to avoid continuing unnecessary modifications or missing an important unmet need. Weight should be checked weekly. Other clinical signs of malnutrition should be looked for in bedridden patients who are difficult to weigh.

SUMMARY

Table 35-3 highlights each stage of the life cycle, describing nutrition concerns and explaining what to look for.

SUGGESTED READINGS

Strongly Recommended

Nutrition and the M.D. (monthly newsletter)
PM, Inc.
14349 Victory Boulevard, #204
Van Nuys, CA 91401

Dairy Council Digest and Nutrition News
National Dairy Council
6300 North River Road
Rosemont, IL 60018–4233

In-Touch (quarterly publication of the Infant Nutrition Institute, Canada)
H.J. Heinz Company of Canada Ltd.
250 Bloor Street East
Toronto, Ontario
Canada M4N 1G1

Food and Nutrition News
National Live Stock and Meat Board
444 Michigan Avenue
Chicago, IL 60611

($2.00 a year outside the U.S.; free in the U.S.)

Other Readings

The American Journal of Clinical Nutrition, volume 36, October supplement #4 and November 1982, contains many articles dealing with nutrition and the elderly.

Series of articles dealing with adolescent nutrition in the Canadian Medical Association Journal, 1983.
129:419–420: Introduction and Summary
129:420–422: Normal Nutritional Requirements
129:549–551: Obesity
129:552–553: Sports and Diet
129:691–692: Pregnancy and Diet
129:692–695: Fast Foods, Food Fads, and the Educational Challenge

B. S. Worthington-Roberts, J. Vermeersch, and S. R. Williams, *Nutrition in Pregnancy and Lactation,* 2nd ed., C. V. Mosby, St. Louis, 1981.
R. A. Lawrence, *Breast Feeding—A Guide for the Medical Profession,* C. V. Mosby, St. Louis, 1980.
P. L. Piper, *Nutrition in Infancy and Childhood,* 2d ed., C. V. Mosby, St. Louis, 1981.
L. Lambert-Lagace, *Feeding Your Child,* General Publishing Co., Toronto, 1982.
K. H. Cooper, *The Aerobics Program for Total Well-Being,* M. Evans, New York, 1983.

Nutrition Reviews' Present Knowledge in Nutrition, 5th ed., Nutrition Foundation, Washington, D.C., 1984.
Infant Nutrition, a guide for professionals available from the Ontario Government Bookstore, 880 Bay Street, Toronto, Ontario, Canada M5S 1Z4.

SOURCES OF INFORMATION

The American Dietetic Association
430 North Michigan Avenue
Chicago, IL 60611

The Canadian Dietetic Association
385 Yonge Street, Suite 304
Toronto, Ontario
Canada M5B 1S1

Nutrition Education Resource Materials
Nutrition Communications—The Ontario Milk Marketing Board
6780 Campobello Road
Mississauga, Ontario
Canada L5N 2L8

Local departments of public health
Provincial or state dietetic associations
Outpatient departments of most hospitals
Nutrition programs at universities and colleges

The Department of Health and Welfare (Canada) and the Department of Agriculture (U.S.) extension services, especially guides for nutrient contents of common foods

AMA Section of Nutrition Information
535 N. Dearborn Street
Chicago, IL 60610

REFERENCES

1 Canada, Department of National Health and Welfare, *Nutrition Recommendations for Canadians,* Canadian Government Publishing Centre, Ottawa, 1980.
2 U.S. Department of Agriculture and Department of Health and Human Services, *Nutrition and Your Health: Dietary Guidelines for Americans,* Home and Garden Bulletin no. 232, U.S. Government Printing Office, Washington, D.C., 1980.
3 Canada, Department of National Health and Welfare, *Canada's Food Guide Handbook,* revised, Canadian Government Publishing Centre, Ottawa, 1982.
4 U.S. Department of Agriculture, *Food for Fitness—A Daily Food Guide,* Leaflet no. 424, U.S. Government Printing Office, Washington, D.C., n.d.
5 Canada, Department of National Health and Welfare, *Recommended Nutrient Intake for Canadians,* National Academy of Sciences, Ottawa, 1983.
6 Food and Nutrition Board, *Recommended Dietary Allowances,* 9th rev. ed., National Academy of Sciences, National Research Council, Washington, D.C., 1980.
7 R. L. Naeye, "Weight Gain and Outcome of Pregnancy," *American Journal of Obstetrics and Gynecology,* **135:**3–9, 1979.

  8 B. S. Worthington-Roberts and L. E. Taylor, "Guidance for Lactating Mothers," in B. S. Worthington-Roberts, J. Vermeersch, and S. R. Williams (eds.), *Nutrition in Pregnancy and Lactation,* 2nd ed., C. V. Mosby, St. Louis, 1981.

  9 G. M. Beazley, "Nursing Bottle Syndrome," *Journal of the Canadian Dietetic Association,* **39:**25–27, 1978.

 10 "Obesity—An Overview," *Diaglogues in Nutrition,* **3**(1):1–10, 1978.

 11 American Heart Association Nutrition Committee, "Rationale of the Diet—Heart Statement of the American Heart Association," *Arteriosclerosis,* **4:** 177–191, 1982.

 12 National Dairy Council, "The Role of Calcium in Health," *Dairy Council Digest,* **55:**1–8, 1984.

 13 M. Krondl and P. Coleman, "Toward Greater Nutritional Adequacy in Advancing Years," *Geriatric Medicine,* **1:**44–48, 1985.

Part Four

Patient Management

Chapter 36

Doctor and Patient

N. H. Hansen, M.D.

When a patient arrives at the physician's office for the first time, expectations of the physician are carried with the patient. Whatever the complaint, patient anxiety and stress are present. The attitudes exhibited by the doctor and office staff will determine whether a comprehensive health care approach is offered to or accepted by the patient. In order to avoid the simple approach of care provision only for the acute problems presented by the patient, the physician must make his or her interest in broader health issues apparent. Alerting systems help remind the doctor of the need to address problems other than the one presented by the patient at each visit. Skill must be gained at recognizing patient needs related to individuals in the context of sex, age, family, and community. These needs require adaptation of physician approaches toward meeting them in individual "difficult" patients, taking into account the physician's personal emotional reactions to such people.

PATIENT EXPECTATIONS

As the chapter on self-care in this book shows, approximately 10 percent of patient-perceived health problems are brought to the attention of a doctor. Thus, the patients we see have made a conscious decision to seek medical help. Patients' satisfaction with a physician's services is influenced by the degree to which that physician's role performance meets patients' expectations.[1] Since patient expectations and worries are not usually mentioned to the physician during this encounter,[2] we must consider and recognize patients' reasons for attending. Then we will be in a position to fully meet their needs.

Although the physician may not do what the patient expected, patient anxiety about unmet needs may be addressed by explaining the different approach adopted.

The reasons for which patients visit the doctor[3] are so important to the doctor's understanding that they are specified here.

Why patients go to doctors

1 *Limit of tolerance*: From minor to severe symptoms, this threshold varies in individuals.

2 *Limit of anxiety*: The implications of symptoms cause distress. This threshold also depends on the individual.

3 *Signal behavior*: The presenting symptom is a "ticket of admission" so that the real reason may be presented.

4 *Administrative*: Forms are required: illness certificate, letters, day care physical form.

5 *Opportunity*: An added symptom or matter is raised (both reason 3 and reason 5 often are presented with the phrase "Oh, by the way, Doctor . . .").

6 *No illness*: Preventive only, e.g., well-baby and breast examinations.

The top three reasons for attendance are reasons 1, 2, and 6 in that order.[4] Physician and patient agree on the reason for visiting in 40 to 70 percent of visits.[5,6]

HIDDEN REASON FOR THE VISIT

The physician should think of a "hidden agenda" or "signal behavior" when a patient attends for any of the following reasons:

Suspect a hidden agenda

1 A minor illness
2 A chronic illness with no change
3 Unorganized symptoms with no suggested organicity
4 Delayed recovery without apparent reason[3]

Judging whether patient expectations have been met is extremely difficult. Before the patient leaves, one should ask oneself questions such as the following.

Questions to ask oneself

Why is the patient *really* here?
Who is the identified patient?
Did the patient receive that for which he or she came?

Frequently, these simple questions will point to a problem that is masked by the patient's presenting symptom (the ticket of admission). Unless this problem is recognized, no investigation or symptomatic therapy will really be helpful. Patients may hide their real problems because of grief, guilt, concern over a family member or friend, latent depression, disease phobia, and a multitude of other feelings and concerns. A few questions from the physician may be sufficient to uncover these problems.

Does the action we've discussed meet your needs?
What have we left undone?
Are there things we have not addressed that we should consider when I see you again?

Questions to ask the patient

EFFECTS OF STRESS

Previous chapters in this book have shown that stressful life crises and particular periods in family development carry a high risk for problems of living and the development of illness. To ignore stress-related symptoms is to ignore the basic etiology of the complaint.

Stress diseases

A disease-oriented physician may see patients undergoing stress, investigate them more or less thoroughly for their physical complaints, reassure them that there is "nothing wrong," and leave them with no resolution of the basic problem. Such patients may return again and again with the same or similar stress-related complaints for symptomatic treatment, which usually takes the form of analgesics, antacid therapy, or psychotropics. An unspoken agreement has been reached between patient and doctor: The patient presents to the doctor, receives a repeat prescription for "nothing wrong," and since the symptom is somewhat controlled, does not press the doctor for more "tests."[7]

Treating "nothing wrong"

There are many situations in which constellations of physical symptoms suggest a functional cause. This "somatization" is a very common way of expressing emotional conflict and stress.[8] A crucial aspect of appropriate management is the need to trust your clinical judgment when such a functional etiology is likely. It is frustrating to patients to have a doctor hear their history, examine them, arrange for investigations, and then say, "We have ruled out any physical problem." This is usually interpreted by patients to mean that the doctor believes they have no problem or that the problem is imagined, neither of which is true.

Thus, when a functional etiology is suspected, trust your clinical judgment and tell the patient, prior to physical examination and investigation designed to rule out physical disease, that stress is the most likely cause. If problem solving with the patient is handled in this way, treatment will follow naturally, not by default.

Rule in stress-related likelihoods early

For example, the family physician may be able to say to a patient with a "painful tightening in my throat": "Okay, I am going to examine you now, but I don't really expect to find any specific physical problem, since most patients I see with the type of pain you describe develop it as a body reaction to stress." The doctor can then describe the relation between stress and muscle tension and the subsequent development of pain resulting from prolonged muscle contraction. If this is done before the physical examination, it ensures that the patient will not come to the conclusion that "the doctor thinks it's all in my head because he couldn't find anything wrong." You can then say, "Now, let's talk about the stressful things in your life. Has that communication problem with your boss improved?" If you do find anything wrong on examination or investigation, you have said "most."

Assuming that you do whatever examination or investigation is necessary to prove your hypothesis and eliminate organic factors, your battle will largely be won. You will then encounter far less resistance to rational treatment of the underlying stress, in preference, for example, to the symptomatic treatment of back pain.

Explain carefully

In this process, it is frequently necessary to hear out the patient in order to see beyond a "medical disease type" history or physical definition of pain as your task. The patient must also understand that you accept the reality of the pain and know that it is not imagined. If you chose to deny the patient's original complaint by saying that everything was normal, your patient will resent your expressed disbelief and will be much less willing to accept the course of therapy you suggest.

Other factors to consider

Finally, visits must include consideration of the patient's reaction to physical illness as well as the patient's social circumstances so that you will be able to choose treatment programs fitting that particular patient—a biopsychosocial approach.[9] Otherwise your approach to patients will be incomplete. This approach integrates medical, emotional, and social aspects of patient presentations in a comprehensive fashion, recognizing the legitimacy of each part as a health care problem requiring assessment and management.[10]

This is the modus operandi necessary for the family physician.

For example, a man with rheumatoid arthritis may be disabled to the point where he is unable to sit at his desk and fulfill his executive position; he cannot wield a pen without pain or get around to visit his associates without extreme fatigue. He is so overtired at the end of his day that he cannot sleep. Understandably, he becomes significantly depressed as he watches his career go down the drain and thinks of the financial implications for his family and himself. There is no point prescribing a difficult therapeutic regimen unless the fears, doubts, and depression are recognized, brought to the patient's attention, and treated directly. If this is not done, your patient may reject a time-consuming, difficult treatment course. Because his situation appears so dismal to him, he may say, "Why try?"

It is often surprising to a physician to receive a patient's answers to the following questions.

Why are you here today?
What do you think is wrong?
What would that mean to you?

These questions apply to any diagnosis you are considering: diabetes, cancer, anxiety attacks, etc.

THE THERAPEUTIC MILIEU OF THE OFFICE

The attitudes of the doctor are reflected in the atmosphere of the outer office. Management begins with patient-staff contact on the telephone and in the waiting area. A restful, relaxed state of mind is promoted by a warm, friendly, concerned, and supportive voice on the other end of the telephone when the patient makes an appointment or seeks advice. A comfortable, well-equipped waiting room with a competent staff attempting to make the waiting time as short and agreeable as possible encourages that impression. This will continue when the staff members (and doctor) are relaxed, caring, confident, and competent.

Office milieu

Think of your personal impression of your surroundings the next time you wait in a professional's office. Ask yourself if you feel welcome and at ease and whether that alters your subsequent attitude toward the professional.

ATTITUDES PORTRAYED BY THE DOCTOR

Students recognize early on that their inexperience makes patients (and themselves) uncomfortable. A relaxed and comfortable interview conducted by an experienced family physician will bring forth a host of information not given to the student. Perhaps the four most significant characteristics that distinguish the experienced practitioner from the student are as follows:

Patient-doctor relationships

1 The physician's knowledge of the patient and the implicit relationship between the two
2 The perception by the physician of subtle signs conveyed by the patient's body language and the way things are said
3 The physician's ability to be an active listener
4 Added confidence from more experience with the uncertainties of diagnosis and treatment (and one's own personal weaknesses)

Figure 36-1   The detached professional approach.

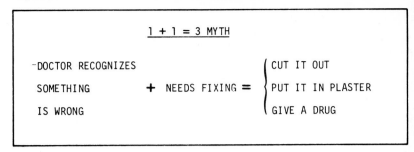

Recognize
needs

A doctor who is basically a technician will use a very direct approach, as depicted in Figure 36-1. This type of physician often fits the description of "detached professional," the end product of training emphasizing high technology and innovation. The result is a physician who acts as a technician, depersonalizing the patient. Such an approach to care is inappropriate for family practice, being "disease-centered" rather than "patient-centered."[11]

> For example, in pregnancy, psychological risk assessment and evaluation of family function, improve prediction of delivery and postpartum risk, while biomedical risk alone is not significantly related.[12] A detached professional is unlikely to recognize the needs of a single pregnant patient who was deprived of love in childhood and was excessively criticized and punished for failure. This patient will be treated in the same way as a secure, married, pleased-to-be-pregnant woman who was loved and supported as a child. Failure to recognize such differences may expose the first woman's unborn child to the later risk of child abuse.

As Gray has commented, "It has been well said that for the general practitioner it is as important to know the kind of person who has the disease as the kind of disease the person has."[13]

Physicians' attitudes and beliefs influence what they look for when seeing patients.[14] However, what is looked for determines what is found and treated. If one looks at the patient's life circumstances, treatment will then be tailored to individual needs in a comprehensive manner; this is what family practice is all about.[11]

THE USE OF ALERTING SYSTEMS FOR COMPREHENSIVE CARE

In order to deal with patient diagnosis and treatment in a biopsychosocial model, the family physician must be as efficient as possible. This means using records and other enabling and alerting methods as a means of organizing the care you wish to provide to the patient.

Appropriately indexed records will refresh the physician's memory regarding a patient, particularly one who may not have been seen for some time. When reviewed briefly at each visit, they will also act as reminders for comprehensive care strategies, including opportunities for anticipatory guidance and preventive interventions. The ideal record is not easily attainable, especially in the psychosocial sphere. Physicians must consciously develop methods that help them trigger actions beyond simple acute care.

Memory aids

Examples of record-keeping techniques that may be used to keep a physician organized and comprehensive are as follows.

1 *A health history questionnaire*: The questionnaire may be used for all new patients. It allows a new patient's waiting time in the office to be fully occupied. The physician is then provided with a capsule summary of past health history at the first visit.

Obtain background

2 *A baseline physical form*: When the questionnaire is combined with a physical examination (and subsequent tests) focused on current health, screening, and prevention soon after the patient enters the practice, a complete entry assessment becomes possible. The recording of a complete problem list, identification of possible risk factors, and age- or sex-related screening and preventive interventions become available up front. This forms a basis for a more satisfying and comprehensive approach which deals with the whole patient.

3 *A recall system*: In addition to the traditionally obvious immunization, chronic organic illness, and drug monitoring, recall systems allow for a review of chronic social or emotional problems.

Provide recall

4 *Review of the problem list*: This is done by the physician before going in to see the patient. It stimulates the physician's memory and helps organize visit time in order to achieve more than acute care for the patient's presenting problem.

Review problem list

Done with the patient on occasion, it may precipitate recognition of unexpected changes or new situations that did not previously require attention. The patient is offered an opportunity to present new problems. This ensures that problems other than presenting ones will be addressed. It may be the basis for suggesting that the patient return for a health risk assessment related to your data on family, age, sex, and risk factors.

5 *Awareness of the life situation*: We are not taught in medical school to consistently report psychosocial problems with the same detail and order that we devote to medical problems. Conceptually, it makes a great deal of sense to record individual life events and life cycles, along with family life cycles. This effort can be very rewarding, especially for problem patients who become difficult to manage. These recording formats offer an organizational framework on which to build information (which often has a direct impact on physical health).

Anticipate

Screening for information in these areas can be most helpful in subsequent patient management. The newly separated, the soon to retire, the alienated adolescent, the recently bereaved, and the physically abused child, spouse, or elder are examples of situations where you may be able to offer support. You may open the door to offer a discussion and display your interest by saying: "Now that you are going through a separation, it is important that you be aware that people who do so may suffer from financial difficulties, loneliness, guilt and depression, or sexual frustration. Do any of these fit you at present? Would you like to tell me about it?"

If insufficient time is available that day, tell the patient, "I would like to set aside a half hour on Thursday to talk about this."

Get comprehensive family data

6 *Family folders*: If individual charts are contained in a family folder which is provided to the doctor when any family member presents for care, there will be numerous new opportunities for comprehensive care. Questions such as the following may be asked of appropriate family members.

How is Mr. Dillon's back pain?
Is Johnny bed wetting as much?
John, how do you feel now about your wife's mastectomy?
Everybody I've seen this past month has stress-related symptoms. Are there some difficulties at home?

If enabling methods and alerting cues are not used, physicians will spend an inordinate part of their time dealing with episodic care rather than discussing preventive measures or physician-recognized problems with their patients.

TIME IN THERAPEUTICS

Time is a factor in any disease process, but it is often neglected by physicians as a therapeutic tool.

A parent may be told, "The findings suggest no more than a viral infection, so I would expect Jimmy to feel much better in another 24 hours. Please call me then if he feels no better, or sooner if new symptoms develop. In the meantime, restrict him to the following clear fluids. . . . Is that acceptable to you?"

Use time wisely

Time may also be helpful when a patient must become accustomed to a particular situation (divorce), disability (paraplegia), or diagnosis (cancer) or must realize his or her need to develop more realistic expectations (an overprotective parent). For the resolution of life crises, a "tincture of time," along with discussion between physician and patient, should be prescribed much more frequently than medication.

The stresses of life are not resolved by a physician in the office even when time is provided for the patient to ventilate, reflect, receive some objective clarification, and consider alternatives. The real improvement occurs between visits. A patient will reconsider some of these elements in that interval in light of the previous office discussion. On the patient's return, problems are frequently resolved, and then the process is repeated with other problems.

Because office time is valuable, it is necessary to have a realistic plan about what one can do for a patient in a brief visit. We must have specific, achievable goals for each patient encounter. The patient and physician together can establish priorities while retaining the option for future change. This will permit them to devise strategies to deal with problems having the highest priority.

Have realistic goals

It is important to tell people explicitly how much of your time is theirs. If 10 minutes is available, this should be stated. If more problems arise than can be dealt with in sufficient depth, one might say: "I would like you to drop by the receptionist's desk and make an appointment for next Tuesday. Tell her I wish to set aside a half hour for that visit so we will have more time to discuss this problem." The patient will have been asked to consider in the interval the subjects raised during your 10 minutes and possibly will have been asked to carry out some specific tasks before returning ("I would like you to consider the pros and cons of Bill's attitude"). Then the patient may come back to see you with that problem solved or better defined.

State how much time you have

In the rapid sequence of patient visits, it is preferable to allow a minute or two between patients so that you can write your notes, think over what has just happened, and then review the next patient's chart. Otherwise, changing gears may occasionally be difficult, especially if the previous patient's problem has been incompletely resolved and you feel uncomfortable about it. It is better to be organized with regard to your approach to the next patient; thus a few moments of scanning the chart will be beneficial. This allows you to give more than episodic care. You will have reviewed the problem list and medication list at least, thereby recognizing topics important to you that may not be brought up by the patient. If you cannot look over the patient's chart beforehand, you may do so during the visit, simply saying, "Just give me a moment to look at your chart so I can briefly review your total health situation." Such maneuvers also help you make the most effective use of the short time you have available.

Allow time between patients

Time constraints may cloud the physician's thinking and cause him or her to reach for a prescription pad as a signal to the patient of the approaching end of the encounter. Another high-risk time is at the end of the afternoon or evening, when one is tired and just wants to get out of the office. This pressure should be recog-

Don't prescribe drugs to save time

nized, especially when a prescription is not the solution and writing one only seems faster than giving a detailed explanation.

PATIENT SITUATIONS REQUIRING SPECIAL CONSIDERATION

A variety of patients require specific talents from the physician to help them with their problems. These patients include the following:

1 Children and adolescents
2 The elderly
3 The family as a unit
4 Patients whose emotional problems classify them as "difficult"
5 Patients whose problems go beyond the "everyday"

Children and Adolescents

When dealing with a child, it often seems easier for the doctor to relate to the child through a parent. This ignores the real patient. Discussion of history, diagnosis, and treatment are just as important to a child, since compliance requires not only a parent but also a cooperative child. Before you start an examination, some time must be spent putting the child at ease. Invest time in developing rapport with the small child. Holding or touching, tickling the child, and asking nonmedical questions (all of which are techniques designed to help the child feel comfortable) contribute to a successful relationship and treatment. Not doing so dooms you to a series of encounters that become unpleasant for parent and doctor, instilling a phobic response to white coats or stethoscopes.

One may ask a girl whether she prefers a liquid medication to a pill. A boy may be asked to confirm a comment made by his father: "Is your father right, Jimmy?" In the majority of instances, questions regarding the type of pain and its occurrence in relation to certain events may be described better by the child than by the parent.

You should ask for a child's agreement to take an unpalatable medicine, since a parent may not persist in forcing medication on a child who objects strenuously. Although discussion with the child in these matters will not always result in reliable information, the effort to treat the child as an individual will virtually always have positive results.

Adolescent attitudes

Communicating directly with children becomes increasingly important as they grow older. If a child has been treated as a separate and worthwhile individual by the doctor, he or she will feel much more comfortable bringing problems to that doctor as an adolescent. Adolescents commonly report that they cannot take their problems to the family doctor (whom they really consider their parents' doctor) because the doctor might tell their parents, having allegiance to them rather than to the child. The prevalence of this feeling suggests that many physicians have difficulty treating children or adolescents as entities separate from their parents.

The young patient may perceive a need to discuss problems with the doctor in private, without the parents being present. When a child reaches the age of 10 to 12, it is useful to suggest to the parents, in front of the child, that the child needs to be treated by the physician as an individual. Later one can seek permission from the parents to discuss problems and their treatment only with the child, in confidence. In my experience, such parental permission has never been refused. — Confidentiality

Once this is done, a child will never fear confiding in the family doctor, being assured that his or her problems will be held in confidence unless permission to share them is given.

Situations arise that should be communicated to the parents. In such cases one is sometimes forced to talk long and hard with the child to encourage the child to discuss an important issue with the parents. The doctor, of course, must then respect the child's confidence, or all the advantages of a good doctor-child or doctor-adolescent relationship will be lost. Once such confidence has been built, one will usually have no major difficulty gaining the patient's agreement for discussion with the parents when necessary, either by the patient or by the doctor. — Respect child's confidence

When the child has become an adolescent, a few more dos and don'ts apply. (See Table 36-1.)

Table 36-1 "Dos" and "Don'ts" for Dealing with Adolescents

Do
Guarantee as arranged that discussions are confidential

Open doors with them regarding the common concerns you recognize, i.e., conflict regarding independence, birth control, sexuality, depression, etc.

Simplify their access to you by saying that you are prepared to discuss any of the above issues if and when they wish

Take any of these opportunities whenever they present, which will most often be in the context of episodic care

Discuss with adolescents the issues you feel they should discuss with their parents

Don't
Moralize or lecture

Involve parents without the adolescents' permission

Try to be a buddy or use their language when it doesn't fit you

The Elderly

Four themes pervade the treatment of elderly patients.

Community
resources

1 *Home or social supports for the ill or the disabled elderly are often insufficient.* Many questions must be asked by the physician caring for such a person. Family care givers often perceive themselves as confined and unable to get relief from their responsibilities. They need supports such as responsible care, elder sitters, nursing, and other supports. They need these aids before a crisis of frustration and burnout occurs that requires nursing home placement. Education of care givers should include an understanding of the needs of the elderly person being cared for tempered with an understanding of the care giver's needs. Family conflicts of long standing, stresses on the care giver, alcohol problems, etc., may be risks for the development of abuse of the elderly.

Activities of
daily living

Many elderly persons live alone and are subject to the loss of their independence in the face of acute or chronic illness. Can the elderly person manage the activities of daily living alone? Dressing, preparing food, getting to the bathroom, and coping with bowel function may be insurmountable tasks without assistance. If the family has dispersed or is unresponsive to the patient's needs, who will help the forgetful person do such necessary things as take medications or shop, bank, and clean—a neighbor, a friend, a homemaker? Community resources are crucial to home care of the elderly, and the family physician must be thoroughly familiar with them.

More problems
per individual

2 *Multiple pathology is common.* In the aged, the coexistence of physical, psychological, nutritional, and social problems makes management much more difficult. Symptoms and signs alter with age. Vague symptoms of fatigue, loss of appetite, and weakness may be the sole indicators of anemia, viral infection, cancer, cholecystitis, depression, hypothyroidism, and duodenal ulcer. Such vagueness may lead the doctor and the elderly patient to accept these warning signs as related to aging. This tendency must be avoided.

Once individual problems have been identified, the elderly person often requires multiple treatments for multiple difficulties. This requirement carries its own problems of iatrogenic illness with adverse effects of medications and drug interactions.

Plan enough
time

3 *Treating the elderly takes more time.* In an elderly person new to a practice, such things as vision, hearing, comprehension, speed of assimilation of information, and short-term memory must all be assessed prior to making a choice of treatment. There is little advantage in expecting a vision-impaired person to read a prescription label. A deaf older person may be sensitive about hearing loss and thus may not ask crucial questions, nodding significantly instead. A person with benign senescent forgetfulness or early Alzheimer's disease may get quite confused by your instructions or forget them on leaving the office (or before).

A visit to the doctor may be an important social event for the patient simply because he or she rarely sees anyone between visits. It may be necessary to involve relatives, friends, or community support services to ensure that treatment is carried out appropriately and that all goes well. This will also provide social contact between visits.

4 *People expect dysfunction to occur with age.* The physician must often seek out symptoms and signs that are ignored by the patient, who often feels that these are attributable to advancing years. The recognition and treatment of such problems often have dramatic effects on improving independent function and quality of life.

However, older patients fear any disability that will require them to leave their familiar surroundings, for example, through hospitalization or placement in a nursing home. The loss of independence and its possible permanence carry a tremendous threat to the individual's perception of the quality of his or her life.

Losses are commonplace for the elderly. They have lost many friends, their jobs, and their social status and may have difficulty performing many physical tasks. Home, spouse, and friends are seen as necessary supports for ensuring social, emotional, and physical well-being in order to retain independence. There is a need to remain in control of one's life. The frail elderly person is in danger of isolation and loss of self-esteem.

The Family as a Unit

Treating the individual is not always enough. In some situations, inclusion of the family is an absolute necessity. The ideal family practice model assumes that the physician cares for all members of the family unit. In practice, there are many variations on this model. Many patients will not be living as part of a local nuclear family. These individuals will benefit from being considered in the context of their "roots."

Living arrangements take many forms, from group-sharing "families" to common-law arrangements, single-parent families, stepfamilies, homosexual relationships, and so on. Each type of arrangement has its own characteristics, but within each type there is great variation from any generalized picture we may have. This variation requires that the contribution of the interpersonal relationships of each patient's current living circumstances, plus that of the patient's family of origin, must be considered when an individual patient is seen. The information on family context is not gained all at once. There will be times when it must be acquired quickly. Then the use of aids such as genograms [15] and the family Apgar[16] will help organize the information gathering.

Many family arrangements prevail

A patient with marital or family difficulties does not often present them as the reason for seeing a doctor.[17] A patient may have persistent complaints of loss of energy, tiredness, headache, or other bodily aches and pains. Accompanying anxiety about these symptoms will often be excessive. The source of the anxiety must be sought by asking about work, home, etc., as sources. Once identified, the source must be addressed, often by means of marital or family counseling.

Despite the doctor's recognition of a need to speak to the spouse, parent, etc., the individual patient's confidentiality should be preserved. Permission must be obtained before any problem is discussed with any other person.

In many "medical" problems as well as "emotional" ones, if treatment is to be comprehensive, it must often extend beyond the solitary patient sitting before you in the office.

Think family unit

For example, if a patient presents with gonorrhea, the sex partner must obviously be treated. If that individual is also a patient, how he or she is approached becomes important. Most family doctors would agree that it is the patient's responsibility to tell the spouse or partner and to make sure he or she comes in for treatment. In situations where the patient simply cannot do the telling, it may fall upon the family doctor to initiate contact. This may then become an ethical problem. Most experienced physicians have at some time been faced with a request from a patient to bring in a spouse for a routine examination, imply that they have found something other than gonorrhea, and treat the spouse without his or her knowledge of the disease being treated. After the patient says that the truth would destroy the marriage, the doctor may feel some responsibility for preserving it.

If the doctor deceives the spouse, the doctor-patient relationship will be destroyed with both patients. Such deceit is indefensible. However, a crisis in the relationship may be precipitated if the doctor insists that the patient tell the spouse or offers to assist in this communication. Our experience indicates that a relationship will probably be helped, not destroyed, by this "blow" unless the relationship is already crippled beyond survival.

Another example of the need to involve the other partner occurs in cases of mastectomy. A woman who undergoes this operation suffers damage to her body image, physical illness, loss of sexuality, and possible depression. In addition, she has to be concerned with her spouse's reaction.[18] Family physician intervention with both partners pre- and postsurgery can be of great help. The key points to be aware of in treating a couple in this situation are as follows.

1 Involve the man in the decision-making process before the operation.

    Arrange for frequent hospital visits.

    Encourage the man to look at the woman's body after surgery.

    Encourage the resumption of sexual relations.

Sexuality and intimacy are severely stressed by a mastectomy. If these problems are not dealt with, the marriage will be severely affected. Once you treat a woman who has not allowed her husband to see her body again and has severely limited any sexual activity because of a loss of sexual esteem, the devastating effect of a mastectomy is never forgotten.

The physician must therefore develop ways of involving other family members when necessary. If a wife has a problem the doctor wishes to address in the marriage context, she will usually say, "He won't come in, Doctor." This is not usually the case. The doctor may, with her agreement, telephone her husband to say: "I want you to come in to talk because I am concerned about your wife's situation. I feel that in order to deal with this properly, you and I must have an opportunity to get together. When can you come in for an appointment?" It is unusual for a husband to refuse this invitation. Of course, it is preferable to ask the patient to make the approach, thus fostering more appropriate communication and encouraging independence rather than dependence. *Getting the spouse in*

Approaching the spouse or other family members may then lead to joint sessions for marriage or family counseling when indicated. Similarly, child behavior problems affecting family dynamics and interrelationships may have to be handled by the family as a whole. The family members will have to consider the effects on the whole unit when a child or spouse has a chronic handicap, when a family member develops leukemia, or when an elderly relative develops needs requiring that they move in.

A plea must be made here for the retention of the house call, which allows the physician to gain a great deal of information about the family in its "natural habitat." The artificiality of the office setting makes it more difficult to get an accurate picture of a family's everyday functioning. In a situation where one needs to appreciate the nuances of the interplay between all members, there may be no satisfactory substitute for a house call. *Home visits help assess the family*

Difficult Patients

"Difficult" patients are described by various doctors with terms such as problem, multiproblem, multiple complainers, chronic complainers, hypochondriacal, dissatisfied, management problems, demanding, thick chart patients, resistive, crocks, turkeys, hateful, and groaners.[19]

There will always be doctor-patient relationships that are not entirely satisfactory. The types of patients each of us identify as difficult will vary. Every physician must identify the types he or she finds "difficult." One writer described six such problem patients for family doctors.[20] The descriptions included numerous medical *Six types of difficult patients* problems, multiple somatic complaints, excessive anger, passivity, dependency, manipulation, and demanding behavior. These problem patients often have difficulty establishing and maintaining interpersonal relationships and may feel that people and conditions outside their control are responsible for their difficulties, whether medical, emotional, or social.

However, it is suggested that this situation should be seen as a problem of the patient-physician relationship. This permits the doctor to choose another mode of relating to the patient, to the benefit of both. Such a focus on communication may allow us to see the problem patient in a context of failure of mutual understanding which relates to physician failure to find out what the patient wants, to recognize how the patient copes, and to ensure understanding of the patient's definition of illness.[21]

To these must be added the physician's failure to think of personal anxieties or emotional reactions to patients as causes of seeing an individual as a problem. The physician must recognize that there are two parts to this equation.

Ask yourself, How does this patient make me feel? In addition to trying to decide what the characteristics of the difficult patient are, the physician must sort out what in his or her own personality causes an emotional reaction. These feelings are usually suppressed because they are seen as unprofessional.[19]

Clarify your feelings about patients

The doctor is often unaware of a reaction to a particular patient except when it is negative. After looking at the afternoon's appointment list, a doctor may say something like, "Not Mr. Sanford again—and followed by Mrs. Fraser—what an afternoon this will be." The likely reaction will be to spend as little time as possible with such patients, while the attractive and enjoyed patients receive extra attention (also a problem).

Some of the danger signs with negatively viewed patients are as follows.

Danger signs

1 Reaching for the prescription pad to close the visit, forestalling further discussion. Other "finishing" techniques include shuffling one's feet, standing up, writing a note, washing one's hands, and reaching for the door handle.

2 Arranging a consultation in order to share your frustration and give yourself a respite.

3 Concentrating on the presenting problem rather than the "real" reason for the visit.

4 Feeling helpless about "where to go from here" in a complex or apparently hopeless situation.

5 Consistently feeling a loss of control over patient visits.

6 Having each visit go overtime (for example, with a voluble patient or one whom the physician finds attractive).

Excessively negative or positive reactions to patients lead to difficulty because the judgment of the physician may be affected.

In these situations, unmet patient needs accumulate, causing further dissatisfaction on the part of both patient and doctor. The essential task is to determine what the patient's unmet needs are, while the physician must look within and assess his or her own personal reactions honestly.

Frustration with Patients Whose Problems Go beyond the Everyday

A helpless feeling is engendered in most physicians by a patient with seemingly insurmountable problems. A physician who feels that he or she must have the answer to everything is the most vulnerable. We must always remember two things: (1) We cannot solve all problems, and (2) the patient is as responsible for improving the situation as we are.

Two things to remember

An insurmountable constellation of problems is illustrated in the following example.

> A new patient, a 56-year-old alcoholic ("dry" for 14 years), has recently developed a degree of angina in addition to chronic bronchitis and emphysema. He also has occasional episodes of neck pain radiating into the left arm, with x-ray findings of degenerative arthritis (many spurs from C2 to C6). He's started to drink again.
>
> His wife has been in to see you and is very much concerned about the return to alcohol, saying that she has been ambivalent about staying home and that she visited her sister twice recently when the going got rough at home. She says she has been eating excessively lately.
>
> The patient presents as a defeated man forced to go on social assistance against his wishes since he was laid off from his job.
>
> "Doc, I don't know where to turn. One son is running with a bad crowd and just lost his license for drunken driving. Another son is separated and living with someone else. My wife is coming and going, is eating like crazy and putting on a lot of weight. My drinking is definitely not a problem, but she worries about it.
>
> "Whenever I try to do anything, I get short of breath or I get that pain in my heart. There is no work for me, but even if there was, my neck is giving me all those problems. I'd just as soon crawl in a hole and die."

Any doctor would be likely to have a severe attack of frustration when faced with this load of impossible tasks. Unless the patient's previous employer gets new contracts, this man is unlikely to return to work. His disease processes apart from the drinking problem are stable but have no great prospects of improvement. Without social or medical improvement, the alcohol problem is not likely to improve.

The problem belongs to the patient

The least frustrating approach for a physician is to *share* the responsibilities with the patient. Agree to work on areas in which early improvement of function can be anticipated, e.g., angina and bronchitis, limiting the problems you deal with at each visit. The patient and physician may then set longer-term goals, e.g., to work on marital problems and alcoholism. Priority setting must obviously be a shared process. Acceptance of only a share of the patient's problems and the communication of this acceptance are basic to an understanding between patient and doctor. Do not vent your anger or frustration on the patient.

For the hostile, the seductive, the uncommunicative, and the unduly verbose, the doctor *must* review the armamentarium of interviewing skills. There are many books on this subject to help practitioners. A variety of approaches are needed in dealing with such patients. Use of them will create more confidence and flexibility in the doctor, and a much improved doctor-patient relationship is likely to result.

On first and subsequent encounters, one must try to evaluate the patient's most prominent character traits, again helped by reviewing interviewing techniques and nonverbal behavior and "body language." Then the style of management may be modified accordingly, accepting the patient as he or she presents. A hysterical or dependent patient should be reassured as soon as possible. An obsessive-compulsive person may be encouraged to retain control. The anxiety of an excessively verbose or reticent patient will be observed and taken into account.

Overly dependent patients

For example, in dealing with an overly dependent patient, one will have to decide whether the initial efforts will be best served by accepting a dependent relationship. If so, as visits continue, it is important for the physician to foster independence by gradually turning over control and responsibility to the patient. Such people will frequently ask the doctor for an opinion on how they have managed a particular problem. The doctor may turn this back to such patients by asking how *they* feel they have done. Self-esteem and a feeling of accomplishment may be stimulated by giving such patients (or any others) support for their feelings. By being nonjudgmental and allowing patients to make decisions that you then actively encourage and support, you can help improve those patients' ability to cope on their own.

Finally, a physician must recognize that he or she cannot be all things to all people. Strategies that suit the doctor will not always work for the patient. The use of techniques that do not fit the doctor's personality may fail, since the doctor cannot honestly believe in them.

If an impasse is finally reached, the doctor-patient relationship may have to be terminated. As in any unwritten contract, the reasons should be discussed, and appropriate referral should be made to a colleague for continuation of care.

REFERENCES

1 D. E. Larsen and I. Rootman, "Physician Role Performance and Patient Satisfaction," *Social Science and Medicine*, **10**:29–32, 1976.

2 B. M. Korsch, E. K. Gozzi, and V. Francis, "Gaps in Doctor Patient Communication," *Pediatrics*, **42**:855–858, 1968.

3 I. R. McWhinney, "Beyond Diagnosis: An Approach to the Integration of Behavioral Science and Clinical Medicine," *New England Journal of Medicine*, **287**:384–387, 1972.

4 M. A. Stewart, I. R. McWhinney, and C. W. Buck, "How Illness Presents: A Study of Patient Behavior," *Journal of Family Practice*, **2**:411–414, 1975.

5 K. Weyrauch, "The Decision to See the Physician: A Clinical Investigation," *Journal of Family Practice*, **18**:265–272, 1984.

6 R. B. Taylor, J. A. Burdette, L. Camp, and J. Edwards, "Purpose of the Medical Encounter: Identification and Influence on Process and Outcome in 200 Encounters in a Model Family Practice Center," *Journal of Family Practice*, **10**:495–500, 1980.

7 M. Balint et al., *Treatment or Diagnosis*, Tavistock Publications, London, 1970.

8 G. Rosen, A. Kleinman, and W. Katon, "Somatization in Family Practice," *Journal of Family Practice*, **14**:493–502, 1982.

9 G. L. Engel, "The Need for a New Medical Model: A Challenge for Biomedicine," *Science*, **196**:129–136, 1977.

10 G. L. Engel, "The Clinical Application of the Biopsychosocial Model," *American Journal of Psychiatry*, **137**:535–544, 1980.

11 E. C. McCracken, M. A. Stewart, J. B. Brown, and I. R. McWhinney, "Patient-Centred Care: The Family Practice Model," *Canadian Family Physician*, **29**:2313–2316, 1983.

12 G. Smilkstein, A. Helsper-Lucas, C. Ashworth, et al., "Prediction of Pregnancy Complications: An Application of the Biopsychosocial Model," *Social Science and Medicine*, **18**:315–321, 1984.

13 D. J. P. Gray, "The Key to Personal Care," *Journal of the Royal College of General Practitioners*, **29**:6666–6678, 1979.

14 P. Williamson, B. K. D. Beitman, and W. Katon, "Beliefs That Foster Physician Avoidance of Psychosocial Aspects of Health Care," *Journal of Family Practice*, **13**:999–1003, 1981.

15 W. Jolly, J. Froom, and M. Rosen, "The Genogram," *Journal of Family Practice*, **10**:251–255, 1980.

16 G. Smilkstein, "The Family APGAR: A Proposal for a Family Function Test and Its Use by Physicians," *Journal of Family Practice*, **6**:1231–1235, 1978.

17 G. Pugh and N. Cohen, "Presentation of Marital Problems in General Practice," *Practitioner*, **228**:651–656, 1984.

18 D. Wellisch, K. Janison, and R. Pasnau, "Psychosocial Aspects of Mastectomy: The Man's Perspective," *American Journal of Psychiatry*, **135**:534–538, 1978.

19 C. E. Evans, "Physician Survival: Should the Doctor Come First," *Canadian Family Physician*, **26**:856–859, 1980.

20 A. B. Schuller, "About the Problem Patient," *Journal of Family Practice*, **4**:653–655, 1977.

21 R. Anstett, "The Difficult Patient and the Physician-Patient Relationship," *Journal of Family Practice*, **11**:281–286, 1980.

Chapter 37

Physician-Oriented Therapeutics and Medication

N. H. Hansen, M.D.

In devising management plans, the family physician has several options, which are usually shared with the patient. These options range from taking no action to prescribing drugs, counseling, surgical intervention, referral, consulting, or a combination of treatments. Ideally, one should avoid being too conservative by using outdated treatments, while being cautious with newer, unproven methods of medical management. In this chapter, the problems of prescribing for minor and major illnesses are discussed along with advice on drug selection, prescription writing, avoidance of drug interactions, and handling of problems in specific situations.

Categories of treatment

The treatment instituted by the family physician should be rational, appropriate to the patient, economic, effective, and safe. Furthermore, the results from the chosen therapy should be clear to both doctor and patient.

Any therapeutic modality falls into one or more of the following categories (Table 37-1):

Curative treatment

1 *Curative*: Unfortunately, except for antibiotics, very few medications fall into this category. Examples of curative therapies are:

a Teaching a patient to deal with chronic constipation by regulating toilet habits and by adding fiber and liquids to the diet.

b Giving a patient with insomnia guidelines for sleep induction other than the use of medication.

c Completing a desensitization program for pollen-related hay fever.

2 *Symptomatic*: Most family medicine treatments fall into this category. Examples are use of analgesics for pain relief, antihistamines for hay fever, splinting for a painful joint, and diazepam for anxiety. The temptation to relieve symptoms, which is strong, falls into two categories:

a Treatment before diagnosis: Symptoms for which relief is available are often treated before the etiology is definitely diagnosed. In these instances, the doctor must always guard against assuming that relief of the symptoms has relieved the disease process. He or she should also ensure that the treatment given will not interfere with subsequent diagnosis (e.g., undiagnosed abdominal pain or anemia). **Symptomatic treatment**

b Treatment after diagnosis: The safest and most reliable form of symptomatic treatment is one that is prescribed after the diagnosis has been made.

For many illnesses, specific diagnosis is impossible in the early stages, and a working diagnosis must suffice. The physician must accept the responsibility for this uncertainty and repeatedly review symptoms treated in this way.

3 *Maintenance and support*: For many illnesses physicians can provide nothing but support until the self-limiting process is over. An extreme example is the use of life-support methods. In many cases, the body's healing capabilities can be supported only by rest. Insulin for the patient with diabetes replaces a frank deficiency, as does thyroid hormone in hypothyroidism. These methods of treatment do not, however, alter the basic disorder. **Supportive treatment**

4 *Preventive*: Until recently, physicians have directed their attention toward acute care. Thus we treat atherosclerotic heart disease with bypass surgery rather than assessing risks and help- **Preventive treatment**

Table 37-1   Therapeutic Modalities

1 Curative
2 Symptomatic
    a Rx prior to diagnosis
    b Rx after diagnosis
3 Maintenance and support
4 Preventive
5 Rehabilitative
6 No active Rx

ing patients make appropriate lifestyle changes to prevent illness. Examples of preventive maintenance are immunization, prophylaxis against malaria for the traveler, and use of aspirin to prevent strokes in a patient with transient ischemic attacks.

Primary prevention by anticipatory guidance

The most difficult changes to achieve are lifestyle changes such as discontinuation of smoking, weight loss, or increased exercise. Consider all the following as therapy: discussions with the teenager regarding sexuality and contraception, education to prevent the empty-nest syndrome in the mother whose family is dispersing, explanations to the patient about to undergo an operation (and to his or her spouse) of possible problems, and teaching the new parent how to cope with infant diarrhea. (Anticipatory guidance strategies are considered in the chapter on the family life cycle and anticipatory guidance.)

Rehabilitative treatment

5 *Rehabilitative*: Once an acute illness or accident has occurred, any disability, physical or emotional, should be recognized and addressed. The post-myocardial infarction patient needs a rehabilitative program but too often does not get one. Supportive treatment may also be a necessary rehabilitation; for example, providing home care assistance for the postoperative patient to allow gradual return to full activity. Another part of rehabilitation is the disclosure to a patient that his or her full capabilities will not be restored, e.g., in the case of a stroke or a disabling accident. Again, support may be needed to help the patient to return to the maximum level of functioning possible, given the disability.

No active treatment

6 *No active treatment*: The doctor who is oriented toward curing disease finds it very difficult to do nothing. "A resident was once heard to say of a patient with lincomycin-induced colitis whom we had helped to recover, 'We did not treat her with anything.' What he meant was 'we treated her with nothing.'"[1] It is most important to avoid prescribing in situations where the prescription may be more dangerous than the disease, e.g., giving phenylhydrazine for superficial phlebitis. The decision to avoid prescribing is often made easier when the doctor includes the patient in the management plan, since a description of the adverse effects of medication may well result in the patient's saying, "Well, in that case, I think I would rather just wait and see how things go." The decision to "wait and see" should include active surveillance when indicated; e.g., if it is decided to avoid oral hypoglycemics for maturity-onset diabetes in an older male at risk for myocardial infarction, the patient should be monitored for weight loss.

PRESCRIBING FOR MINOR ILLNESS

Strategy for minor illness

When patients have very little wrong with them, the best course of action for a physician is to tell them that they do, indeed, have very little wrong and then give them nothing for it! The family doctor should avoid prescribing drugs for self-limiting illness, since the patient will get better no matter what. Many illnesses seen by the family physician fall into this self-limiting category.

The physician who feels abused by patient visits for minor illness can deal with the problem by patient education (see chapter 40). Once satisfied that the presenting problem represents a minor, self-limiting illness and is not a "ticket for admission" to discuss other concerns, the physician can discuss with the patient methods of managing the problem, thus anticipating the next occurrence. The patient should be alerted to danger signals that would indicate the need to be seen by the doctor. This approach has been successfully used in practice, leading to major reductions in prescription writing and an increase in physician satisfaction. Health professionals have found it easier to incorporate general health education in their routine practice.[2] An example of patient education is found in Table 37-2.

Patient education

PRESCRIBING NONDRUG THERAPIES

Prescribing involves not only medication but also other forms of treatment, which are at least as potent and should be handled just as carefully.

Lifestyle Changes

Motivation is the key to success, but it is difficult to influence the asymptomatic patient, particularly if the lifestyle change required

---

Table 37-2 Prescription for Handling Acute Viral Upper Respiratory Infection in Children

1 Reassure that nothing threatening is present.
2 Describe the clinical course of the viral illness.
3 Provide symptomatic and supportive measures.

a	Fever:	Remove clothes to lower temperature. Tepid sponges (aspirin—acetaminophen only when recovery begins).
b	Cough:	Honey and warm milk, cough drops.
c	Nasal congestion:	Remove nasal mucus by suction *or* phenylephrine ⅛% nose drops. Bed rest and fluids (to avoid dehydration). Humidity if appropriate.

4 Explain situations requiring physician contact.
5 Avoid patent medicines such as antihistamines, decongestants (oral), polypharmaceuticals, e.g., cough syrups, and antibiotics.

is dramatic or is seen as more inconvenient than the far-off threat. Even where the risk is more immediate, change is not easily accepted. For example, a recommendation to a 55-year-old dockworker with chronic obstructive lung disease and angina to seek lighter work may result in the doctor quickly being told, in no uncertain terms, how impractical that is.

Involve family

Success in initiating lifestyle changes will permit further changes. Family support must be sought and encouraged; there is greater success in post-myocardial infarction exercise programs when the wife expressed support (80 percent adherence) compared with 40 percent adherence when the wife had a neutral or negative attitude.[3]

Rest

Rest is helpful, and sometimes essential, for recovery in many illnesses and injuries. However, cost is often a serious consideration. Doctors should find out what compensation their patients will receive for time off work so they can prescribe accurately and practically. The uninsured laborer with back pain may suffer great hardship if he follows medical advice, and may therefore wait until the weekend to have the sorely needed rest.

The prescription of rest should be utilized only when absolutely indicated. When rest is necessary, this fact must be presented forcefully to both the patient and the family; e.g., the spouse must be prepared to do the work, clean the house, and wash the dishes, and the children must learn to fetch and carry. The social worker can be of immense help in suggesting avenues of assistance.

Nutrition

Utilize nutritionist

Dietary modifications are commonly prescribed in particular illnesses and for particular reasons (see Chapter 35). High-potassium diets, low-sodium diets, high-protein diets, low-protein diets, low-fat diets—the list is very long. The assistance of a nutritionist can be invaluable to both doctor and patient. The doctor may know the general guidelines for a particular diet, but the nutritionist is better equipped to give specific descriptions of just how the patient can comply. The nutritionist can show the patient how to make a diet palatable, how to allow some flexibility in the diet, and how to tailor a restrictive diet to an individual lifestyle.

Many of the diets we prescribe are unpalatable. For example, a totally salt-free diet is not likely to be adhered to by any patient for a meaningful period of time. It is usually necessary to compromise, prescribing a no-added-salt diet—more appropriate in almost all such situations. One can expect short-term compliance with high-potassium diets by an individual on diuretics, but unless the individual really enjoys foods such as bananas, molasses, cola drinks, and fruit juice, compliance falls off.

The family doctor must take diet into consideration when medications are prescribed, and medications when diet is advised. Some dietary adjustments are absolutely necessary; for example, for patients on MAO-inhibiting medications, tyramine-containing foods must be avoided. Other medications will be inadequately absorbed when taken with food; for example, tetracycline is poorly absorbed when taken with milk. Thus, effects of diet on the absorption of medication must always be considered.

Illness-medication-diet interactions occur as well. An example is the patient in borderline cardiac failure on a low-sodium diet; the use of phenylbutazone may cause sodium retention and push this patient into overt heart failure. The patient with hypertension combined with peptic ulcer must be counseled to avoid high-sodium antacids such as sodium bicarbonate. The patient with epilepsy taking diphenylhydantoin (Dilantin) may develop folate deficiency unless this is anticipated and folate prescribed in diet or pill form.

Food and drug interactions

Dietary restriction and obesity go hand in hand. Obesity is the ninth most common problem seen in family practice.[4]

Hospitalized patients are faced with particular problems. The foods served are often unfamiliar, and the patient's appetite is often poor. Food may be served at times when the patient is otherwise occupied and thus becomes cold. The patient may be so ill that he or she does not make the effort to eat. Mistakes may be made, such as serving salt when restriction is necessary.

It is, therefore, essential that family physicians arrange for a nutritionist to visit appropriate hospitalized patients to determine their likes, dislikes, and special needs. In all difficult problems a direct doctor-nutritionist dialogue is desirable and should be sought. Nutritional deficiency is a hospital problem that is commonly overlooked by physicians.

Physical Measures

The family physician who makes a diagnosis of a musculoskeletal disorder must be prepared to use specific physiotherapeutic modalities. Traction, massage, heat, cold, and isotonic and isometric exercises hold mysteries unless one has a practical knowledge of how and when to use them.

Although some severe injuries will not be treated solely by the family physician, his or her role is important. For example, a patient who has been diagnosed as having a torn medial meniscus will quickly be referred to an appropriate surgeon, but the family physician must, at the time of diagnosis, prescribe strengthening quad-

Physiotherapy

riceps exercise to prepare the patient for surgery. This will prevent a prolonged convalescence resulting from preoperative or postoperative weakness in these muscles.

Physical methods are useful as both preventive and curative techniques. Some practical examples follow.

Sports
medicine

Pretrauma In athletics, prevention of trauma includes the use of proper equipment, adequate conditioning, and preventive bandaging or taping. (While equipment may not be considered physiotherapy, its proper use may prevent the need for this type of treatment.) The family physician can reduce the incidence of amateur-sports trauma in the community by ensuring:

1 *Use of proper equipment*: League and school officials should be made aware of the need for proper equipment both in practice and in games. All hockey eye injuries and most head injuries are totally preventable if proper helmets with eye protectors are worn; injuries to the face and head exceed those to other parts of the body.[5,6]

2 *Conditioning*: Preseason conditioning and pregame warm-ups provide efficient muscle strength and ligamentous flexibility to decrease the incidence and severity of strains, sprains, and contusions.[7] The weekend athlete and the beginning jogger in particular require advice regarding the need for warm-up before participation, and for graduated introduction to new effort after a long interval of relative inactivity.

3 *Preventive taping and bandaging*: Repeated injury to ligaments around joints may be decreased by the use of taping to prevent re-straining of the damaged part. The joint is positioned and supported to put minimum stress on the ligament being protected, and tape is applied. The tape replaces some of the function of the ligament.

Posttrauma For the first 48 hours after an injury, *i*ce, *c*ompression, and *e*levation (ICE) are the key elements for trauma not requiring surgery or casting. Regrettably, physiotherapy principles are easily neglected in the postinjury period, with considerable adverse effects, whether or not casts are applied or surgery is performed. For example:

1 Healing of a second-degree sprain to an ankle is improved by ice, compression, and elevation for the first 48 hours, rest with crutches until the pain settles, and a program to regain function (heat, muscle-strengthening exercises, and proper footwear).

2 An elderly woman who has fallen on her wrist and suffers a Colles's fracture may find that the fracture heals when placed in a cast. However, if exercises for her hand and shoulder are not prescribed, she may have secondary complications of weakness of the hand and pain or stiffness in the shoulder.

3 A high incidence of phlebitis is found in elderly persons who are confined to bed for whatever cause. This may be avoided by appropriate bed exercises.

Rehabilitation There is no better example of the need for rehabilitation than that of a stroke. An active rehabilitation program should begin 1 to 2 days after a stroke,[8] and the patient should be hospitalized if community physiotherapy services are inadequate. Passive exercise and proper positioning of limbs are essential. Footboards and splints for the paralyzed leg prevent foot drop and contractures. When the patient is out of bed, an affected upper limb should be supported by a sling to prevent excessive shoulder traction. Passive exercises prevent fixation of joints and shortening of tendons, which otherwise lead to severe limitation of function, are painful to overcome, and are almost impossible to correct later.

Poststroke

Such exercises may be administered by anyone, after being taught by a physiotherapist. A family member may contribute his or her newly learned skill.

Learning to walk again may be a frightening experience, requiring patience and proper equipment for support. Retraining in activities of daily living is essential—even for a simple thing like hair grooming. Physical conditioning for both affected and unaffected limbs is necessary to prevent undue fatigue from ambulation.

Attention must be paid to reevaluation to ensure that easily solved problems that contribute to disability are not overlooked.[9]

The family physician must accept physiotherapists as active colleagues on the health care team. Physiotherapists receive extensive training, which includes more than a technical ability to administer specific types of exercise programs. They should be supplied with a diagnosis for the patient, and told of any limitations and contraindications. Close contact is essential to ensure that physiotherapist and physician are aware of each other's levels of expertise and judgment.

Community Services

When initially locating in a community, a physician would do well to arrange to meet with representatives of professional and volunteer agencies. This allows the doctor to learn what community support systems are available to patients and how to gain access to them. A personal introduction will facilitate later communication regarding patient problems. The physician must develop contact

Utilize local help

points—people he or she may telephone to get information quickly about resources or referral for a particular patient problem.

Depending on the size of a community, a variety of public health and volunteer agencies may be available. In large communities, enormous numbers of special interest groups may have developed. In small communities, although specific organizations may not exist, there is usually an informal system of support. For example, a neighbor who is also a practical nurse may be delighted to have an opportunity to help. The man living next door may be willing to carry an elderly invalid up and down stairs morning and night to encourage patient convalescence or to permit the patient to eat meals with the rest of the family. In a farming community, friends may band together to cut hay for an individual recuperating from a surgical operation.

Further information on community resources may be found in Chapter 40.

Unmet Needs   There is an extreme shortage of home care services in North America. Expensive hospital care has developed to fulfill society's perceived need that the best possible care, whatever the cost, be available to all. It would be preferable to concentrate on increasing the supply of support systems to keep people at home. Good home care support permits early discharge from hospitals and prevents overutilization of their facilities by occasional admissions for social reasons. Moreover, such support has proved to be an acceptable alternative to long-term institutional care for the permanently seriously disabled, many of whom are elderly. Finally, home care is considerably less costly than inpatient services.[10]

Hospital Treatment

Reasons for hospitalization of patients vary widely. Severe illness, emergency trauma, and urgent surgical intervention all require admission. Occasionally the need for a speedy resolution or an intensive investigation warrants in-hospital care.

Alternative
strategies

The decision to admit a patient may be one of convenience—either for the patient or for the doctor. Social circumstances may make it advisable for a child to be treated for pneumonia in the hospital, for example, when a doctor recognizes that the mother is unreliable or incapable of supplying the care needed. However, as an alternative, a social agency may be able to provide a home care worker to help out. An elderly person who lives alone and who must have bed rest may be unable to get that rest if he or she has to prepare meals, and this may result in either nutritional deterioration or lack of bed rest. Moreover, if such an individual stays in bed and does not have intensive physiotherapy, he or she risks the complication of deep vein thrombosis.

Such considerations must be weighed against the fact that hospitalization may result in disorientation as to time and place. An evaluation must always be made of the severity of the illness, the availability of support systems, and the possible adverse effects of either hospitalization or home care.

Unnecessary Hospitalization   It is important that the inexperienced physician recognize the tendency to admit patients because the physician feels the need for full control of care. For example, an unwillingness to treat otherwise uncomplicated congestive heart failure at home is often a function of the comfort of the physician rather than the patient's need.

PRESCRIBING "THE DOCTOR"

Frequently the family doctor must be prepared to give of him- or herself to help a patient, and in this case part or all of the prescription is the doctor's time and interest.[11] As in any prescription, the amount needed must be calculated. How much time is to be spent and the frequency of the dosage must be taken into account—more in crises, less for maintenance. Again, the physician's attitudes and feelings may interfere, whereas self-understanding helps to avoid loss of objectivity. If treatment consisted only of prescribing the right medication, the doctor's task would be relatively simple.

Listening, developing rapport, demonstrating understanding, and providing reassurance and support are a part of every patient contact for the thoughtful family physician. Whatever the problem, these basic needs are always present.

Behavioral interaction

Essence of the Family Doctor Approach to Emotional Problems

A problem is brought by the patient to the family doctor under circumstances different from those encountered by other therapists. In the ideal physician–patient relationship, problems of both a physical and an emotional nature may be brought up, often at the same visit. The continuity of this "any problem" relationship allows the family physician a more intimate glimpse of the life, in health and illness, of the individual and the family unit, and of their social circumstances, than can be gained by a consultant who deals with a specific part of the person at a specific point in time. No other therapy situation is comparable.

The nature of family practice imposes short visits, and therapy is altered by this constraint, although not necessarily adversely. Although short visits at intervals over an extended period of time may accomplish much, it is extremely important to have realistic expectations and goals. The experienced family physician accepts the lack of immediate "cure" at the end of every encounter. With experience, the interval between visits can be used to make the most of treatment. The patient reviews matters discussed, makes decisions, carries them out, and returns with a report of success (or failure). Thus change is produced by the patient, not the doctor, in these intervals. A doctor who is aware of this fact will provide appropriate tasks and goals so that this time can be used effectively. "The components of psychotherapy related to change are basic, non-esoteric elements of communication."[12]

Family dynamics

In many situations, inclusion of other members of the family will be necessary for therapy to be successful. Indeed, the root of the problem presenting in a patient may be a family problem. A family conference may be advisable to assess family functioning, and much can be gained from an observation of family dynamics.

Interviewing and assessment skills are required in dealing with the family as a group. The family physician may see various family members in many isolated visits before recognizing the need for family intervention. The physician also sees families in partial units—a mother and child, both parents, a son and elderly parent.

Techniques

Interviewing skills

For further guidance, refer to basic texts on interviewing,[13,14] and on counseling techniques in brief psychotherapy[15,16] and family therapy[17] to gain skill and versatility in using varied approaches for different patients. The following points are emphasized:

1 *Listening*: Simply because it allows a person to tell his or her troubles to someone, listening is therapeutic. It offers an opportunity to think out issues and to explain them to another. *Active* listening aids this process by inquiry and encouragement and by demonstrating empathy and understanding. A simple indicator of success is to compare the amount of talking time taken up by the patient with the time taken up by the physician. Generally the more the patient speaks, the more the physician learns, both from what is said and from the manner of presentation (e.g., body language).

2 *Supportive*: A warm supportive climate allows the patient to feel enough trust to be honest. Such a climate can be created by reassurance (e.g., "Most people in this situation feel as you do") or by a positive attitude (e.g., "While you are painting everything black, there are many positive things you are playing down").

3 *Confrontation*: Essential to change, confrontation may be positive or negative in its impact. It cannot be effective without preexisting rapport. Perceptions gained by listening may be disclosed (e.g., "You mention respect for your boss, but then you clench your fists"). Confrontation may best be used to point out areas of strength and competency in order to counter low self-esteem.

4 *Immediacy*: The initial focus should be the problem at hand. Definition of this problem and initial steps to diminish or resolve it may need to precede the exploration of underlying problems. Medication, as a temporary crutch, may be necessary, but often rapport, empathy, and support will suffice. Once the immediate problem is dealt with, one may seek *some* understanding of precipitating factors, *some* recognition of the personality problems involved, *some* understanding of past experiences, and *some* assessment of the home, work, and social relationships that will affect long-term adjustments.

Caution

As in all areas of practice, in individual and family therapy the physician must be conscious of his or her limitations. One must be willing to seek further knowledge and skill and appropriate consultative advice or referral for patient problems that one is not equipped to handle.

FACTORS INFLUENCING THE DECISION TO PRESCRIBE

A variety of factors influence both the decision to prescribe and what is to be prescribed. These factors are summarized in Figure 37-1.

Explosion in Drug Consumption

Perhaps the most important factor is the explosion in drug consumption. In the United States in 1977 the total expenditure on health care amounted to $162 billion (around $650 per capita). Of this, consumer expenditure on drugs was $14 billion—$9.6 billion on prescription drugs and $4.4 billion on over-the-counter (OTC) medications.[18] In the past decade this has probably increased considerably.

Consumer expenditure

It seems difficult for many doctors *not* to prescribe for patients, probably because it is quicker and easier to write a prescription than to give a long explanation of why medication may not be necessary. The natural consequence of prescribing to terminate an interview is the patient's assumption that the prescription is indicated for the presented problem. It further implies that the visit was appropriate and that the problem required treatment. If the visit was for a minor illness, the patient would probably consider it appropriate to return to the doctor if similar symptoms occurred and

Figure 37-1   Factors influencing physicians' prescribing.

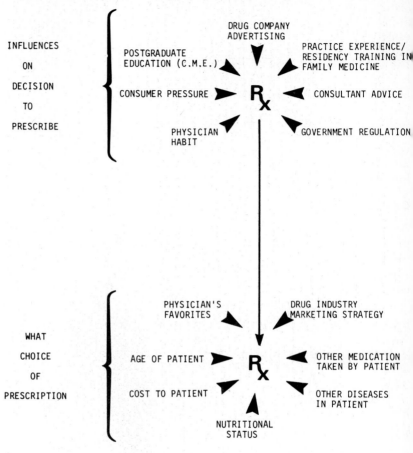

again expect a prescription. Such a sequence of events can only be altered by appropriate educational intervention by the physician, in lieu of a prescription.

Problems in Choosing Drugs

The number of drugs prescribed by family doctors varies considerably—from 84 to almost 500.[19-21]

From the over 22,000 drugs available in the United States, the top 200 made up 68.8 percent of the almost 1.5 billion prescriptions written in 1977. Generic prescriptions were written for only 10.5 percent of the total number.[22] Since the marketing costs of the U.S. drug industry are estimated at over $4000 per year per doctor,[23] the influence of this industry must be considered.

Table 37-3   Outline of Information and Sources Required for the Safe Prescribing of Drugs

Information required	Sources*
Generic name	
Trade names and bioavailability	1, 2, 3, 5, 10, 11
Costs of each	1, 11, 12
Indications	2, 3, 4, 5, 6, 11
Contraindications	
Absolute, relative	1, 2, 3, 4, 5, 7, 8, 10, 11
Precautions in use	1, 2, 3, 4, 5, 6, 7, 8
Action on target organs	1, 2, 3, 4, 5, 6, 7, 11
Pharmacokinetics	1, 2, 3, 4, 5, 7, 10, 11
Absorption—Promotion and interference	
Distribution—In what tissues, bound to protein, access to target organ(s)?	
Duration of action—Peak effect, half-life, accumulation	
Metabolism—Where? Active metabolites, excretion	
Adverse effect—Frequent, occasional, rare, and dangerous	1, 2, 3, 4, 5, 6, 7, 10, 11, 12
Abuse potential	1, 3, 5, 6, 7, 10
Overdose	2, 3, 4, 6, 7, 9, 10
Drug interactions—Significant, common or uncommon	1, 2, 3, 4, 5, 6, 7, 8, 10, 11
Preparation forms available	1, 4
Dosages	1, 2, 3, 4, 5, 6, 7

*Sources of information
1   Pharmacists
2   Medical journals
   a   Drug reviews
   b   Research studies
3   Medical letter
4   **a**   *Physicians' Desk Reference (PDR)*—United States
   b   *Compendium of Pharmaceuticals and Specialties (CPS)*—Canada
5   AMA drug evaluations
6   Therapeutic texts
7   Texts on pharmacology
8   Texts on drug interactions
9   Poison control centers and texts on poisoning
10   Drug information centers
11   Drug manufacturer
12   Patient

    In spite of the plethora of available products, the prudent family physician restricts prescriptions written to a limited number of medications that are well known, in most instances eliminating even the minor variations in available products. Obviously, an approach to the accumulation of complete information on each drug used is necessary. Such an approach is shown in outline in Table 37-3, which includes information sources.

It is recommended that physicians accumulate this information gradually for each medication utilized in their practices, noting situations in which one drug would be preferred over another. The physician should also remember that at least as many OTC drugs are taken by patients as drugs prescribed by physicians.[24] Because of this it is advisable for the family physician to keep handy an up-to-date publication on OTC drugs, such as the American Pharmaceutical Association's *Handbook of Non-Prescription Drugs*.[25]

PRINCIPLES OF PRESCRIBING

Rationalize
decision to
prescribe

Before a drug is prescribed, the physician should consider the following questions:

1 Is the medication chosen really *necessary*? The physician must guard against putting pen to prescription form without considering this question carefully.
2 Is the medication chosen really *effective*? Just because a drug is acceptable for a condition does not mean its prescription is useful. Controversy rages around simple choices such as deciding between an expectorant and a suppressant for a cough.
3 Is the medication chosen really *safe*? No drug appears to be completely free of harmful effects. Do these outweigh the benefits in this case? Would the prescription do more harm than good?
4 Is the medication cost *warranted*? Perhaps there is a less expensive way of solving the problem as effectively.
5 Is the medication chosen *appropriate for this patient*? Have age, concurrent disease, pregnancy, idiosyncrasy, other medications, etc., been considered?

Adding New Drugs

In making the decision to add new drugs to your pharmaceutical armamentarium, you should ask the following questions:

1 Why a new drug? Does it represent a new approach? If the same generic family, does it have
    a A broader spectrum?
    b Lowered toxicity?
    c Convenient packaging, dosage, and route?
    d Lower cost?
    e Increased patient acceptance?
2 What drug will it replace?
3 Do randomized double-blind controlled trials show clear effectiveness?

Evaluate drug
trial evidence

To identify appropriate drugs, one must evaluate the information available on therapeutic effectiveness. The ideal study is one that uses the double-blind method; e.g., the medication and comparison drug or placebo are administered randomly without anyone knowing who is getting which. Assessment of levels of compliance should be carefully reviewed, and drug use should be observed for adverse effects and interactions over a long enough period to warrant accurate conclusions. All data should then be subject to careful statistical analysis. Family physicians should acquire the needed skills in critically evaluating the medical literature.

Sadly, most drug studies do not meet these standards. It is not enough to demonstrate that a medication works, since placebos also work to a significant degree. One must be able to show a *significant difference* using appropriate statistical analysis. In addition, comparative studies should be made of other preparations used for the same conditions. These should also demonstrate an advantage that is statistically significant before any decision is made.

A recurrent theme in the doctor's mind should be "What real benefit will my patients obtain if I change my prescribing habits?"

An enormous amount of useful drug information is available to the family doctor, most of which cannot be discussed in this book. Our choice therefore has been to focus on areas in which individual physicians appear to have had difficulty when adjusting to the daily requirements of family practice. The four main areas chosen are therapeutic failure, adverse effects of drugs, drug interactions, and a practical guide to prescribing.

THERAPEUTIC FAILURE

In most clinical situations, there are many potential causes of therapeutic failure. The role of bioavailability in causing failure has been grossly exaggerated. More important factors are listed in Table 37-4.

Table 37-4   Important Causes of Therapeutic Failure

Cause	Example
Improper choice of drugs	Sulfa in lobar pneumonia
Inappropriate dose	Digoxin in congestive failure
Concurrent disease	Insulin need in hyperthyroid diabetic
Drug interaction	Tetracycline taken with antacid
Patient idiosyncracy	Penicillin in allergic patient
Lack of compliance	Forgotten doses, etc.
Individual variability	Absorption, distribution, etc.

A demonstration of statistically significant differences in the bioavailability of equivalent drugs from different manufacturers does not prove that the therapeutic effects of the drugs will differ in a clinically important fashion. Moreover, the differences are even less important for drugs for which the effective dosage is highly variable, e.g., diuretics used for hypertension. Physicians are accustomed to titrating the dosage of such drugs against pharmacological effects and establishing an effective and safe dosage for each patient. In contrast, the family physician must be aware of the need to identify medications with a narrow range of safety—e.g., cardiac glycosides, anticoagulants, cytotoxic drugs—and carefully consider bioavailability in these cases.

Prescribing generically

A U.S. congressional investigative body concluded that 85 to 90 percent of clinically equivalent products presented no problems in therapeutic equivalence and could be used interchangeably.[26] Thus generic products should be prescribed more frequently than at present.

It is important to recognize that regulatory standards have been set up in Canada and the United States for all new drugs introduced. These standards require reasonably equivalent bioavailability of competitively marketed drug products.

ADVERSE EFFECTS OF DRUGS

Every drug has adverse effects. Because of this simple fact, consideration of a medication must include how frequently specific adverse effects occur and how dangerous they are when they do occur. The physician must judge whether a particular illness warrants the use of a drug with adverse effects that may be more dangerous to the patient than either going without medication or substituting a less therapeutically satisfactory but safer drug.

Iatrogenic diseases

In reviewing the magnitude of this problem, reports indicate that between 18 and 30 percent of all hospitalized patients have a drug reaction and the duration of their hospitalization is doubled as a consequence.[27] Of all admissions to the hospital, 3 to 5 percent are primarily the result of a drug reaction, and 30 percent of patients admitted for this reason have a second reaction during their hospital stay. A drug reaction is defined as any unwanted consequence of drug administration, including administration of the wrong drug to the wrong patient and the wrong dosage (form, amount, route, or interval) at the wrong time and for the wrong disease.[27] Any single "wrong" may result in unwanted effects. Classic reactions (e.g., hypersensitivity, idiosyncracy), or the inevitable risk of toxic drugs, make up less than 20 to 30 percent of drug reactions. This means that the remaining 70 to 80 percent are predictable, and thus largely avoidable.[27] The physician must always consider that the use of a drug may cause a disorder to which the patient would not otherwise be subject (ulceration of the bowel may develop from potassium chloride, cardiac failure from propranolol).

Unfortunately little information is available to quantify the frequency of adverse reactions in ambulatory settings. Drug reactions are generally poorly reported by physicians. In the absence of accurate information, a constant awareness of potential adverse effects is necessary.

Classifying Adverse Reactions

In the relative isolation of family practice, in which most doctor-patient interactions occur in the office, the physician needs to be able to organize his or her thoughts on adverse reactions so as to prescribe thoughtfully and appropriately.

Dose-Related Reactions

1 *Excessive therapeutic effect*: This is most likely to occur as an exaggeration of the normal therapeutic effect and is especially important if a precise dose is needed, e.g., in the use of oral anticoagulants, potent antihypertensives, or digoxin.
2 *Side effects.*
   a Pharmacological: Because most drugs have more than one action, effects other than the therapeutically desired one occur. For example, antihistamines usually have an anticholinergic effect, decreasing secretions and depressing the central nervous system and thus causing drowsiness. At times, side effects are a reason to use the drug; e.g., aspirin can be used to decrease platelet adhesiveness in transient ischemic attacks, and codeine, which has the adverse effect of constipation when used as an analgesic, may be helpful in the treatment of diarrhea.
   b Toxic: Most drugs, if used in large enough doses, have toxic effects. Occasionally, the therapeutic level and the toxic level are quite close, which makes toxicity difficult to avoid, e.g., in the case of digoxin.
   c Secondary: The use of a medication may result in problems because it may pave the way for another illness; e.g., corticosteroids may lower defense mechanisms, predisposing to activation of latent tuberculosis; and broad-spectrum antibiotics, such as tetracycline and ampicillin, eliminate normal flora, encouraging the development of candidiasis.

Non-Dose-Related Reactions

1 *Idiosyncratic*: These reactions occur in a few individuals, and are probably due to some genetically determined abnormality. While their precise mechanisms are usually unknown, it is important to remember the problems they can cause. For example, one of the most common inherited enzyme defects in black patients is glucose-6-phosphate dehydrogenase (G6PD) deficiency. Here, hemolysis may be precipitated by many drugs and chemicals because of impaired red cell stability in this deficient state. Commonly used medications such as sulfonamides and aspirin may present problems in this condition.

2 *Allergic*: Drug allergy occurs through antigen-antibody reaction. A necessary ingredient is sensitization by previous exposure to the drug or a chemically related substance. High-molecular-weight medications can act as a complete antigen. Most drugs are small molecules and therefore become antigenic after they combine with body proteins. Atopic individuals are especially likely to develop drug allergies. Sensitization may be produced by any route of administration, even on the skin. Thereafter very small doses may produce a reaction, with clinical manifestation determined by the antigen-antibody reaction. Examples are penicillin causing anaphylaxis, thiazide causing thrombocytopenia, phenylbutazone causing agranulocytosis, and serum sickness from the use of sulfonamides or long-acting penicillin. Drug fever and urticaria are other examples.

Long-Term Effects   With the passage of time it is often more difficult to detect reactions to a long-term medication. If, as sometimes occurs, the reaction manifests itself clinically after the medication has been stopped, the relationship is even harder to establish. Even more important, reactions may be irreversible by the time they are detected. Long-term reactions can be divided into two types:

1 *Cumulative overdose*: This type of effect is usually dose-related, and is sometimes associated with deposition of the drug in specific tissues, which can happen, for example, with chloroquine if it is given for prolonged periods in the treatment of rheumatoid arthritis. This drug is deposited particularly in the cornea and retina and may be detected in tissue for several years after it has been discontinued. Only early detection of these asymptomatic changes in retinal function can prevent visual loss. Cumulative effects can also be seen with the use of topical drugs; e.g., fluorinated steroids used on the face have been related to skin atrophy and perioral dermatitis.

Think of drug effects
  2 *Delayed effects*: A number of effects that occur months or years after the use of drugs are well documented, e.g., hypothyroidism after treatment with radioactive iodine, retroperitoneal fi-

brosis with prolonged use of methysergide for vascular headaches, and hypertension with use of an oral contraceptive.

The point has already been made that detection of adverse effect of drugs may occur only after prolonged clinical use. The responsibility for reporting such reactions when they occur in medical practice cannot be overemphasized. The incidence of many adverse effects is unknown, partly because doctors do not take this responsibility seriously. Suspected associations between the use of a medication and an illness should always be reported.

Report adverse drug effects

Practical Pointers for Minimizing Adverse Effects: The Patient

Individual Variation   Each patient has his or her own unique response to any medication. While one individual may experience no drowsiness after taking 25 mg of chlordiazepoxide, another may be totally unable to function with 5 mg.

Age   Special risks occur with age. The effect of the doses and the distribution of drugs in the body vary for the neonate, infant, child, adult, and the aged. Particular care should be paid in prescribing at the extremes of age. Care of the newborn has been well described, but care of the elderly is not so well understood. The percentage of adverse reactions rises from 3 percent in the 20-to-29 age range to 21.3 percent in the 70-to-79 age range.[28] There are particular reasons why elderly patients are more likely to develop adverse reactions to drugs, and tailoring drug dosages for the elderly must take these into account. (See Table 37-5.)

It is extremely important to remember that drugs are not the answer to many elderly patients' symptoms and problems. Instead, changes may have to be made in the elderly person's lifestyle. Lack

Precautions with the elderly

Table 37-5   Practical Pointers for Minimizing Adverse Drug Effects

The patient.
1   Individual variations.
2   Age.
3   Diet.
4   Altered physiological states, e.g., pregnancy and breast feeding.
5   Patient information.
6   Concurrent illness, e.g., liver, kidney, GI.

The drug.
1   Limit your drug armamentarium.
2   Know individual drug pharmacokinetics.
3   Limit polypharmacy.
4   Have therapeutic objectives (cure or palliation?).
5   Be aware of interference with chemical tests.

of physical and mental exercise, combined with poor nutrition, may increase the patient's rapid downhill course. Furthermore, it should be noted that people frequently do just what is expected of them. A daughter may say to her mother, "Just relax, Granny, we will do everything." If Granny does just that for a couple of years, the daughter will have a problem on her hands, and she may then demand medical help. The physician who sees a patient at this point often finds multiple pathological conditions, with multiple symptoms and signs. This situation may invite polypharmacy, increasing the likelihood of drug interaction.

Loss of cerebral reserve, with gradual failure of cognitive function, imposes severe constraints on the use of many drugs, particularly for the individual who lives alone. Barbituates, like other tranquilizers, may produce nocturnal restlessness rather than sedation. Furthermore, elderly people are often unsteady on their feet and liable to fall, particularly if they are on any drug that causes clouding of the consciousness, increased tendency to sway, or postural hypotension. Codeine may increase a tendency toward constipation. Tricyclic antidepressants may cause urinary retention. Such adverse effects may precipitate a crisis in an older person.

Since few tools are available to help one to precisely evaluate an elderly person's physiological status, good judgment is essential. Smaller doses of all drugs should be given initially. An acceptable practice is to start the older patient on one-half of the usual dose of the drug and then monitor the response.

In addition to being careful when adding medication, it is important to know when to take patients off their drugs. A "drug holiday" may be indicated for the elderly patient who has been confused, incontinent, or "chairfast" while taking a large number of drugs. At the end of the drug holiday, medications can be reintroduced one at a time and the patient monitored carefully for adverse reactions. Only those drugs that are absolutely necessary should be reintroduced.

Diet   Quite often, the physician is unaware of the patient's diet. Salicylate levels are 50 percent lower when ASA is taken with a meal rather than before or after. However, this level may be acceptable if one must avoid gastric irritation. It should be recognized that ASA is the second most common drug (first is digoxin) implicated as the cause of hospital admission, principally for gastrointestinal bleeding.[29]

When they are taken with food, the absorption of some antibiotics (e.g., penicillin G, tetracycline) is impaired. Individual foods may further markedly reduce absorption (e.g., tetracycline with milk). To prevent adverse effects for patients on an MAO inhibitor, it is essential to eliminate tyramine-containing foods (e.g., cheese, Chianti wine).

Altered Physiological States Requiring Special Considera-tion *Pregnancy* ⎯ The concept of the placenta as a barrier to drug transfer should have disappeared with the disaster of thalido-mide. One of the major problems in identifying drug reactions in pregnancy is the fact that prospective studies on drug use are not carried out in pregnant women. Since occasional prescribing will occur prior to the time a woman is aware of pregnancy, the physi-cian should be aware of the need to restrict medication use in women who use no satisfactory method of contraception unless the medication is absolutely necessary. It may be that this risk must be run if the medication is needed to treat a maternal disorder. Stud-ies have indicated that every mother consumes one drug in normal daily dosage throughout 60 percent of her pregnancy, and on the average 10.3 drugs are taken in the course of the pregnancy.[30,31]

Placental transfer

The duration of consumption of drugs and the timing of drug administration during pregnancy are important if the doctor is to ascertain clinical effects on the fetus. Table 37-6 shows that there are tendencies to use particular medication at particular stages of pregnancy.[32]

In fact, it is likely that 75 to 80 percent of all medications, as a low estimate,[33] should *not* be prescribed in pregnancy, since conclu-sive evidence for this population is not available. There are no safe drugs in pregnancy, only calculated risks!

At the time of labor and delivery, a variety of medications are commonly utilized—narcotics, anesthetics (local and inhaled), bar-bituates, and numerous tranquilizers—all of which may depress the fetus's central nervous system so that respiration is not adequately

Table 37-6   Drugs Prescribed or Self-Administered during Pregnancy

Early pregnancy	Late pregnancy	Throughout pregnancy
Antiemetic	Antacids	Antibiotics
Antihistamines	Analgesics	Cough medicine
Appetite depressants	Barbituates	Iron
Bronchodilators	Diuretics	Tranquilizers
Hormones	Hypnotics	
	Sulfonamides	
	Vitamins	

Source: Yaffe.[32]

established at birth. In addition, addiction of the mother to morphine, heroin, or alcohol may result in withdrawal symptoms.

Breast Feeding   In recent years women have been increasingly choosing to breast-feed their offspring, with the result that a growing number of babies have become the passive recipients of drugs, prescribed or otherwise. However, little research has been done on the presence of drugs in breast milk and the effect on young recipients. It is generally agreed that any substance taken by the lactating mother will to some extent be found in her milk. If drugs must be prescribed to the lactating mother, one must weigh the drug benefits against the known and unknown risks to the child.

Drugs in
mother's milk
Some drugs are excreted in the mother's milk in greater quantities than others, and the cumulative effect of drugs on the development of the baby's organs is not known. In any event, one might consider advising mothers who are taking medications that may not be easy for the immature liver and kidney to handle that breast feeding is contraindicated. For example, steroids have such broad effects that they contraindicate breast feeding. Antimigraine agents such as ergotamine cause severe reactions in infants, such as vomiting, diarrhea, and even shock.

Prescribing any drug during lactation should be approached with caution.

Patient Information   Doctors often seem to avoid telling patients that the use of a potent medication may have unwanted side effects. Even though the physician may be uncomfortable discussing these possibilities, this is no excuse for avoiding the subject. It is often argued that such discussions will result in the patient's imagining adverse reactions. But we are not nearly as reluctant to discuss the pros and cons of an operation or other therapeutic measures and to disclose the risks involved. If informed consent is important in one situation, it is important in the other. The risk is that the patient may refuse to use the medication, but reason demands that the patient should have this right. Full disclosure must always be tempered by the physician's knowledge of the patient.

Concurrent Illness   Great care must be taken in prescribing drugs for patients with both liver and renal disease, since most drugs are first inactivated in the liver prior to excretion by the kidney. In patients with severe liver disease, increased sensitivity to sedatives and hypnotics occurs due to slower breakdown of these drugs. Patients with renal failure will often develop symptoms related to either excessive therapeutic effect (e.g., with barbituates) or accumulation of metabolites due to poor renal excretion (e.g., with diazepam).

It is easy to forget that tetracyclines may cause a rise in blood urea if renal function is poor; potassium-sparing diuretics may cause hyperkalemia in the elderly patient with a decrease in renal function who is unable to excrete potassium. In addition, many drugs are toxic to the kidney and are therefore more likely to cause damage in renal function that is already compromised.

Many illnesses alter either drug availability or tissue sensitivity. The patient with hypothyroidism has increased sensitivity due to slower elimination and may have problems with digoxin. Congestive failure may be aggravated by the use of phenylbutazone, producing sodium retention. Bronchospasm may be induced in patients with asthma when beta-adrenergic blockers such as propranolol are used.

Every time a drug is prescribed, the patient's problem list *must* be perused.

Practical Pointers for Minimizing Adverse Effects: The Drug

Limit Drug Armamentarium   Doctors are legally responsible for being knowledgeable about the drugs they prescribe and must ensure that a potent medication with recognized severe adverse effects is not used in situations in which less dangerous medications (or no treatment at all) may suffice. The potential harm of a drug should not prevent the doctor from prescribing such a drug if the calculated risk is justified, but the risk *must* have been carefully considered. In addition, the patient should be aware of both the therapeutic benefits and the dangers of the drug.

Individual Drug Pharmacokinetics   Pharmacokinetics may be defined as a study of the factors which must be considered to ensure that a safe, consistent, predictable, therapeutically effective level of drug results from drug administration. Such factors determine the absorption, distribution, metabolism, and excretion of a drug and/or its metabolites. The absorption of drugs across the intestinal mucosa is governed largely by the lipid solubility of the compound, and the more lipid-soluble it is, the more readily it will pass by passive diffusion.

Body weight and thickness may modify the effect of a drug. Since any nonionized compound is more lipid-soluble, it is more likely to distribute in adipose tissue. An obese patient may demonstrate relatively little effect from this type of drug for a fairly long time. However, once effects are seen, they may persist even after administration is terminated as the drug slowly migrates from fat stores to receptors. Conversely, a thin person may demonstrate a pronounced effect rather quickly after a low total dose of a drug with high lipid solubility (e.g., pentobarbital, diazepam).

In excretion, the renal clearance of some drugs is remarkably influenced by changes in the pH of urine. In urine of low pH, weakly acid drugs such as sulfonamides or phenobarbital are found in relatively low concentration. The opposite is true if the urine is alkaline. Using such information in prescribing not only helps make the drug more effective but also may help to eliminate drug overdose.

Multiple drug prescriptions

Polypharmacy Multiple drug prescriptions should be avoided whenever possible. This is especially true at the initiation of therapy. Most physicians are familiar with the elderly patient who arrives with a bag filled with pill bottles, all with directions to be taken at different times throughout the day. The best approach in these circumstances is to attempt to reduce the number of pills or the number of times a day they are taken.

Despite the frequent denunciation of fixed combinations of drugs, they may have a valid use in cases where effective dosage levels have been established. The vast majority of drugs prescribed individually are used in standard dosages. The same dosages are sometimes (but not always) available in combinations.

Therapeutic Objectives   The use of a drug entails the need to consider the specific aims of the therapy. This is particularly necessary for two categories of drugs—antibiotics and psychotropics that are extensively used by family physicians.[19-21] The aim of antibiotic therapy should be to cure an infection. However, there is a tendency to use antibiotics when one has evidence only of a viral infection.

The prolonged use of psychotropics without addressing the underlying problems is also commonplace.

Drug Interference with Clinical Chemistry Laboratory Tests   When testing a patient taking medication, the possibility of drug interference should always be kept in mind. For example, methyldopa administration interferes with measurement of catecholamine excretion in the urine; aspirin will often cause a decreased serum albumin due to technical interference with the test, while small doses of aspirin may also increase uric acid level through biological interference.

These examples show that medications alter laboratory tests by either pharmacological or technical mechanisms. Either because of its primary action or incidentally, a drug may cause a *true* change in the concentration of the substance being measured.

Technical interference stems from chemical or physical problems that the drug creates in the methods used for analysis. Physicians must keep in mind that unexpected or even contradictory laboratory results may be due to the effect of prescribed or self-administered drugs. When unusual or unexpected results occur, further information should be sought.

When blood tests are being considered, the physician should always ask what drugs patients are taking on their own initiative. Like ASA, oral contraceptives may be overlooked, since patients do not consider these medications. Birth control pills are notorious for causing an increased serum thyroxin test result by increasing the concentration of serum thyroxin–binding globulin.

DRUG INTERACTIONS

Polypharmacy generates additional adverse reactions. One study showed that the average medical inpatient in the United States receives about nine different drugs per hospitalization.[34] If the incidence of adverse reactions per drug is 5 percent, on the average, it is evident that enormous numbers of hospital patients will statistically show drug reactions and interactions. The tremendous number of possible drug interactions and the pharmacological complexities involved make it impractical, if not impossible, for family physicians to depend on their memories for full information on drug interactions.

Drug interactions are usually the direct result of therapeutic decisions. If the physician does not have a good record system, the patient can easily be exposed to higher risks of interactions. Prescribing a drug without an adequate medication list for the patient also increases the risks. This is particularly likely to happen when the physician on call is in a group practice. Some drug interactions are shown in Figure 37-2.

Keep good records

Adverse effects of one medication may lead to the use of another to treat these effects. Take the example of a patient with multiple problems of chronic arthritis, severe chronic obstructive lung disease, and hypertension. Such a patient may be on phenylbutazone, which causes some degree of indigestion. An antacid mixture is prescribed to treat the indigestion. The physician on call the following weekend sees the patient in relation to a flare-up of the chronic obstructive lung disease. Tetracycline is prescribed, but the antacid interferes with absorption of the medication. Moreover, additional sodium may be provided in the antacid, compounding the effect of phenylbutazone in promoting sodium retention. The blood pressure, previously under reasonable control with hydrochlorothiazide and methyldopa, worsens. The patient is tipped into cardiac failure, and digoxin is then added to the regimen. Unfor-

Figure 37-2 Examples of drug interactions.

	Coumadin (Warfarin)	Hydrochlorothiazide	Glyburide (Diabeta)	Penicillin G.	Tetracycline	Aspirin	Digoxin	Propranolol	Ampicillin	Ferrous sulphate	Birth Control Pill	Insulin	Ibuprofen	Maalox	Quinidine	Vitamin C	Probenecid
Coumadin (Warfarin)						*							*				
Hydrochlorothiazide							*	*									
Glyburide (Diabeta)								*					*				
Penicillin G.																	*
Tetracycline										*							
Aspirin	*																*
Digoxin		*						*						*			
Propranolol		*					*					*					
Ampicillin											*						
Ferrous Sulphate					*												
Birth Control Pill										*							
Insulin								*									
Ibuprofen	*		*														
Maalox						*	*										
Quinidine																*	
Vitamin C.															*		
Probenecid						*											
Lab Test		1				2	3				4					5	

1. Hydrochlorothiazide - Increases serum glucose, uric acid and decreases serum potassium
2. Aspirin - Decreases serum albumin, increases serum uric acid
3. Propranolol - Decreases serum glucose
4. Birth Control Pill - Increases serum thyroxine
5. Vitamin C - False negative urine glucose

tunately, the patient becomes depressed by this turn of events and is placed on a tricyclic antidepressant, which further worsens the chronic obstructive lung disease by its anticholinergic effects.

Nonprescribed medications must *not* be forgotten. Alcohol content in numerous cough syrups, tonics, and so on may interact with other medications. Since it is related to disulfiram, metronidazole can cause a severe reaction if alcohol is consumed. Metronidazole, in fact, is used as adjunctive therapy in the treatment of alcoholism, since intensely uncomfortable symptoms result when alcohol is taken.

What Can Be Done about Reducing Interactions

Short of never prescribing more than one medication, how can a family physician effectively cope with the problem of multiple drug usage? Since our knowlege of drug interactions is severely limited, access to more information is obviously necessary.

Examples of publications that provide such information are *Evaluations of Drug Interactions*, published by the American Pharmaceutical Association,[35] and *Drug Interactions* by Hansten.[36] *The Handbook of Non-Prescription Drugs*, published by the American Pharmaceutical Association,[25] is also useful with regard to OTC preparations. There is a variety of regional drug information centers in North America that may be consulted for information when necessary. Physicians living near such a center should seek further information from the center.

PRACTICAL GUIDE TO PRESCRIBING

At this point in the discussion, it is useful to summarize the elements necessary for sensible prescribing, since they need to be reviewed each time a prescription is written.

1 Look critically at the need to prescribe at each visit.
2 Use prescriptions only when the medication will (*a*) cure, (*b*) relieve symptoms, or (*c*) slow the progression of the disease.
3 Remember that short-term, self-limiting illness is not cured by medication.
4 Consider whether the risks of the medication outweigh the risks of the illness.
5 Write prescriptions for restricted intervals or with few repeats, so that monitoring of therapy can occur, to review (*a*) compliance, (*b*) adverse effects, (*c*) response, and (*d*) the continuing need for the medication.
6 Encourage patients to get rid of medications that may have lost their potency because their expiration dates have passed.
7 Use the least expensive medication that has comparable therapeutic efficacy; i.e., know about costs!

8   Give your patients instructions on the how, why, and when of taking medications.

9   Avoid polypharmacy if possible, but when necessary simplify treatment regimens.

10   Recognize special circumstances of prescribing (age, pregnancy, abuse potential, etc.).

11   Use accurate, legible prescription writing.

12   Do not trust your memory when prescribing information.

13   Restrict the variety of drugs used.

14   Collaborate with the pharmacist.

15   Consider your patient's lifestyle.

Writing Prescriptions

An appropriate prescription pad should contain all the elements shown in Figure 37-3, which is self-explanatory.

Using the Prescription Form

1   *Physician's name, address, and phone:* Have prescription forms imprinted so that (a) your signature can be interpreted accurately and (b) a pharmacist may easily contact you. Remember that a prescription is a legal document.

2   *Patient's name and address* should be clearly legible.

3   *Medication name, form, and dosage strength* should be clear to the pharmacist.

4   *Quantity:* Figures alone may be satisfactory (e.g., 50). However, in cases of drug abuse, prescriptions have been altered after leaving the physician's hands. To prevent this, the amount to be prescribed should be both spelled out and expressed as a figure (e.g., "diazepam tabs 5 mg. Quantity—50—fifty"). This is especially important during an on-call rotation or when dealing with individuals new to the practice.

5   *Renewal:* If repeat prescriptions are indicated, it is essential to specify the number of times and the intervals at which they may be renewed. While this is most important with prescriptions that may be abused, it is also pertinent when one needs to see patients at regular intervals to monitor compliance, response, adverse effects, and continuing need for medication. Initial prescriptions are best written with no repeat. "As necessary" (prn) repeats should not be written. (This topic is discussed more fully in a later chapter.)

6   *Safety cap:* A childproof safety cap is indicated when small children are in the house. However, it may be contraindicated for the elderly, a person with arthritis of the hands, or the occasional individual who cannot make it work.

7   *Drug name on label:* In some regions of the United States and Canada, the law demands that pharmacists place the name and dosage strength of the medication on the label. Where the law does not require it, common sense does (e.g., penicillin VK tabs 300 mg). In addition to the patient, other physicians who may see the patient will find this information useful, and sometimes essential.

Figure 37-3   A typical prescription form.

D Dalhousie University
Family Medicine Centre
5599 Fenwick Street
Fenwick Towers
Halifax, Nova Scotia B3H 1R2

Phone: 424-7010

Date: _____ 19 _____

For: _____

Address: _____

Rx

Label as to contents   YES ☐   NO ☐
Safety Closure   YES ☐   NO ☐
No Repeat ☐   Repeat ☐ X   at   intervals
Product Selection Authorized   YES ☐   NO ☐

_____
Physician's Signature

_____
Print Physician's name

---

8   *Substitute least expensive generic drug:* In situations where bioavailability is not a problem, the patient should receive the least expensive equivalent. If "least expensive" is not inserted, the pharmacist may substitute any product in stock, which could be more expensive than necessary.

9   *Expiration date:* Insertion of this information makes it more likely that patients will not take unused portions of prescriptions that may have declined in effectiveness.

10   *Signature:* Be sure that your signature is legible.

11   *Patient directions:* Wording a prescription "as directed" is unsatisfactory. The patient's memory is no better than yours. The need for specific directions cannot be overemphasized. Patients may be confused about directions but reluctant to ask the pharmacist or the physician for clarification. Table 37-7 illustrates pa-

Table 37-7   Frequency Distribution of Patient Interpretations of Instructions on Prescription Labels

Prescription label	Interpretation	No.	%
Tetracycline "Every 6 hours"	Every 6 hours	24	35.8
	Every 6 hours for three doses only	17	25.4
	Four doses unevenly spaced Other	13	19.4
Penicillin G "Three times a day and at bedtime"	After meals and at bedtime	60	89.5
	10 a.m., 2 p.m., 6 p.m., and 10 p.m.	3	4.5
	No response	3	4.5
	Morning, noon, evening, and bedtime	1	1.5

Penicillin G
  "30 minutes before meals and at bedtime
  on an empty stomach"
	Correct	61	91.0

	Incorrect	6	9.0
Nitrofurantoin "With meals"	Before meals	36	53.7
	With meals	22	32.8
	After meals	9	13.4

Nitrofurantoin
  "To be taken immediately after food 4 times
  a day"
	Correct	57	85.1

	Incorrect	10	14.9
Propoxyphene "Every 4 hours as needed for pain"	Correct	54	80.6
	Incorrect	13	19.4

Propoxyphene
  "Every 4 hours as needed for pain" (What is
  the maximum number of doses that can be
  taken in 24 hours?)
	Six	35	52.2

	Four	22	32.8
	Five	4	6.0
	Two	2	3.0
	Three	2	3.0
	More than six	1	1.5
	No response	1	1.5

Source: Mazzullo et al.[37]

tient understanding of specific common directions.[37] Be sure your directions are clearly understood, and avoid abbreviations.

Special Considerations

Pointers to aid compliance

1 *General:* Remember to write in metric terms. The form of medication should be considered—tablets and capsules are difficult to swallow for some adults and for most children under 10 years of age. These individuals will invariably gag, spit, or refuse to swallow.

2 *Liquids:* Liquid preparations have their own problems. For example, accurate doses can be difficult to administer. A survey of 1000 households revealed that 15 percent of those interviewed did not know a teaspoon from a soupspoon or tablespoon. Moreover, teaspoons varied in size from 2.4 to 7.2 ml.[38] Many pharmacies will supply calibrated dose cups, and this should be encouraged. Where the proper dose is one-half or one-quarter teaspoonful, it is often easier to use a diluent to bring the individual dose to a 5-ml teaspoon.

3 *Topicals:* Topical preparations require special consideration, and their use should be reviewed. Only three points will be mentioned here: (*a*) remember that lotions and creams are advisable for erythematous, weepy lesions, while ointments retain moisture in dry ones; (*b*) the classic division between topical and systemic drugs may not apply with impaired skin, which may allow systemic effects when ulcers, burns, and lesser injuries are treated; (*c*) patients have the tendency to feel that if some is good, more will be better. Write "Use sparingly" in directions.

4 *Lifestyle:* A careful consideration of a patient's lifestyle makes it possible to adjust medication taking to suit that patient's daily schedule. This requires familiarity with the chosen drug's duration of action to ensure that intervals are appropriate. For example, deterioration in compliance will obviously occur if one prescribes a rapid-acting morning diuretic for an individual with a fairly active morning schedule. To assist the patient, one may suggest that morning medications be placed by the toothbrush or denture cup; mealtime medications can be placed on the table. Older, confused patients may be assisted if one arranges for another individual to lay out their medications with clearly marked directions. The person with recent memory loss will appreciate this help, since he or she will easily be able to tell whether or not a particular dose has been taken.

5 *The telephone in treatment and prescribing:* The role of the telephone in a modern North American family practice is extremely important. In one Canadian practice, telephone contact (considering only clinical calls involving the doctor) represented 28 percent of all doctor-patient encounters outside the hospital, or 20 percent of total practice contact with patients.[39] The time required for these calls represented a daily average of 30 minutes. Many physicians find that telephone time consumes a much higher proportion of their work life. In one pediatric practice, up to 1½ hours per day was devoted to telephone consultations with mothers.[40] Since many doctors do not charge a fee for a telephone consultation, the saving in money to the patient treated on the phone can be quite considerable. One physician estimated that if all patients contacted by telephone were seen in the office, his workload and resulting gross income would rise over 20 percent.[38]

The physician or nurse is faced with a special set of circumstances in telephone management. It is first necessary to decide if the patient must be seen. If the patient need not be seen, treatment by telephone may result, for example, when the physician or nurse considers the diagnosis relatively clear or when the symptom presentation does not seem serious. A wait-and-see approach may also be decided on.

Depending on how well the patient is known, a decision to prescribe advice or phone a prescription to a pharmacy may result. This requires accepting the patient's presentation of the problem as accurate and trusting in his or her responsibility.

The variability in the way physicians deal with problems on the telephone suggests that each of us must look carefully at our use of this powerful communications tool. Telephone treatment is deplored by some, but in a busy family practice it offers the patient quick access to the physician, and vice versa.

Added Patient Directions

More directions than can be placed on a prescription label are often required. The pharmacist will sometimes include extra labels, e.g., "Shake well before using" for suspensions, or "Refrigerate" if necessary. In some cases, the physician must also include special directions to the patient. For nitroglycerin prescriptions, for example, one must inform the patient of the need for keeping tablets dry, cool, and out of direct light. The patient also needs a small amber pocket vial to be carried for use as needed (the amber color of the vial prevents the medication from being gradually broken down by exposure to light). This is because the active ingredient is depleted by frequent opening of a larger vial, since the cotton pledget absorbs considerable medication. The patient should also be instructed to replace the stock vial every 3 months.

Instructions printed as handouts

Other precautions include giving the patient prepared handouts with the prescription form. Two examples are displayed in Figure 37-4.[41]

Many other prescriptions require special directions because of the method of administration. Vaginal preparations are supplied in packages appropriate for the usual course of therapy, which contain instructions for use. Products sold in an inhaler form also have a patient leaflet. Since inhalers are often misused, additional directions may be advisable; an example is given in Figure 37-5.

Eye preparations are supplied both as ointments and liquids;

Figure 37-4 Patient instructions.

```
TORONTO GENERAL HOSPITAL, PHARMACY DEPT.

            DIAZEPAM



Unless otherwise directed by your physician,
Alcohol should be avoided while on this
medication.

Do not exceed the dose prescribed by your
physician.

This medication may make you drowsy.
Therefore exercise caution when driving
or when operating machinery.
```

```
TORONTO GENERAL HOSPITAL, PHARMACY DEPT.

         HYDROCHLOROTHIAZIDE



Take this medication with food.

If your diet allows, drink plenty of
fruit juice (orange, grapefruit, or
apple) or eat a portion of fruit
(bananas or oranges) daily.

While on this medication, avoid excessive
exposure to sunlight, as this may result
in a skin rash or irritation.  If this
occurs, contact your physician.
```

Figure 37-5 Patient instructions for therapeutic effectiveness.

TORONTO GENERAL HOSPITAL, PHARMACY DEPT.

BECLOMETHASONE DIPROPIONATE AEROSOL

To assure proper use of inhaler, follow
instructions outlined in the "Patient's
Leaflet" enclosed with inhaler.

After each dose (either 1 or 2 "puffs"),
thoroughly rinse out mouth with water.

If no relief in symptoms is obtained after
2 weeks of therapy at the prescribed dose,
notify your physician.

Store inhaler at room temperature away
from stove, radiators or other sources
of heat.

Figure 37-6 Instillation of eye drops.

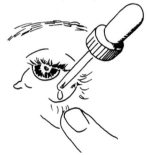

1. Open eye and tilt head backward and look toward ceiling.
2. Gently pull down the lower lid to form a pouch.
3. Approach the eye from the side and hold the dropper or bottle-
    dropper near the lid but do not touch the eyelids or eyelashes.
4. Drop the prescribed number of drops into the pouch.
5. Close the eyes (do not rub the eyes) and blink several times.
6. Apply gently pressure for a few minutes with your fingers to
    the bridge of the nose to prevent the medication from being
    drained from the eye.
7. Blot excess solution around the eye with a tissue.
8. Do not use solution if it is discolored or has changed in
    any way since being purchased.
9. Never contaminate the dropper and solution by touching the
    eye or eyelid with the dropper.
10. If possible, have another person administer the eye drops
    for you.

☐ If this medication causes blurred vision, do not drive a car
   or operate machinery.

☐ For external use only.

ointments are usually preferred because they are longer-acting. Putting eye drops into the tightly closed eye of a squirming child is a job for two or three people, and many parents give up the struggle. The use of such medications may be facilitated by demonstration or the provision of clear, special printed instructions. The example in Figure 37-6 saves repeated explanation of basic instructions, which takes precious time. Such aids are available from a variety of sources.[42]

SUMMARY

This and the preceding chapter constitute an overview of patient management, a subject in which the family physician must be particularly expert. The chapters provide only pragmatic advice, and the added depth needed by the family physician must be gleaned from the many excellent sources available, some of which have been referred to in the text.

REFERENCES

1 W. Watson, "The Cures and Treatment of Non-disease," *Canadian Medical Association Journal,* **114:**402–403, 1976.

2 T. Marsh, "Curing Minor Illness in General Practice," *British Medical Journal,* **2**(6097):1267–1269, November 12, 1977.

3 F. Heinzelmann and R. Bagley, "Response to Physical Activity Programs and Their Effectiveness on Health Behaviour," *Public Health Reports,* **85:**905–911, 1970.

4 D. W. Marsland, M. Wood, and F. Mayo, "Content of Family Practice," *Journal of Family Practice,* **3**(1):3, 1976.

5 D. Hastings et al., "A Study of Hockey Injuries in Ontario," *Ontario Medical Review,* **41:**686–692, November 1974.

6 D. Hayes, "Hockey Injuries: How, Why, Where and When?" *The Physician and Sports Medicine,* **3:**61, January 1975.

7 D. Kovach, "Helping Hockey Players Avoid Groin Pulls," *The Physician and Sports Medicine,* **4:**110, May 1976.

8 B. Howard, "The Clinical Stroke Team," *Stroke Diagnosis and Management: Current Procedures and Equipment,* Warren H. Green, St. Louis, 1973.

9 F. H. McDowell, "Rehabilitating Patients with Stroke," *Postgraduate Medicine,* **59**(3):145–149, 1976.

10 T. Hunt and R. Crichton, "One Third of a Million Days of Care at Home, 1959 to 1975," *Canadian Medical Association Journal,* **116:**1351–1355, 1977.

11 M. Balint et al., *Treatment or Diagnosis: A Study of Repeat Prescriptions in General Hospitals,* Tavistock Publications, London, 1970.

12 A. J. Fix and E. A. Haffke, *Basic Psychological Therapies: Comparative Effectiveness,* Human Sciences Press, New York, 1976, pp. 15–20.

13 L. Bernstein, R. Bernstein, and R. Dana, *Interviewing: A Guide for Health Professionals,* 2d ed., Appleton-Century-Crofts, New York, 1974.

14 A. Benjamin, *The Helping Interview*, 2d ed., Houghton Mifflin, Boston, 1974.

15 P. Castelnuevo-Tedesco, *The Twenty-Minute Hour: A Guide to Brief Psychotherapy for the Physician*, Little, Brown, Boston, 1965.

16 A. Hodges, *Psychological Counselling in General Medical Practice*, Heath, Lexington, Mass., 1977.

17 V. Satir, *Conjoint Family Therapy*, rev. ed., Science & Behavior Books, Palo Alto, Calif., 1967.

18 R. Thurlow, "Annual Consumer Expenditures," *Drug Topics*, **122**(12):31–42, June 20, 1978.

19 A. Dixon, "Drug Use in Family Practice: A Personal Study," *Canadian Family Physician*, **24**:345–353, April 1978.

20 D. Skegg, R. Doll, and J. Perry, "Use of Medicines in General Practice," *British Medical Journal*, **1**(6076):1561–1563, June 18, 1977.

21 P. D. Stolley et al., "Drug Prescribing and Use in an American Community," *Annals of Internal Medicine*, **76**(4):537, 1972.

22 "1977: Top 200 Drugs," *Pharmacy Times*, April 1978, pp. 41–48.

23 J. Goddard, "The Medical Business," *Scientific American*, **229**(3):161, 1973.

24 R. Kohn and K. White, *Health Care—An International Study*, Oxford University Press, London, 1976.

25 *Handbook of Non-Prescription Drugs*, 5th ed., American Pharmaceutical Association, Washington, 1977.

26 "How to Pay Less for Prescription Drugs," *Consumer Reports*, January 1975, p. 48, based on *Resisted Prices: A Study of Competitive Strains in the Antibiotic Market*, Council of Economic Priorities, New York, 1976.

27 K. Melmon, "Preventable Drug Reactions—Causes and Cures," *New England Journal of Medicine*, **284**:1361–1368, June 1971.

28 O. Wade and L. Beeley, *Adverse Reactions to Drugs*, 2d ed., William Heineman Medical Books, London, 1976.

29 R. Miller, "Hospital Admissions due to Adverse Drug Reactions," *Archives of Internal Medicine*, **134**:219, 1974.

30 R. Hill, "Drugs Ingested by Pregnant Women," *Clinical Pharmacology and Therapy*, **14**:654, 1973.

31 J. Forfar and M. Nelson, "Epidemiology of Drugs Taken by Pregnant Women—Drugs That May Affect the Fetus Adversely," *Clinical Pharmacology and Therapy*, **14**:654, 1973.

32 S. Yaffe, "A Clinical Look at the Problem of Drugs in Pregnancy and Their Effect on the Fetus," *Canadian Medical Association Journal*, **112**(6):728–733, March 22, 1975.

33 S. Milovech and B. Van den Borg, "Effects of Prenatal Meprobamate and Chlordiazepoxide Hydrochloride on Human Embryonic and Fetal Development," *New England Journal of Medicine*, **291**(24):1268–1271, December 12, 1974.

34 H. Jick, "Drugs, Remarkably NonToxic," *New England Journal of Medicine*, **291**(16):824, 1974.

35 *Evaluations of Drug Interactions*, 2d ed., American Pharmaceutical Association, Washington, 1976.

36 P. D. Hansten, *Drug Interactions*, 3d ed., Lea & Febiger, Philadelphia, 1975.

37 J. M. Mazzullo, K. Cohn, L. Lasagna, and P. F. Griner, "Variations in Interpretation of Prescription Instructions," *Journal of the American Medical Association*, **227**:929, 1974.

38 M. Mattar, J. Makelo, and S. Yaffe, "Pharmaceutic Factors Affecting Pediatric Compliance," *Pediatrics*, **55**(1):101–108, 1975.

39 R. Wenbury, "The Electric Speaking Practice—A Telephone Workload Study," *Canadian Family Physician*, **20**(2):69–76, 1974.

40 M. Greenlick et al., "Determinants of Medical Care Utilization: The Role of the Telephone in Total Medical Care," *Medical Care,* 11(2):121–134, 1973.

41 *Patient Drug Information,* Toronto General Hospital Pharmacy Department, Toronto, 1977.

42 D. L. Smith, *Medication Guide for Patient Counselling,* Lea & Febiger, Philadelphia, 1977.

Chapter 38

Self-Care

N. H. Hansen, M.D.

The medical encounter is only one step in the sequence of health care. Before seeing a physician patients have usually, on their own or others' advice, undertaken self-diagnosis and self-treatment. The experienced physician asks, "And what have you done for your problems before coming to see me?" Many factors bear on patient behavior at this stage of illness. Taking preconsultation self-care behaviors into account may make a considerable difference in the physician's choices of diagnostic and subsequent treatment strategies. Patients' self-management education concerning their acute and chronic illnesses should then become an integral part of everyday office practice.

Self-care is a fact that has been with us forever. Hundreds of "family health care" books have been published in the last 300 years.[1] It has been suggested that preconditions for the emergence of self-care as a social movement exist.[2] Only lately has the medical profession begun to pay any real attention to its ubiquitous presence. This is surprising when one considers some international facts. Symptoms do not require a visit to the doctor in roughly 90 percent of their occurrences. This is fortunate, since we would obviously be swamped if the proportion we now see was increased to any degree.

Most symptoms avoid doctors

Figure 38-1 Patient perception of ill-health in the 2-week period preceding interview.

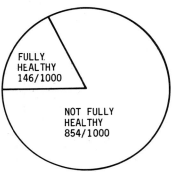

Parker[3] has conservatively suggested that if the Canadian elderly were to consult a physician for just one out of five health problems they now handle themselves, the annual result would be:

14 million more visits to physicians' offices
2.6 million more hospital emergency room visits
$650 million increase in health care costs

Given these realizations, we should reconsider how to view diagrammatically the pyramid of health care. (See Figure 38-1.)

Some evidence for this prevalence follows:

Diary keepers

1 In a New Zealand population-based health diary study,[4] 61 percent of individuals had "upset" days within a 2-week period. The response to symptoms by medical consultation was one person in six in the highest-income third of the population, one in twenty in the middle third and one in fifty in the lower third, with an average of one in twenty (5 percent) overall. Home remedies were used for 59 percent of symptoms.

2 In Sweden, a health diary study of young families[5] showed that a health problem was perceived in an individual approximately every 4 days. Actions were taken for 63 percent of spontaneously reported symptoms. Only 10 percent of all problems were cared for with professional consultation.

3 In Britain, a family practice study[6] found that only one in thirty-seven symptoms was taken to the doctor (less than 3 percent).

4 In Canada, a family practice health diary study[7] of symptoms for a 3-month winter period demonstrated that 140 (5.2 percent) of 2716 diaries reported "sore throat." Of these only 11 (7.9 percent) contacted their doctor who then recorded a respiratory diagnosis. It was found that the rate of contact increased with symptom severity.

5 Results from six North American centers (four U.S. and two Canadian) extracted from a comprehensive international study by Kohn and White[8] show that over 85 percent of the population did not consider themselves fully healthy in a 2-week period of study. Of this group, 13.3 percent visited a physician for a variety of reasons during that period, including some unrelated to the period of surveillance.

We will review self-care from a variety of perspectives that have practical importance for family physicians. This will include:

1 The sequence from illness perception to self-care
2 Patient sources of information on self-care
3 Self-medication
4 The collaborative role for physicians and patients in self-care for common acute and chronic illnesses

THE SEQUENCE OF ILLNESS PERCEPTION TO SELF-CARE

The term *self-care,* as used here, describes patient actions in the diagnosis and treatment of a health problem without seeing a physician for its review. This choice of definition emphasizes the point that patients currently may consult multiple sources of information and advice which they may then follow before deciding to see (or after seeing) a physician.

Disease is a term applied by physicians. Disease is an objective biological phenomenon, measurable through observation, physical signs, and laboratory and other tests. Patients do not usually come to the physician with a disease, but with perceived symptoms of possible impaired health. *Illness* refers to these more subjective of psychological dimensions (perceived symptoms and signs) of non-health, generally of more immediate concern to the person experiencing them.[9] Examples are pain, fever, weakness, indigestion, and changes in appearance such as redness, pallor, or swelling. | Symptoms, disease and illness

Kleinman[10] suggests, "The illness process begins with personal awareness of a change in body feeling and continues with the labelling of the sufferer by family or self as 'ill.'" Such changes are variably perceived, evaluated, and acted upon or ignored by different kinds of people and in different social situations. These actions may be called *illness behavior.*[11] | When illness begins

What individuals then choose to do about being ill is based upon experiences based in their society, culture, subculture, community, peer group, and family, among their school or work companions, etc. All of these elements tend to influence response to a particular symptom at a specific level of severity. However, any theoretical assumption about how an individual Puerto Rican, Jewish | Response to illness is variable

Canadian, Irish-American, steelworker, or nurse may react to a symptom must be recognized as subject to great individual variation.[12]

Many other factors contribute to the ways in which individuals determine their health needs. Some of these include knowledge of illnesses and of the health care system, the availability of health care and access to it, and personal health beliefs.[13] These and other issues and their influences on patient actions are addressed in chapters on illness behavior and transcultural health.

In summary, people choose self-care because of a degree of confidence in their own information level or that of their sources of advice about what to do in response to certain symptoms of illness.

PATIENT SOURCES OF INFORMATION ON SELF-CARE

Other providers of care

Self-care information is available from many sources. Western medicine is superimposed on other traditional or alternative forms of health care provided by folk cures, spiritual healers, herbalists, chiropractors, acupuncturists, and many others not usually included by physicians in management plans and often totally ignored. A host of other health professionals as well may be sought out for advice before or after we have seen the patient.

Doctors aren't uniform

There is also great individual variation between the approaches of physicians to identical problems in the same person and patients expect this. For example, a family physician will frequently hear a patient say something like "I was seen on the weekend by the doctor on call and he gave me a prescription, but I didn't fill it. I thought I should see if you felt I should take it." Patients will also present to their family physician with requests for alternative (nonmedical) health care referral.[14]

Information sources

The information sources available to patients for self-care decisions may be summarized in five categories:

1   Family, friends, co-workers: "I've got . . ." is frequently responded to by "Well, why don't you try . . . ?" In some areas specific folk remedies will be well known. For example, in the state of Vermont there is a popular folk acceptance that a regular dietary supplement of honey and apple cider vinegar (commercial product: Honegar) will ensure good health and long life.[15]

Trusted home remedies are likely to be used when there is a belief that the illness situation is not too serious, a home remedy is known, there is faith in the home remedy for this illness, and perceived barriers exist to accessibility (including costs and availability) of medical services.[16]

2   Publications: A variety of resources are available to meet

the North American public's insatiable thirst for health care information.

A recent personal visit to a typical shopping-mall bookstore showed on display 225 different books on psychological matters, 159 more on health subjects, and an added 35 books describing diets. Selling well were such health titles as *The New Peoples Pharmacy*,[17] *Non Prescription Drugs and Their Side Effects*,[18] Dr. Spock's *Baby and Child Care*,[19] *Readers Digest Family Medical Adviser: An A-Z Guide to Everyday Ailments, Their Symptoms, Causes and Treatment*,[20] and *How to Raise a Healthy Child in Spite of Your Doctor*.[21] Magazine articles on health subjects range from advice on acne to solutions for sexual problems. The April 1985 issue of *Good Housekeeping*[22] contained health and behavior information on 31 subjects.

3 Advertising: Television currently contains numerous commercials aimed at over-the-counter (OTC) medication use, particularly for the headache market, emphasizing "new" and "extra strength" and showing satisfied actors relieved of their pain. Many products for the common cold get heavily advertised as providing fast relief from symptoms. In a June 1985 issue of a popular Canadian monthly women's magazine 10 ads for OTC medications were found.[23] Quick weight-loss programs are also ubiquitous, with their claims of a health diet that produces special "guaranteed results" and with marketing methods often making physician and dietician mistrustful.

4 Nonprofessional contacts: Use abounds of advice from herbalists, masseurs, medicine men, folk healers, faith healers, and, recently, health food stores. Quackery is prevalent, with many unsubstantiated claims for cancer cures and nutritional supplements.[24] The May 1985 issue of *Consumer Reports* magazine listed 42 companies offering products that violate major provisions of the U.S. Food, Drug and Cosmetic Act. It also quotes the U.S. House Subcommittee on Health and Long-Term Care as reporting that quackery is now a $10 billion business in the United States and growing at a rate of probably more than 12 percent a year.

Use of nonprofessional advice on health matters is almost universal but is most obvious where there is opportunity for cross-cultural misunderstanding. A notable lack of understanding of alternative health behavior traditions may be seen in the traditionally trained physician. Use of alternative health care may also be related to a language barrier.[25] "Culture brokers" may not only translate language and interpret health care (similarities and differences as compared to the subculture) but also provide access to the health care system.[26] Do not discard alternative health care practices without close scrutiny. A close examination of practices in Spanish-American immigrant care in New York demonstrated striking similarities in psychiatric and spiritualist approaches.[27]

5 Professional contacts: Health professionals other than physicians give advice to patients. Nurses, pharmacists, optometrists, opticians, podiatrists, and chiropractors were contacted by North Americans at a rate of 114 per 1000 population in a 2-week period.[8] In addition, physiotherapists, homeopaths, osteopaths, orderlies, nursing assistants, receptionists, and a host of other individuals in and around the health care system may offer professional or experiential advice.

From a British physician's perspective, Elliott-Binns[28] found that 88 percent of patients visiting his general practice for new problems had received some advice prior to visiting. The major sources were relatives, 36 percent; friends, 22 percent; nurses, 7 percent; and pharmacists, 5 percent.

SELF-MEDICATION

Information from the six North American centers that were part of Kohn and White's comprehensive study[8] shows that an astonishing 55 percent of the population had taken medication in the previous 2 days, and 36 percent had used nonprescribed medications (see Figure 38-2).

High usage of nonprescribed medication

In a large 1-year U.S. study, Rabin and Bush[29] reported that, for a 2-day period, 19.9 percent of those interviewed used OTC pain relievers, 5.7 percent took cough-cold preparations, 4.9 percent applied skin ointments, and 4.2 percent administered stomach remedies. Elsewhere,[30] they confirmed that in a 2-day period 36 percent of the population studied used OTC drugs, with an average 1.1 drugs taken per illness (1.4 including vitamins).

There is variation in national patterns of use of the most popular OTC groups: analgesics, vitamins, cough medicines, skin preparations, and OTCs for gastrointestinal complaints (Table 38-1).[8]

Figure 38-2 Patients who took medications in the 2-day period preceding interview.

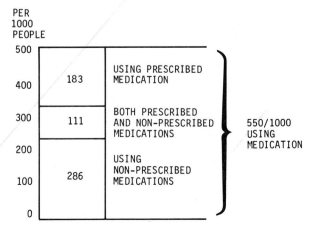

Table 38-1   National Variation in Self-Medication

Medication	Highest	%	Lowest	%
Vitamins	Finland	29	Yugoslavia	2
Analgesics	Yugoslavia	69	Finland	33
Cough-cold	Finland	16	Brazil	8
Skin preparation	Canada	18	Brazil	3
Laxatives	Britain	16	Yugoslavia	2

Source: Kohn and White.[8]

Skinner[31] reviewed 22 studies on the use of OTC medications and concluded that well over 90 percent were used appropriately, with possible misuse occurring in only 1 to 2 percent. As one example, a British study reported on pharmacy sales and advice from pharmacists and physicians for selected complaints. For coughs and indigestion, only a small number of physician consultations followed visits to the pharmacy, with or without the pharmacist's advice. Using that as an indication of treatment success, for coughs and indigestion, self-medication works very well.[32]

Self-medication can be effective

Not only is self-medication with OTC medications prevalent and apparently effective, it is also enormously profitable for drug companies. In 1983, the U.S. population spent well over $7 billion on OTCs. The big four were analgesics, $1.6 billion; cough and cold remedies, $1.5 billion; vitamins, $1.3 billion; and digestive aids, $1.2 billion. In addition to OTCs, a combined total of $2 billion was spent on home health care products and first-aid merchandise.[33]

THE PHARMACIST'S ROLE

The pharmacist is called upon as a community health counselor and is expected to recommend OTC medications. Twenty or more primary care services per day per pharmacist have been recorded, with 80 percent resulting in a recommendation for an OTC medication.[34]

Especially in a small community the family physician may expect a great deal of cooperation from the pharmacist. It is worthwhile for the physician moving to a community to include the pharmacist(s) when identifying community resources. In recent years, pharmacy schools have been emphasizing more information on pharmacist-client relationships and counseling. Hospital pharmacists in particular are becoming much more active in advising physicians on the efficacy, adverse effects, and interactions of medications, as well as in providing patient education. Both physician and pharmacist will benefit from better communication, since each will reinforce the other's advice.

Desk references on OTC's

Canadian Self Medication[35] contains information on the major product and/or symptom areas and many brief monographs. While this is intended as a reference for pharmacists, it is equally valuable for physicians, who are taught little about OTC medications. A superb U.S. counterpart is *The Handbook of Non-Prescription Drugs,*[36] published by the American Pharmaceutical Association for pharmacists. There is also a U.S. OTC reference for physicians, the *Physicians' Desk Reference for Nonprescription Drugs,* in recognition of self-medication as a significant factor in health care.[37]

The Over-the-Counter Drug Information Program in Nova Scotia[38] consists of 24 patient counseling sheets on OTC drugs, displayed in community pharmacies to be available for review at the time of product selection.

Physicians, recognizing self-care and self-medication as important parts of the health care of patients, may wish to repair their educational deficits by reviewing some of these or other sources.

COLLABORATION OF PHYSICIAN AND PATIENT IN SELF-CARE

Education for self-care reduces doctor contacts

A majority of physicians believe that at least 25 percent of visits were for conditions that people could care for themselves.[39] This belief requires an answer to the question, "Does self-care education have a positive effect by decreasing utilization of health services?" While earlier studies were equivocal,[40–42] two more recent studies are resoundingly positive. A controlled trial of education for the common cold reported a 40 percent reduction in visits for upper respiratory infections (URI).[43] Vickery et al.[44] undertook a prospective randomized and controlled study in a health maintenance organization. Self-care educational references and a newsletter were distributed. One subgroup was offered an individual counseling conference by a nurse. This was attended by high utilizers, who subsequently displayed a greater than average decrease in visits. In all experimental groups significant decreases were observed in both total visits (17 percent) and those for minor health problems (35 percent). This project was also cost-effective, with savings of $2.50 to $3.50 for each dollar spent.

Education for self-care reduces hospitalization

Self-care education has also been described as having significant effect in chronic illness. For example, family monitoring of blood pressure produced a lower dropout rate for treatment.[45]

Also, a group of diabetics[46] underwent a program including monitoring their blood glucose themselves, insulin adjustment, and an exercise program, with emotional support in group meetings. While 7 out of 10 had been hospitalized within the year prior to the program, none were admitted in the two years after its inception. Physicians involved felt the burden of responsibility had shifted from themselves to the patients, while the doctor assumed the role of consultant and adviser.

With these confirmations of its value, patient self-care education emerges as an important role and responsibility for family physicians. Such education can be aimed at

1 Self-management of minor illnesses
2 Maximization of health
3 Illness prevention
4 Major acute and chronic illnesses

This brief list recognizes that most major risk factors in, for example, coronary artery disease involve a certain behavior on the part of the individual associated with the risks. When patients become more active collaborators in treatment planning, goal setting, and health maintenance, compliance with medical regimens is enhanced.[47]

EXAMPLES OF SELF-CARE EDUCATION

Two examples are offered, one for an acute, minor illness (URI) and one for a chronic illness (diabetes). The specific areas to consider are briefly described. For a review of patient education in the context of all aspects of practice, see the chapter on patient education.

Planning education for patient self-care

Upper Respiratory Infection Advice

1 The clinical causes of upper respiratory infections (URI) as well as ways to avoid them
2 The limitation of medications to symptom relief only
3 The recognition of complications requiring medical attention, e.g., otitis media
4 Available supportive measures: nebulized water (vaporizer, steam), bed rest, avoidance of overtiring

    5 Appropriate and inappropriate medication choices for symptom relief

    6 Potential problems with OTC medications, e.g., antihistamines with drowsiness and drying of secretions

    7 Limitations of remedies; avoidance of overuse or overdose

    8 Need for storage away from child access, to avoid poisoning

Self-Care Advice for Insulin-Dependent Diabetics

After diabetics have worked (or have been helped) through the stages of reaction in relation to their diagnosis—denial, aggression, anger, depression, to acceptance or adaptation—they are ready to accept responsibility for their own self-care.[48] This outline will assume that the patient's initial illness experience involved introduction to basic issues such as insulin administration in rotating sites and that such information will be reviewed from time to time. "Teachable moments" must then be sought for the following:

1. Problem definitions: Basic description of diabetes, diagnostic methods, causes, and risk factors.
2. Methods of basic control: Diet, exercise, and insulin effects as they interplay; goal setting for control; meaning of glycosylated hemoglobin measurement.
3. Living with diabetes.
   a. Physical: Activities of daily living; work effects; how to deal with ill days; recognizing insulin reactions and hyperglycemia-ketoacidosis; when to take sugar, how to use glucagon; blood (or less satisfactory, urine) monitoring with a view to learning adjustment of diet, insulin, and exercise (regular, sporadic, and aerobic).
   b. Patient concerns: Addressing feelings, beliefs, and attitudes allows misconceptions and fears to be dealt with to improve self-image. Stress management and self-image improvement can enhance control. Clarifying misinformation and fears concerning sex, infertility, and heredity is a priority.
   c. Problem prevention: Foot and skin care methods; avoiding recurrent urinary tract and vaginal infections; routing monitoring methods for higher risks; eye, heart, etc., and when to see the doctor or when to call.
4. Self-help: Books to read for information; groups for peer support; diabetic association assistance.
5. Family education about diabetes including use of glucagon, ill-day management, general understanding of diabetes, and the

patient's need for support in accepting responsible collaborative management.

REFERENCES

1 P. Curtis, "Three Hundred Years of Family Health Care: Some Perspectives," *Journal of Family Practice,* **12:**323–327, 1981.
2 P. L. Schiller and J. S. Levin, "Is Self-Care a Social Movement?" *Social Science and Medicine,* **17:**1343–1352, 1981.
3 W. A. Parker, "The Canadian Experience in Patient Self-Care—Extending the Role of the Pharmacist in Community Medicine," in *Proceedings of the Pharmacy Practice Foundation Symposium on Self Care,* University of Sydney, Sydney, 1985.
4 S. R. West, "Everyday Health, South Auckland, 1980–81," *New Zealand Medical Journal,* **96:**472–476, 1983.
5 G. Dahlquist, S. Wall, J. Ivarsson, et al., "Health Problems and Care in Young Families—An Evaluation of Survey Procedures," *International Journal of Epidemiology,* **13:**221–228, 1984.
6 D. Morrell and C. Wade, "Symptoms Perceived and Recorded by Patients," *Journal of the Royal College of General Practitioners,* **26:**398–403, 1976.
7 C. E. Evans, A. H. McFarlane, G. R. Norman, et al., "Sore Throats in Adults: Who Sees a Doctor?" *Canadian Family Physician,* **28:**453–458, 1982.
8 R. Kohn and K. White, *Health Care—An International Study,* Oxford University Press, London, 1976.
9 A. C. Twaddle, "Sickness and the Sickness Career," in L. Eisenberg and A. Kleinman (eds.), *The Relevance of Social Science for Medicine,* D. Reidel Publishing Co., New York, 1980, pp. 111–133.
10 A. Kleinman, "Culture, Illness and Care," *Annals of Internal Medicine,* **88:**251–258, 1978.
11 D. Mechanic, *Medical Sociology,* 2d ed., Macmillan, New York, 1978.
12 A. Segal, "Sociocultural Variation in Sick Role Behavioral Variations," *Social Sciences and Medicine,* **10:**47–51, 1976.
13 J. G. Bruhn and F. M. Trevino, "A Method for Determining Patients' Perceptions of Their Health Needs," *Journal of Family Practice,* **8:**809–818, 1979.
14 S. Poole and R. Anstett, "Patients Who Request Alternative (Non-medical) Health Care," *Journal of Family Practice,* **16:**767–772, 1983.
15 P. Atkinson, "From Honey to Vinegar: Levi-Strauss in Vermont," in P. Morley and R. Wallis (eds.), *Culture and Curing: Anthropological Perspectives on Traditional Medical Beliefs and Practices,* Peter Owen, London, 1978, pp. 168–188.
16 J. Young, quoted in F. Wolinsky, *The Sociology of Health: Principles, Professions, and Issues,* Little, Brown, Boston, 1980, pp. 146–148.
17 J. Graedon and T. Graedon, *The New Peoples Pharmacy,* revised ed., Bantam Books, New York, 1985.
18 R. J. Benowicz, *Non Prescription Drugs and Their Side Effects,* Berkeley. New York, 1982.
19 B. Spock and M. B. Rothenberg, *Baby and Child Care,* Simon & Schuster, New York, 1985.

20 *Readers Digest Family Medical Adviser: An A-Z Guide to Everyday Ailments, Their Symptoms, Causes and Treatment*, Readers Digest Association, London, 1983.

21 R. S. Mendelsohn, *How to Raise a Healthy Child in Spite of Your Doctor*, Contemporary Books, Chicago, 1984.

22 *Good Housekeeping*, April 1985.

23 *Chatelaine Magazine*, June 1985.

24 "Drugs in Disguise," *Consumer Reports*, pp. 275–283, May 1985.

25 L. R. Marcos, L. Urcuyo, M. Kesselman, and M. Alpert, "The Language Barrier in Evaluating Spanish-American Patients," *Archives of General Psychiatry*, **29:**655–659, 1973.

26 R. Laurens, "Culture Brokers and Medical Behavior in the Puerto Rican Community of Cleveland," presented at North American Primary Care Research Group Annual Meeting, Lake Tahoe, 1981.

27 P. Ruiz and J. Langrod, "Psychiatry and Folk Healing: A Dichotomy?" *American Journal of Psychiatry*, **133:**95–97, 1976.

28 C. P. Elliott-Binns, "An Analysis of Lay Medicine," *Journal of the Royal College of General Practitioners*, **23:**255, 1973.

29 D. L. Rabin and P. J. Bush, "Who's Using Medicine," *Journal of Community Health*, **1:**106–117, 1975.

30 P. J. Bush and D. L. Rabin, "Who's Using Nonprescribed Medicines," *Medical Care*, **14:**1014–1023, 1976.

31 D. Skinner, "Consumer Use of Nonprescription Drugs," *Canadian Pharmaceutical Journal*, **118:**206–214, 1985.

32 R. Jones, "Self-Medication in a Small Community," *Journal of the Royal College of General Practitioners*, **26:**410–413, 1976.

33 "36th Annual Report on Consumer Spending—1983, 'It Was a Very Good Year,'" *Drug Topics*, **128**(13):22–88, 1984.

34 M. Bass, "The Pharmacist as a Provider of Primary Care," *Canadian Medical Association Journal*, **112:**60–62, 1975.

35 *Canadian Self Medication*, 2d ed., Canadian Pharmaceutical Association, Toronto, 1984.

36 *The Handbook of Non-Prescription Drugs*, 7th ed., American Pharmaceutical Association, Washington, 1982.

37 *Physicians' Desk Reference for Nonprescription Drugs*, Medical Economics Co., Oradell, N.J. 1980.

38 I. Sketris, D. Frail, *Over the Counter Drug Information Programme*. Dept. National Health & Welfare, Canada. Distributed by Pharmacy Association of N.S., Halifax, 1982.

39 K. Dunnell and C. Cartwright, *Medicine Takers, Prescribers and Hoarders*, Routledge & Kegan Paul, Boston, 1972.

40 S. H. Moore, J. P. LoGerfo, and T. S. Innui, "Effect of a Self Care Book on Physician Visits," *Journal of the American Medical Association*, **243:**2317–2320, 1980.

41 K. Lorig, K. G. Kraines, C. Broccich, et al., "Take Care: A Study of the Cost Effectiveness of Minimal Health Education in the Workplace," *Presentation at the American Public Health Association Annual Meeting*, Los Angeles, 1981.

42 D. W. Kemper, "Self-Care Education: Impact on HMO Costs," *Medical Care*, **20:**710–718, 1982.

43 C. R. Roberts, P. B. Imrey, J. D. Turner, et al., "Reducing Physician Visits for Colds through Consumer Education," *Journal of the American Medical Association*, **250:**1986–1989, 1983.

44 D. M. Vickery, H. Kalmer, D. Lowry, et al., "Effect of a Self-Care Education Program on Medical Visits," *Journal of the American Medical Association*, **250:**2952–2956, 1983.

45 S. M. Stahl, C. R. Lelley, P. J. Neill, et al., "Effects of Home Blood Pressure on Long-Term BP Control," *American Journal of Public Health,* **74:**704–709, 1984.

46 C. M. Peterson, S. E. Forman, and R. L. Jones, "Self-Management: An Approach to Patients with Insulin-Dependent Diabetes Mellitus," *Diabetes Care,* **3:**82–87, 1980.

47 R. B. Haynes, D. L. Sackett, E. S. Gibson, et al., "Improvement of Medication Compliance in Uncontrolled Hypertension," *Lancet,* **1:**1265–1268, 1976.

48 S. Popkess-Vawter, "The Adult Living with Diabetes Mellitus," *Nursing Clinics of North America,* **18:**771–789, 1983.

Chapter 39

Cultural Factors Influencing Compliance: Toward Transcultural Family Practice

P. N. Stern, D.N.S., R.N., F.A.A.N.

CULTURE

Health beliefs

Culture can be defined as a system of values and beliefs which influence behavior. Beliefs about how to become or stay healthy are culturally determined. When the patient's beliefs about health care differ from those of the family physician, the patient may not comply with the physician's management proposals because the patient's culture forbids her or him to do so. The patient's health beliefs may be those of a visible or nonvisible minority group, or they may be those of the general lay population. To surmount the gap in beliefs or expectations, the family physician must show cultural elasticity and respect for the patient's beliefs, working within the patient's cultural framework and trying to establish rapport.

Cultural differences

Cultural beliefs influence both the search for health and health maintenance behavior. The patient who comes to the family physician's office almost certainly holds at least some beliefs about health care which differ from the physician's. This is true whether the patient belongs to a clearly different cultural group or simply holds lay (as opposed to professional) cultural beliefs. What the patient believes about becoming or staying healthy influences his or her ability to follow the physician's program of care. Noncompliance, then, may result from asking a patient to do something which he or she is simply unable to do, because the patient sees the treatment as valueless or actually harmful. This discussion deals with some situations which may arise from the existence of opposing belief systems, some diverse cultural beliefs, and some processes which allow physician-patient rapport to transcend cultural barriers.

Culture has been described by Olien[1] as a system, and by Tylor[2] as a complex whole encompassing knowledge, beliefs, art, morals, law, and custom. Leininger[3] writes that *"culture* refers to the learned, shared, and transmitted values, beliefs, norms and lifestyle practices of a particular group that guides thinking, decisions, and actions in patterned ways."* Arguing about beliefs with a patient makes as much sense as arguing politics. Patients observe particular health practices because to them they are *right.*

CULTURAL HEALTH REASONING

A study involving patients and their beliefs about care[4] identified the process used by individuals in making decisions about themselves. This process, termed *cultural health reasoning,* involves a series of decisions about care, based on the individual's cultural background.

Culture Shock

When a patient enters the world of professional health care, that individual is confronted by sights and sounds which seem vastly different from those of the outside world. Several authors have pointed out that the patient goes through a kind of culture shock when confronted by foreign beliefs (the physician's) and a foreign language (medical jargon).[5-8] Culture shock is characterized by disorientation, confusion, anxiety, and loss of control. Physicians themselves may experience a kind of culture shock at the patient's behavior or lack of compliance. Each of the persons involved, patient and physician, has difficulty understanding why the other is behaving in what seem to be inexplicable ways. When we are unaware of the beliefs and values which guide behavior, we can be left with feelings of shock and disbelief.

Being aware of patient's beliefs

Power Struggles

Trying to change belief-based behavior is doomed to failure. Whether the physician presents the plan of care verbally, in writing, or both, compliance depends on the value the patient places on the instructions. Attempting to force the issue engenders greater patient resistance. Threatening, entreating, or cajoling does no good. When the patient walks out of the office, she or he is in control.

Withdrawal

Avoid power struggles

When power struggles reach a critical level, one or both of the participants may withdraw from the conflict. The patient may formally withdraw from the physician's care or may adopt subtle forms of withdrawal such as "bending the truth" or avoiding the subject of controversy.

Physicians may also withdraw in the face of noncompliance. They give up on patients in formal or subtle ways. They may refer the patient to someone else, or end their attempts to maintain a warm, caring relationship with the patient.

The family physician may be more aware of possible cultural differences when a patient looks or sounds different from the physician, but the wise clinician knows that differing beliefs are just as common in individuals who look and sound familiar. Some indicators of opposing cultural health reasoning will help the physician identify problems.

A study of Filipino immigrants[9] showed that Filipinos find it rude to disagree with persons in authority. Unable to say "no" because of cultural prohibitions, they solve the problem by delaying their "yes" answer. To Filipinos a delayed "yes" means "no":

"Did you understand the instructions?"

Detecting a silent "no"

"Ah . . . yes." The delayed "yes" means something like "I don't understand because my mother told me that to do what you advise is harmful."

A comparison between Filipinos and North Americans showed that the latter also use the delayed "yes" to bend the truth when responding to an authority figure such as a physician:

"Have you been checking your breasts?"

"Ah . . . yes." The delayed "yes" here may mean, "Yes, sometimes, but I'm really too busy to bother," or "I haven't been, because it could bring on cancer."

Other indicators of disagreement include frowning, avoiding eye contact, or maintaining contact but going out of focus: a blank expression.

CULTURAL BELIEFS ABOUT CARE: EXAMPLES

Short of taking a graduate course in anthropology, the family practice physician will have little opportunity for studying the culture of her or his patients. Some examples of differing cultural beliefs may help the physician to identify an existing cultural problem. The examples which follow include the Filipino culture, the black culture of the American south, and rural culture. Similar problems exist in relating to additional cultures.

Filipino Immigrants

I began a study involving Filipino immigrants[10] when my nursing students in maternity practice found difficulty communicating health teaching to their Philippine-born patients. Besides the delayed "yes" cited above, students were puzzled by their patients' unwillingness to behave in (to the students) normal ways. We were able to determine that allowing for individual differences, some Filipino immigrants hold general beliefs concerning safe child-bearing practices which differ from North American beliefs. Some Filipino immigrants, for example, believe that it is harmful to bathe for a period of 2 to 4 weeks following birth. Sponge baths are safe, but their mothers have told them that showers or tub baths are dangerous. (We learned later that Chinese nationals hold this same belief. When they bathe too soon after delivery, they believe they develop a condition called postpartum arthritis.) Some Filipinos who originate in the area around Manila believe that colostrum is "old stock" and harmful to the baby. For this reason, they delay breast feeding until "the milk comes in," and for the first day or two either feed their baby a bottle or give it to a wet nurse.

Another belief concerns taking medications while pregnant. Many Filipinos consider even vitamins a medication to be avoided.

Culture Shock   We found that Filipinos were often shocked when nurses asked them to do things they believed would be harmful. When nurses asked them to take their own baths, they either thought that the nurse was lazy and unwilling to take care of them or felt the nurse must dislike them—why else would the nurse try to harm them?

Withdrawal   The individuals in our study avoided open confrontation with their nurses. They withdrew from the nurse's instructions in artful ways:

"The nurse insisted that I take a shower so I just turned the water on and stood outside the shower. Then I wet the towel so she would feel good." The Filipino was able to observe her own beliefs and still maintain an image of compliance.

The following data come from a nurse's report at the change of shift:

"Mrs. Aquino said she was going to breastfeed her baby, but

when I tried to help her, she said she would do it later. Now she tells me she wants to bottlefeed. I just don't understand." In this example, Mrs. Aquino maintained her image of compliance by asking for a bottle of formula. This left her free to breast-feed when "the milk comes in" after discharge from the hospital.

A pregnant woman had this to say: "The doctor wanted me to take vitamins, but my mother said no medicine when I am pregnant. So I take some, but when the nurse asks am I taking them, I say yes. When my mother asks, I say no." This woman was forced into dishonesty in order to balance her physician's and her mother's opposing beliefs.

Northern Louisiana Black Women

Traditional practices

Scott found that northern Louisiana black women hold some beliefs about health care which differ from those of the dominant culture.[11] Some of these women, for example, believe that a cure for thrush involves having a male who never knew his father blow in the mouth of the infant. As thrush tends to be a self-limiting disease, individuals were able to report that this treatment method works. Other women practiced what they considered preventive care when they taped a silver dollar over their baby's umbilicus. This treatment is designed to avoid umbilical hernia, a condition common in black people. Another prescription involved menstruation. Many young black women are advised to avoid washing their hair during their menstrual period "because you'll get sick."

Culture Shock   The black women in Scott's sample experienced culture shock when their physicians called their beliefs "old wives' tales." This lack of respect for the advice given them by wiser older women caused them pain or offense. They often practiced some form of withdrawal as a consequence.

Withdrawal: The "Ethno Market Theory"   Scott developed what she called the "Ethno Market Theory" to describe these black women's reaction to professional health culture. She found that the women fell into three major groups. Some women, depending on their treatment in the office or clinic and often because of their exposure to the media, became what Scott called "corporate buyers"; that is, they bought the whole professional health cultural package. At the other extreme were the "cultural buyers," those women who rejected professional advice and followed the teachings of respected older women. In between fell the "careful shoppers," those who followed a part of the teachings of each health culture.

Rural Beliefs

"Rural," as it is used here, refers to areas in comparative isolation. This can vary from settlements just a few miles outside of Halifax, on the one hand, to townships 200 miles north of San Francisco on the other. The factor distinguishing rural from urban is the insularity of life. The examples in this section come from observations made by my colleagues who practice in areas of relative isolation.

Because of the parochial quality of their life, rural individuals rely heavily on the advice of the "lay referral system," as Chrisman[12] calls it. They tend to place more faith in folk remedies than in so-called scientific advice given them by someone "from away." A professional may regard the rural individual as quite ignorant of scientific health care knowledge. The outsider, however, does well to remember that these people act on the advice of relatives and neighbors because it has always worked for them. Or so it seems.

Lay referral system

A major strength rural individuals usually enjoy is the mutually supportive system in which they live. A sick person can count on the help of neighbors for food, care, and acceptance. For generations, country people have relied on the help of one another for survival.

Culture Shock The professional who moves to a rural area to practice because of a desire to help the poor unfortunates who live there may be shocked to find that the natives consider her or him to be lacking in common sense. "Why should I go to the doctor for a checkup every year when I ain't sick? That just don't make good sense."

Withdrawal Individuals in rural areas use strategies common to all culturally different groups when confronted by a professional from a health culture they fail to understand and value. They either stay away or do not follow the doctor's advice.

TOWARD TRANSCULTURAL FAMILY PRACTICE

Transcultural practice involves transcending differing health culture beliefs. When faced with opposing health beliefs, the physician can overcome cultural barriers by showing respect for the patient's beliefs and by using cultural elasticity, that is, by working within the patient's cultural framework.

Showing respect for patient's beliefs

Showing Respect

The beliefs of individuals *must* be treated with respect. No matter how foreign a patient's ideas may seem to you, remember that they are the product of the teachings of a respected individual. To insult those beliefs is to insult the patient and the person who taught the patient those beliefs.

Most individuals faced with differing cultural behaviors make allowances when they perceive a respectful attitude. A physician will be forgiven for not knowing everything about another person's beliefs if the patient can see that the physician is trying to be culturally sensitive. Kleinman, Eisenberg, and Good[13] advise that physicians must try to discover how the patient views her or his illness: "Clinicians need to be persistent in order to show patients that their ideas are of genuine interest and important for clinical management." Interest is a way of showing respect.

A good rule of thumb to follow regarding a health belief is to leave it alone if it is not harmful. The patient may be persuaded to follow one of your beliefs in addition if the patient in turn considers that your belief is not harmful.

Cultural Elasticity

Working within the framework of the other is an interactional process involving the physician and the patient. The patient must be persuaded to accept some of your framework before a given treatment plan will be adhered to. Brigitta[14] illustrates this concept when she writes about nurses working with native citizens in the Yukon:

Using local
references

> The nurse is most likely to be understood when using a cultural approach to nutrition with clear concrete examples. She or he would say, "This bush was eaten by the elders and they had clear skin."

Kleinman, Eisenberg, and Good[13] suggest a number of questions which will help the physician develop a transcultural treatment plan:

1 What do you think has caused your problem?
2 Why do you think it started when it did?
3 What do you think your sickness does to you? How does it work?
4 How severe is your sickness? Will it have a short or long course?
5 What kind of treatment do you think you should receive?

Kleinman et al. suggest these additional questions:

6 What are the most important results you hope to receive from this treatment?

7 What are the chief problems your sickness has caused for you?

8 What do you fear most about your sickness?

Consultation

When you are faced with a particularly difficult or puzzling problem which you think is culturally based, consultation is in order. A university health science center, department of medical anthropology, or university school of nursing may be able to provide that missing piece of information that you need to practice transculturally. A cultural consult can be as important as any other special advice for the successful management of patient problems.

Cultural consult

REFERENCES

1 M. D. Olien, *The Human Myth,* Harper & Row, New York, 1978.
2 E. B. Tylor, *Primitive Culture,* Harper & Row, New York, 1958. Originally published 1871.
3 M. M. Leininger, "Transcultural Care Diversity and Universality: A Theory of Nursing," *Nursing and Health Care,* **6:**209–212, 1985.
4 P. N. Stern, *Women, Health and Culture,* Hemisphere, N.Y., 1985.
5 K. Oberg, *Culture Shock,* Bobbs-Merrill, Indianapolis, 1954.
6 M. Brein and K. H. David, "Intercultural Communication and the Adjustment of the Sojourner," *Psychology Bulletin,* **76:**212–230, 1971.
7 P. J. Brink and J. M. Saunders, *Cultural Shock: Theoretical and Applied.* P. J. Brink, *Transcultural Nursing,* Prentice-Hall, Englewood Cliffs, N.J., 1976.
8 R. Taft, "Coping with Unfamiliar Cultures," in N. Warren (ed.), *Studies in Cross-Cultural Psychology,* vol. 1, Academic Press, London, 1976.
9 P. N. Stern, "Solving Problems of Cross-Cultural Health Teaching: The Filipino Childbearing Family," *Image,* **13**(2):47–50, 1981.
10 P. N. Stern, V. P. Tilden, and E. K. Maxwell, "Culturally Induced Stress during Childbearing: The Filipino American Experience," *Issues in Health Care of Women,* **2:**129–143, 1980.
11 M. D. S. Scott and P. N. Stern, "Ethno Market Theory: Factors Influencing Childbearing Health Practices of Northern Louisiana Black Women," *Health Care for Women International,* **6:**45–60, 1985.
12 N. J. Chrisman, "The Health Seeking Process: An Approach to the Natural History of Illness," *Cultural Medicine and Society,* **1:**351–377, 1977.
13 A. Kleinman, L. Eisenberg, and B. Good, "Culture, Illness and Care: Clinical Lessons from Anthropologic and Cross-Cultural Research," *Annals of Internal Medicine,* **88:**251–258, 1978.
14 A. Brigitta, "Yukon Medicine: The Vital Role of Public Health Nurses," *Canadian Medical Association Journal,* **130:**492–496, 1984.

Chapter 40

Patient Education and Community Resources

B. Prime-Walker, B.Sc.N

Patient education is gaining recognition as one of the most important aspects of family practice. The outcome of many primary health problems is dependent on patient behavior, and patient education offers everyone an opportunity to participate in the management process. During the office or home visit, the family physician is in an ideal position to facilitate learning which can enhance the patient's understanding of health problems, improve compliance, and possibly even reduce risks from lifestyle factors. This chapter presents guidelines for the development of patient education skills and resources within an office milieu which is conducive to effective patient-doctor communication.

Patient education is not a new concept in health care. Physicians, like other health professionals, have traditionally been involved in patient teaching to some degree for many years. Prior to 1970, however, few controlled research trials existed, and formal training in health education skills was limited. Most clinical teaching grew from intuition or trial-and-error experiences rather than any pre-planned systematic approach. Controversy arose among disciplines concerning who should teach what and whether patient education really had any significant impact on health care outcomes. Today, there is sufficient evidence in the literature to substantiate the efficacy of patient education, while its unlimited potential in the primary care setting is becoming widely recognized.[1] Patient education is compatible with the general philosophy of family medicine because it is prevention-oriented, family-centered, and participation-directed (see Common Problems and Principles, pp. 73).

A national Task Force on training family physicians in patient education was established in the United States in 1977. One of its accomplishments has been the publication of a patient education handbook for teachers, designed for use in residency programs in family medicine.[2] Patient education sessions are also being integrated into short courses as well as many practice management seminars today. Clinical settings and communities were two of the target priorities chosen by the U.S. government for health education in the 1980s.

WHAT IS PATIENT EDUCATION?

> Patient education encompasses any health education experience planned by physicians, professional health workers and the patient himself to meet the patient's specific learning needs, interests and capabilities which is offered as an integral part of the patient's total health care.[3]

Patient education is a process of education and advocacy based on a purposeful exchange and sharing of information with patients. It differs from health education and patient teaching in that it encompasses much more than the simple transfer of factual information; ultimately, the individual's behavior must be positively affected. It is best explained as a communication activity occurring within the context of a patient-doctor encounter, which influences patient behavior toward improved health. Patient education includes a variety of strategies not only to facilitate behavioral change but also to help people identify their social supports, and to help them maintain their achieved behavior over a long period of time. It is much more complex than the printed handouts, audiovisual aids, and modern-day gadgetry so often associated with it. Personal interaction is the important varying factor. In addition to scientific medical facts, patient education incorporates basic principles of human psychology, social theory, and adult learning from the behavioral sciences.

The purpose of patient education is "to provide people with enough information and motivation to help them understand the factors that promote and/or threaten health so that they may have a better opportunity to make informed choices in their lives; also, to provide the support as well as the technical assistance necessary

Information sharing

Facilitating change

Personal interaction

Monitoring behavior

to help them carry out their choices."[4] The focus of patient education is on behavior, rather than knowledge or personal beliefs.

RATIONALE FOR PATIENT EDUCATION

Social forces

Patient education activities are widespread today. Social forces such as the consumer movement, human rights legislation, and self-help programs, together with holistic and prospective medicine, have greatly influenced a renewed interest in health education issues.[5] People are not so much uninformed as they are misinformed. With the focus of health care services gradually shifting toward reduction of environmental and personal health hazards and long-term management of chronic disease and disabilities, the demand for patient education continues to grow. Universal anxiety over the ever-increasing costs of modern-day health services has further intensified the interest in patient education and the need to document its effects.

The advantages of patient education for the patient, health care financers, and the physician are summarized in Table 40-1.

Cost

Most discussions of patient education become controversial whenever the topics of time, cost, and effectiveness arise. According to Dr. Larry Green, there is sufficient evidence available today to justify patient education against the arguments of time and dollar constraints. He recommends that future research energies be directed toward evaluating quality assurance.[6] A variety of clinical trials involving patients with diabetes, asthma, and congestive heart failure have demonstrated that patient education can have a positive effect on health outcomes and reduce utilization of health services.[7]

Positive outcomes

Compliance

Patients' compliance with treatment regimens may break down for a number of complex reasons. Several of these are related to the patients' comprehension, personal beliefs, and attitudes. Sackett and Haynes,[8] Svarstad,[9] and others have described a correlation between patient education efforts and improved patient compliance.

Consent

One of the primary goals of ambulatory care is to ensure that patients consent to treatment with full understanding and a realistic information base. Patients have the right to refuse education; however, health care providers have a legal and ethical as well as humanistic responsibility to give patients the opportunity to choose.

Self-care

Patient education also performs another critical function—enhancing patient responsibility and encouraging self-care. It helps

Table 40-1 Advantages of Patient Education

For patient
  Supports basic human right to knowledge of personal health
  Promotes positive "wellness behavior"
  Allows "active" participation by patient and family
  Provides an understood "informed consent"; decreases anxiety through understanding

For funding source
  Reduces financial cost by placing more responsibility on the patient
  Reduces lifestyle health risks
  Helps the "worried well" to cope
  Promotes appropriate utilization of services

For physician
  Strengthens physician-patient understanding and communication (a major factor in reducing the risks of legal action)
  Improves quality of primary health care
  Increases patient compliance for treatment
  Facilitates interdisciplinary sharing of responsibility; team approach

to clarify responsibility by differentiating the patient's role from what really needs to be contributed by health professionals.[10] Recognizing the patient's family and community network as also being members of the health care team reinforces the potential of care givers as an important part of the solution and not merely part of the problem.

The family physician's office is a logical setting for promoting patient education, since it is usually the initial, and often the only, contact with the health care system for most of the population. Only a small percentage of people require admission to a hospital during their lifetime; thus hospital-based education programs reach only a select few. The office visit provides an ideal teaching opportunity, since persons seeking health care advice are more highly motivated to learn during the diagnostic stage. The family physician has the opportunity to reach people before they become ill. In contrast to the specialist who provides tertiary care for episodic illness or injury, the family physician serves a diversified population with a wide range of health problems over many years. Continuity of care provided across generations gives the family physician insight into background social and lifestyle information—a history which may prove crucial for planning management in times of stress or crisis.

Advantages of office setting

Initial contact

Continuous care

Family physicians often use patient education techniques to provide anticipatory guidance for various life-cycle stages or events—birth, adolescence, marriage, death—which may threaten

Anticipatory guidance

family health. (See chapter 4, Family Life Cycle and Anticipatory Guidance.)

Symptoms of disease can create different reactions in different people at different stages in life. Daily exposure to the growth and maturation of families helps to develop the physician's sixth sense—ability to perceive potential stresses ahead of time and prepare the patient to cope before they become full-blown.

Incurables and "worried well"

Patient education is also therapeutic for monitoring incurable conditions as well as helping the "worried well" to cope. Patients who feel ill because of psychosocial stress rather than organic disease respond positively to the interpersonal support provided through patient education. Teaching the patient how sick is sick and when to seek medical help reduces precious time often lost to inappropriate calls about trivial problems, or no calls on important issues which in time may reach emergency proportions.

Prevention

Large corporations, third-party payers, and patients themselves are beginning to recognize prevention as a means of saving money as well as saving lives. In some countries, group insurance programs are financing patient education as an extended benefit. Several kinds of health professionals today (e.g. dentists, nutritionists, and some physicians) are incorporating patient education into their practice routine, charging on a fee-for-service basis. Many studies reveal that consumers want more information and education than is currently being provided by health care professionals.[1] As the demand for prepaid services increases, patient education will be more commonly seen in community as well as institutional settings.

INCORPORATING PATIENT EDUCATION INTO FAMILY PRACTICE

Getting started. . . .

How can a busy practitioner make simple changes in his or her present methods of teaching to provide a more effective learning environment for patients? Where does one begin?

Set goals

An ideal starting point is to develop an operational definition of your particular patient education philosophy and write it down. Review available literature on various strategies to determine possible goals, and discuss your ideas with experienced physicians who have developed office programs. Share your interest with staff members to raise group consciousness, then form a working committee to thrash out a draft blueprint. It is important for all persons involved to understand the desired outcomes of the model which

Table 40-2   Questions to Help Assess Practice Targets for Patient Education

Objective questions
1   What is age and sex distribution of your patients? How many children? How many geriatrics? How many women in the fertile age group? How many single parents?
2   How many deliveries per year?
3   How many emergencies?
4   How many nursing home and hospital visits?
5   Is your practice rural or urban?
6   How accessible are specialized services?
7   What is the level of education, cultural background, socioeconomic status of the community?

Subjective questions
1   Are your patients exposed to any environmental or occupational health hazards which might put them at risk for unhealthy lifestyles or certain diseases (e.g., asbestos workers, computer programmers)?
2   Do you have a large number of young families with a high rate of pregnancies?
3   What are the most common problems in your practice?
4   What is the incidence of chronic disease and handicaps?
5   Is there a high prevalence of psychosocial family problems?
6   What effect do community resources and the news media have on the health care expectations of your patients?
7   What is the general coping ability of your patients, and what is their perception of sickness or good health?
8   Are your patients accustomed to being involved in self-care and playing an active part in promoting good health?

is being developed to avoid confusion, false expectations, or lack of interest later on.

Practice Targets for Patient Education

It is unrealistic to assume that the physician could adequately educate everyone under his or her care. Concentrate on priority problems and the greatest health risks to begin with.[10] The questions presented in Table 40-2 depict some variables which affect health status. The answers to these provide general information on the scope of your patient population and practice trends as well as important demographic characteristics of the community served. You may also wish to determine the knowledge level of your patients.[11] A medical-knowledge quiz, conducted in the waiting area, was tried in England.[12]

Practice profile

Next, identify clinical conditions for which patient education is frequently indicated. Review the study done in the state of Vir-

Establish a baseline

Questionnaires
and health
hazard
appraisals

Home visits

ginia.[13] Prepare a list of the most common problems presented during the past 2 years or more, ranking them according to frequency seen, severity of condition, and the likelihood of improvement with patient education intervention. Figure 40-1, from *Patient Education: A Handbook for Teachers*, is a sample format for quantifying factors to be considered in needs assessment.[2] Self-administered health questionnaires can provide basic patient information, but are of little value unless social and attitudinal questions are included and the results explained. Health hazard appraisals are commonly used to measure potential risks from certain lifestyle habits or behavior. Finally, home visits on those patients who cannot come to the office will help to clarify their coping ability and future needs.

A practice profile is a useful guide to determine the level of need in a particular practice and highlights areas of essential content to be developed.

Practice
variations

Patient education programs evolve slowly over time with unique variations in different practices depending on the type of practice, staff complement, patient needs, and professional preferences. For example, one physician may wish to begin by teaching about administrative aspects such as office policies and procedures, instructions to new patients, and referral protocol. Another may focus on a clinical aspect of patient care such as chronic home care, health prevention strategies, or a behavior modification program for dieting, stress control, or smoking cessation.

Assessing Patient's Needs

Problem
orientation

The most challenging task in the patient education process is calculating what the patient actually needs to know or do. The American task force developed a structured approach to help physicians analyze a presenting problem or risk in terms of behavioral causes and to determine the educational technique most appropriate for the treatment goals and desired outcomes. (See Figure 40-2 "Steps In Patient Education".[2]) The problem-oriented medical record (POMR) system provides an ideal mechanism for developing an educational diagnosis with the patient. The shift in focus from diagnosis to problem orientation is the advantage of this approach. A combination of factors, rather than a single cause, is considered with various combinations of strategies tried in order to arrive at a satisfactory management plan.[14] Educational objectives are based on patient behaviors, or absence of behaviors, that influence or cause a particular health problem. If the individual's health-related behavior is appropriate, reinforcement may be the only patient education intervention required. However, if some deficiency is obvious, it will be necessary to identify that behavior and appropriate actions which may help to resolve it.

Figure 40-1 Sample practice survey to determine priority areas for planning patient education packages.

PROBLEM	Column 1 FREQUENCY ENCOUNTERED IN YOUR PRACTICE Rare 1 2 3 4 5 Freq.	Column 2 SEVERITY Minor 1 2 3 4 5 Severe	Column 3 LIKELIHOOD OF IMPROVEMENT BY EDUCATION INTERVENTION OR PREVENTION OF COMPLICATIONS OR RECURRENCE Unlikely to Help 1 2 3 4 5 Treatment of Choice	SCORE Col. Col. Col. 1 x 2 x 3
UPPER RESPIRATORY ILLNESS	3	2	3	18
BIRTH CONTROL ADVICE	4	2	4	32
DEPRESSION	3	3	3	27
URINARY TRACT INFECTION	4	3	4	48

Source: Report of The National Task Force on Training Family Physicians.[2]

Figure 40-2 Steps in patient education.

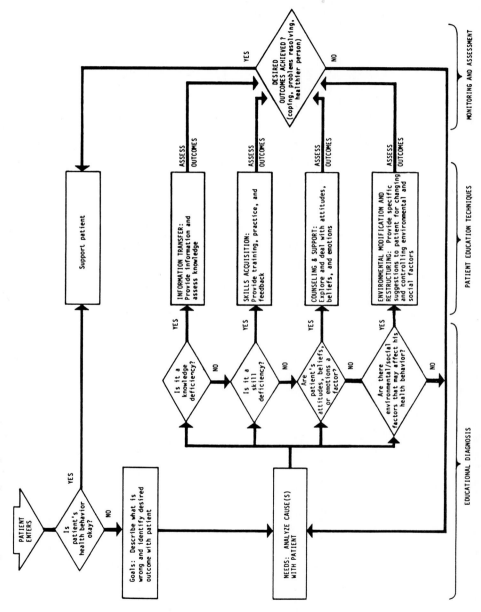

Establishing the cause of the performance deficit is most important. Is it due to knowledge gap, skills deficiency, an emotional factor, a social or environmental variable, or some combination of these? The patient who is giving an incorrect insulin dosage because of diminished eyesight has a skills deficit. A procedure review, practice demonstration, and follow-up supervision are required to improve performance. On the other hand, misinformation or lack of knowledge may explain why the hypertensive patient on a low-salt diet continues to eat smoked fish and luncheon meats. It is important to know the educational level of the patient as well as his or her general level of intelligence. Bear in mind that the studies on compliance mentioned earlier show no correlation between the number of university degrees a patient has and commonsense behavior in health care. The knowledge base of the patient's family is also relevant in the management of child care or the elderly. Sound methods for assessing the knowledge, wisdom, and tradition handed down through generations have not yet been developed.

Causes of
performance
deficit

Skills deficit

Information
gap

The patient's attitudes, beliefs, or emotions may also be a predisposing factor interfering with appropriate health behavior. A patient may be governed by religious or cultural doctrine or may be so preoccupied with "peripheral" concerns (e.g., attractive figure or physique, career aspirations or a romantic relationship) that he or she ignores warning signs of ill health. If the physician and staff are not perceptive of these personal traits, they may cloud patients' priorities, block learning, and interfere with motivation.

Emotional or
social factors

The physician has a legitimate interest in the social and environmental constraints that influence health behavior. He or she cannot create ideal environments for patients or dictate what they should do. They can, however, help patients to recognize factors which weigh the pros or cons for change, identify alternative options, and guide patients in gaining more self-control over their personal environment and life.

Environmental
factors

Patient Education Techniques

Learning facts and skills is a necessary prerequisite to successful involvement of the patient in the maintenance of good health. The basic educational principles for transferring information and teaching new skills are listed in Table 40-3.

Teaching facts
and skills

Counseling and psychological support of patients are receiving much more emphasis today than in the past. Most patients take the scientific competencies of health professionals for granted and often judge them instead in terms of counseling skills, receptive personality, and the type of information given. Social support, family therapy, self-care instruction, and ongoing reassurance are com-

Counseling

Table 40-3   Basic Principles of Information Transfer and Skills Acquisition

1   Patient education cannot accomplish more than a behavioral change.
2   A combination of strategies is required for all learning.
3   Health affects many; the patient cannot be taught in isolation from family, friends, peers, employers.
4   Audiovisual and printed aids cannot be substituted for personal instruction.
5   Sophisticated techniques and fancy gadgetry do not ensure success.
6   Begin where the patient is *now*, relate new information to previous knowledge and adapt available aids to individual needs.
7   Value the KISS principle—"Keep it simple, stupid." Be specific, brief and direct; avoid overkill.
8   Illustrate anatomy and physiology with pictures, graphics, or models.
9   Encourage patients to write down critical or complex information and repeat it.
10   Practice skills in simulated settings, supervise in real-life situations.
FOLLOW-UP IS ESSENTIAL.

mon interpersonal skills performed daily by the physician and office staff during patient encounters. The personal interaction itself is highly therapeutic.[15] The doctor-patient relationship usually continues for several years; therefore not everything needs to be resolved in a single brief visit.

Coping strategies

Physicians have been warned by psychiatrists not to become overinvolved in a patient's home life or work setting. Environmental modification and restructuring are the patient's responsibility; the health care team merely introduces coping strategies and supports efforts made by the patient to solve the problem.[16] Appropriate expertise may be sought for complications outside the realm of family medicine, but the family physician continues to provide supportive maintenance care.

Evaluation of Outcomes Achieved

Evaluation is important for patient satisfaction, staff development, and justification of the overall patient education program. Positive reinforcement is one treatment with no side effects. Patients need objective assessment of their performance as well as the opportunity to provide feedback to staff on teaching methods and aides. A number of evaluation trials are available today to measure knowledge, skills, and behavioral changes of patients. Patient interviews are, or course, the most important. Questionnaires, group discussions, suggestion boxes, and patient newsletters all facilitate shared input and brainstorming for new directions toward quality care. Regular staff meetings with progress updates and peer review are also essential to maintain a health program and happy staff. Chart documentation of patient education intervention is crucial for au-

Patient interviews

Staff meetings
Chart recording crucial

dit and research purposes as well as future program development. The problem-oriented record format is ideal for retrieving information quickly, since "SOAPing" behavioral problems includes patient education outcomes.[14] Flow sheets, such as those used for pediatric, prenatal, diabetic, or hypertensive patients, help to provide a check of what has been done and future needs. If the POMR system is not being used, the physician will have to develop an effective shorthand system of recording. Further investigation needs to be done in evaluating the impact which recording patient education strategies on the chart has on subsequent teaching efforts during follow-up visits.

POMR

Flow sheets

CREATING A LEARNING ENVIRONMENT

Team Cooperation

Who does what?

The physician of the future must be prepared to provide patients with more information; however, he or she will have to rely heavily on other health professionals to share this responsibility. The report of the American task force recommended the team approach, since no single profession or individual possesses the requisite skills to undertake patient education independently. All health personnel with direct patient contact influence it to some degree. To realize the full impact of patient education, the teaching potential of all available staff should be assessed and expanded wherever possible, be it a solo practice, group clinic, or large teaching center. New services will prove neither cost- nor time-efficient if existing resources are not being used effectively.

Team approach

Assess staff potential

Improving patient education in any practice necessitates bringing all staff together to decide what should be accomplished and to collectively develop objectives and establish priorities. Building a practical model which is comfortable for the staff and clinically realistic for the patient population is most important. The physician's role in this process is crucial.

Design program

Extent of Physician's Role

As manager of patient care, the physician acts as *coordinator* and *facilitator* for all patient teaching. His or her primary responsibility is to involve patients in the educational process, to oversee maintenance of patient education in the practice on an ongoing basis, and to evaluate practice performance and outcomes. The physician must demonstrate a genuine interest in patient education in order to motivate patients to become involved, as well as foster team spirit among co-workers. It is the physician's attitude and commitment to patient education which sets the office tone and establishes cred-

Initiates program

Supports others

M.D.'s attitude crucial

Needs
assessment

ibility for strategies and programs implemented by others. The most important decisions made by the physician are *who* and *what* is to be taught *when*. Much less important is who will teach and how what is to be taught is accomplished. The physician weighs the problems seen in the practice to determine high priorities, or sift out situations for which improvement is likely with patient education intervention. Interpersonal communication skills will not be discussed in detail in this chapter. It is sufficient to say that exploratory and listening skills are an essential component of the physician-patient encounter when eliciting health care needs.

The problem-oriented medical record system introduced by Dr. Lawrence Weed lends itself easily to recording the need for patient education on the "problem list" and the inclusion of an education prescription under the "plan" in each progress note. Its design also facilitates team communication by enabling several health workers to read and act on the goals outlined in the chart.[14]

Reinforcement

Although all physicians provide the traditional medical content necessary during the office visit (e.g., anatomy, physiology, drug interactions, etc.) each individual must clarify any additional areas of personal interest which he or she would prefer to teach. One physician may choose to handle sports injuries, another geriatric problems, another prenatal education, depending on personal and professional experience as well as research interests. Educational *follow-up* by the physician during future visits is as important as the initial patient "overload" so often attempted during the first visit. Many things change over time. Periodic review and reinforcement of input provided by both the patient and staff aid compliance and help to keep everybody's interest and motivation up.

Provides
perspective

The physician must determine *when* to teach for two reasons. First of all, disinterested patients make up approximately 5 percent of the average practice population. A protocol should be established outlining how much time will be invested in those patients who want supermarket medicine without becoming involved. Second, the physician makes a unique contribution to patient education by providing *perspective* on the patient's problem—that sixth sense mentioned earlier.[17]

Optimal
teaching
moments

The intensity of the patient's reaction to the disease must be considered as well as the disease itself. Acute diarrhea in the young child, middle-aged executive, and elderly person each requires a different educational approach. Timing is very important. A patient with cancer requires more complex education than the patient with strep throat; however, any condition may be considered potentially serious by the patient until experience or a good teacher provides a proper perspective. Determining optimal teaching moments enables staff to provide highly personalized patient education at a time most meaningful and therapeutic to the individual.

The heavy smoker adolescent whose father has chronic emphysema is an ideal target.

Dr. Gayle Stephens, chairman of the American task force, outlined three types of patient problems which are best resolved by direct physician intervention.[17] One is the spontaneous question occurring at a time when least expected, presented with some sense of urgency, and requiring a sophisticated explanation. A patient says, "Am I a hypochondriac?" or "Doctor, I know I have cancer!" Also, there is the well-educated patient who exhibits unhealthy coping mechanisms through disease denial or intellectualization; apprehension may be so great as to prevent learning. These, as well as incurable patients—who for a variety of reasons do not wish to or cannot change—require careful management by the family physician, who has in-depth knowledge and understanding of their personal needs.

M.D. handles complex problems

The physician should initiate periodic review and evaluation of patient education with all persons involved. Keeping a watchful eye for negative feedback and patient dissatisfaction is particularly important. Often patients do not complain unless the physician draws comments out, but unresolved problems may become the source of future misunderstanding, wasted time, or errors. The physician can also keep abreast of new trends and growing needs by enlisting support from the local medical society, participating in continuing education programs, and working closely with service community agencies.

Role of the Nurse

Nurses have a professional interest and commitment to patient education. Trained as patient *teachers, counselors,* and *advocates,* they guide patients through the treatment process assuming responsibility for implementation of much of the treatment plan. Information sharing, skills demonstrations, group instruction, psychosocial counseling, monitoring family caregivers, and ongoing reinforcement are educational strategies which can be effectively performed by a nurse. Nurses also play a vital role in helping to standardize practice protocols, flowcharts, and patient information handouts. Nurses often train office assistants, receptionists and volunteers in certain patient education responsibilities. See the next chapter for a more in-depth job description. Physicians who do not have a qualified nurse in their practice may obtain assistance by contacting community health department nurses, retired nurses, or those unemployed due to child rearing. Many are adept at maternal and child health. Often they are willing to assist with specific teaching sessions on an hourly basis or as volunteers. Nursing students show a keen interest in providing direct patient teaching in

Direct teaching

Patient advocacy

Counseling

Training staff

Sources outside office

Student nurses

Clinical
consultants

exchange for clinical experience. Nurses trained in clinical specialties such as diabetes, hypertension, home care, or palliative care
may also provide patient teaching on a consultant basis.

Role of the Receptionist

PR
responsibility

Promotes
learning
atmosphere

The receptionist greeting the patient, both on the telephone and
in the office, plays a vital *public relations* role in transmitting the
health team's interest in promoting patient education. He or she
triages requests for medical intervention, explains practice protocol, and oversees completion of heath questionnaires on initial visits. Maintaining an educational tone in the waiting room through
appropriate pamphlet, poster, and magazine distribution is important. The dissemination of patient information leaflets, practice
brochures, and patient newsletters in a positive manner can also
have a powerful impact on the quality of patient education
provided.

Role of the Patient

On the team!

Contractual
agreement

Family involved

Emotional
support

Evaluating
materials

Enlisting the participation, cooperation, and support of patients in
health care is the crux of patient education. Dr. L. Weed encouraged physicians to make patients *partners in care,* helping to develop
the problem list and to determine realistic priorities. Some physicians establish a written contractual agreement with the patient.[18]
       The range and depth of teaching skills potentially available to
physicians through patients and their families is often underestimated. Experienced patients may volunteer to share information
by serving as models or *lay therapists* to those facing a new situation.
They also function extremely well as *group facilitators* for therapeutic or emotional support sessions. Retired individuals (e.g., health
professionals, teachers, librarians) are capable assistants in patient
teaching as well as editing or evaluating printed materials. Those
who are actively involved in community agencies are usually eager
to share their knowledge with both patients and staff.

Facilities and Logistics

Appearance of
practice

Reception area

Putting it all together. . . .
       Most medical offices have not been designed with patient edu-
cation activities in mind; however, any facility can be adapted to
such use without major structural changes. Take a critical look at
the office atmosphere which the patient enters. Are the layout, de-
cor, furnishings, lighting, and sound effects conducive to relaxation and learning? Or do people sense a sterile atmosphere with
noise, frenzied activity, and disorganization? Do staff always appear
overwhelmed and hurried? Consideration must be given to the

general impression created by the reception area. Ensure that yours is a positive one!

The examination room is the area where most patient educa- tion in the physician's office occurs. Materials appropriate to the type of care provided there should be available for both patients and staff (e.g., infant feeding and child care information in a pe- diatric room, prenatal and gynecologic information in a female ex- amination room). In a surgical treatment room, facts on cast care, wound care and accident prevention would be appropriate. It is extremely important that the physician take advantage of teaching opportunities during the history and physical examination. To realistically accomplish patient education in a 15-minute time frame, activities must be performed simultaneously and educa- tional aids easily retrieved when needed.

Examination room

EDUCATIONAL AIDS—THEIR USE IN FAMILY MEDICINE

What to Use, Where?

The introduction of certain educational aids into the reception area and throughout the office will reinforce the physician's sensitivity toward good general health and self-care.

Books, pamphlets, and posters provide "food for thought" and often motivate patients to seek more information. Educators be- lieve that there is some limited potential for health education dur- ing the "downtime" when the patient, family and/or escorts are waiting for service. Table 40-4 lists a variety of educational aids suitable for the reception area.[2] Not all will be appropriate or rele- vant to every practice.

Printed materials

Selecting magazines for your patient population is no easy task. Some controversy still exists over the amount of scientific infor- mation to which patients should be exposed. Health-focused mag- azines are plentiful today, while many household magazines carry health sections written by professionals. Choosing is purely a mat- ter of personal preference. The important point is that all printed materials, including posters, be rotated periodically and grossly outdated editions discarded. Staff must keep abreast of new ma- terials and programs. Failure to display current health information could imply lack of interest or outdated medical care.

Magazines

Pamphlet racks appropriately placed throughout the office present patients with a variety of topics from which to choose read- ing materials. Again, keep them updated and neat.

Pamphlet racks

Schedules and pamphlets on local services available should be posted in areas easily accessible to the patient. In Canada and the United States, government educators as well as the news media fo-

Schedules and pamphlets

Table 40-4   Educational Aids for Reception Area

1   MAGAZINES.
Provide variety, ensure appropriateness for patient population.

Keep attractively displayed, current, and tidy.

Many health publications for public available (e.g., *Family Health, Family Safety, Listen, American Health*).

2   BULLETIN BOARD DISPLAYS.
Specific health topics associated with seasons of year, media promotion of current health issues, or campaigns of voluntary agencies (e.g., frostbite, picnics and food poisoning, handicapped olympics, heart disease in February, childhood immunization in November).

New programs in local area (e.g., first aid program for seniors, stress telephone line for parents).

Health article of the month (e.g., AIDS, alcohol and adolescents).

Critical health issues, the "big killers" (e.g., cancer, heart disease, highway accidents).

Upcoming TV or radio programs on health (e.g., Alzheimer's disease, family violence).

Newspaper clippings of community projects involving staff or patients.

Research projects in family medicine.

Book displays or equipment displays (e.g., library or commercial company).

3   PAMPHLET RACKS.
Schedules and lists of available community resources (e.g., equipment loan service for home care, handicapped bus service, prenatal classes, home nursing services).

New services in area (e.g., stroke club, transition house, premarital classes).

Self-help and family support groups (e.g., bereavement, child abuse, mastectomy visiting program).

Lifestyle information (e.g., nutrition, smoking cessation, elderobics, stress management).

Safety and accident prevention (e.g., sports helmets, pediatric car seats).

4   SPECIALIZED BROCHURES.
Office brochure.

Patient newsletter or health letter.

Patients' bill of rights.

Government and insurance company mail-outs or inserts (e.g., fitness).

5   EDUCATIONAL TOYS.
Doctor's kit, nurse's kit.

Anatomic models.

Hand puppets with injuries.

Doll's house or hospital.

Coloring books, puzzles, quizzes on health.

6 "HEALTH LINE" TELEPHONE INFORMATION SERVICE.
Install a direct line in reception area.

Provide a list of available audiocassettes on health topics with the telephone number.

Checklist evaluation form for feedback on program.

7 AUDIOVISUAL DISPLAYS.
Cassettes.

Slide-tape presentations (lifestyle information, facts on ages and stages).

Hand-operated filmstrips (e.g., skills demonstration).

Provide earphones to ensure privacy and avoid disturbance to others.

Maintain equipment in good repair.

Checklist on value of program.

8 SUGGESTION BOX.
Encourages anonymous input into practice performance.

9 CATALOGUES.
Information on sources and costs.

ALL EDUCATIONAL AIDS PROMOTE DISCUSSION. BE PREPARED.

---

cus on particular health issues throughout the year. Providing similar information simultaneously in the office, on a bulletin board, reinforces health teaching and increases audience exposure. Local libraries, commercial companies, or consumer bureaus may set up book displays or equipment demonstrations in the office periodically.

Educational toys, games, and coloring books for children are very popular, with a wide assortment available today. Anatomically correct dolls or puppets with injured parts are being used in many schools and hospitals. No doubt there is a role for them in the ambulatory care setting as well.

Many physicians design patient information brochures to supplement verbal instructions and explain practice philosophy, office procedures, and patient responsibility.[19] Patient newsletters, usually published quarterly, are being developed by an increasing number of family physicians to provide ongoing patient education. Emphasis is placed on preventive care and common problems presented in the office.[20] Health letters, an expanded version of this, are also being offered to the general public on subscription by several university health departments as well as other sources. *The Harvard Medical School Health Letter* and *Health News* from the Faculty of Medicine, University of Toronto, Canada, are two popular publications (see Figure 40-3).

Book displays

Toys, games, dolls

Office brochures

Newsletters

Health letters

Suggestion box

Resource
catalogues

Audiocassettes

"Health line"

Audiovisual
technology

Home video
machines

Limitations

Microcom-
puters

Self-care
products

Monitoring
home
diagnostic kits

A suggestion box in the waiting area allows patients the opportunity to have input into practice activities. Access to resource catalogues also enables them to selectively choose further information
independently.

The telephone is another office tool which can be used effectively for patient education. Telephone contacts are beneficial for
just keeping in touch with patients—to give verbal progress reports, provide supervisory follow-up care, and explain or interpret
some aspect of treatment.[21] They are commonly used for recall
purposes (i.e. periodic health checkups, Pap smears, immunization) and the scheduling of patient flow. Isolated patients such as
handicapped persons and senior citizens rely on the telephone as
their "lifeline" with the health care system. Providing recorded
health information from audiocassettes via the telephone is a popular system available in some metropolitan cities today. The University of Wisconsin's "Health Line" is one which offers the public
a wide range of general health subjects for easy listening in the
privacy of home. Health centers and clinics often have a direct line
from the waiting room or patient education library to a health information source.

Audiovisual technology has exploded in the last few years, providing many options for patient teaching. Until recently, the cost
of equipment and media has not been economically feasible for the
average solo practitioner. However, studies have shown that as the
price goes down and versatility of material increases, more physicians are getting involved.[22] Patient acceptance of this type of learning has been universal, since viewing in the office or at home is
convenient, entertaining, and economical. A number of excellent
health games, quizzes, and documentaries are available for home
video machines today. It is most important that audiovisual equipment in the office setting be placed in a location readily accessible
to patients with limited mobility—those in wheelchairs, in braces,
or on crutches. Hearing and visual defects may limit the usefulness
of the audiovisual approach with some patients.

The novelty associated with microcomputers has also increased
physician interest in their potential for patient education.[23] The
concept remains intriguing but not really cost-effective for patient
education, unless the computer can also be used for administrative
and clinical tasks in the practice.

An area where health professionals need improved patient
education aids is that of self-care products. The misuse of non-
prescription drugs is well documented. The misuse of accessory
health care products and home diagnostic kits is becoming a problem as well. Home diagnostic kits can be a useful adjunct to care,
providing a cheap method of monitoring or screening (home pregnancy tests, glucose or blood pressure monitoring, fecal blood tests,

Figure 40-3

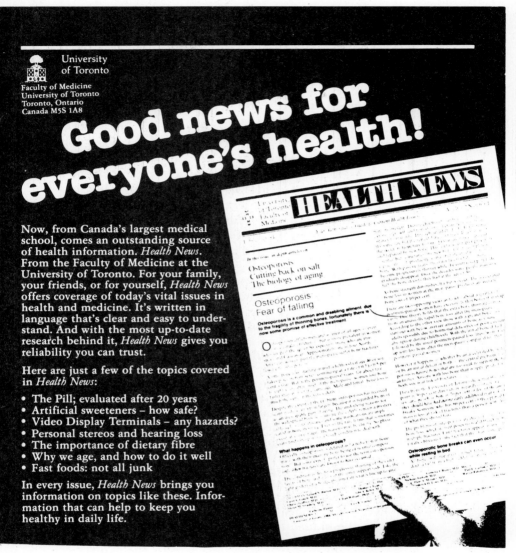

etc). However, as the number of products available increases, so do the risks of improper usage and misinterpretation of results. In one study on home pregnancy test kits only 32 percent of users complied with instructions, while 24.3 percent of the test results were false negatives.[24] Care must be exercised that patients receive reliable products with accurate instructions, and also that they do not become victims of fraud or quackery.

Quackery

Selection and Development of Printed Resources

Aside from direct oral instruction in professional encounters, printed materials remain the most popular and most adaptable educational aids for many types of situations presented in family medicine. Guidelines for the use of printed aids and their adaptation to the office setting are outlined in Table 40-5.

Appropriate Usage

Effective
presentation

Timing

Printed aids can be used effectively to create awareness, to provide factual information, or to review and reinforce key points. Do not attempt to present written materials to depressed or overanxious persons, to those in emotional crisis, or to illiterate or visually impaired patients. Patients who frequently change physicians or react negatively to suggested treatment goals are also poor candidates for written information. Timing of presentation is very important. If the patient is in a poor state of mind, any educational effort will prove ineffective. Printed aids will not stimulate motivation or interest in behavioral change; a combination of strategies must be used beyond the mere presentation of facts. Specific aspects of family practice for which printed aids prove helpful are:[25]

Prehospital and
posthospital

1 *Hospitalization:* Patients should receive sufficient prehospitalization instruction to eliminate any false expectations or embarrassment, particularly for first admissions. Discharge planning helps to ensure adequate follow-up during their transition back to the community, so that patients do not feel lost or abandoned.

Diagnostic tests

2 *Diagnostic procedures and laboratory tests:* Many diagnostic procedures are repeated unnecessarily because health professionals have not given adequate pretest instructions to the patient (e.g., bowel evacuation regimes for barium enema, fasting procedure for basal glucose levels).

Health system

3 *Health care system protocol:* Patients should know how to seek care when needed. Office policy statements or practice brochures explain office procedures and tell patients when to call the physician and what to do in emergencies. Many patients complain about the hidden costs of services about which they were not informed but which they are expected to pay (e.g., extra billing, consultation fees, or diagnostic services not covered by health insurance programs). Some government agencies provide free booklets that explain services and costs. Patients are often confused by complexities of the referral or consultation process. It is most important that they understand what to expect, where to go, and what arrangements have been made for follow-up care.

Self-care

4 *Home care or self-treatment:* Written instructions can guide patients and families in the provision of self-care. Helping them to understand their responsibilities and limitations in performing

Table 40-5   Guidelines for Use of Printed Aids

Organization

Outline the responsibilities of co-workers in patient teaching; assign one employee the task of organizing, sorting, and ordering materials.

Design a form letter for ordering purposes.

Set up a filing system that facilitates accessibilty and quick retrieval; code each item.

Determine best locations for displaying aids—one central area or dispersed throughout treatment areas.

Prepare an inventory of educational materials available in your office.

Discard outdated material; periodic evaluation keeps information current and up to date.

Document patient's level of comprehension and motivation to learn.

Establish standardized method of recording the use of aids on the patient's chart—on problem list, progress notes, or educational flow sheets; maintain consistency.

Ensure that your receptionist knows which staff handle questions regarding educational resources.

Evaluation

Review and evaluate all material before distribution to ensure that information is suitable for physician's clinical approach.

Utilize staff, family, or selective patients to pretest appropriateness of material.

If material is designed for a general audience, adapt it to suit individual needs or prepare your own written handout.

Personalize aids whenever possible (with patient's name, physician's name, added notations, etc.).

Consider accuracy, content, language, and appearance.

Avoid aids that are lengthy or highly scientific or technical, as well as those that present controversial information or lack illustrations.

Presentation

Introduce early in medical management, not as a postscript to patient interview.

Explain purpose, allow for questions, supplement with follow-up discussion at a later time.

Aids must not replace interpersonal communication or be presented in isolation without discussion.

procedures such as the administration of drugs or use of equipment is crucial (e.g., insulin injections, inhalation therapy).

Common
conditions

5 *Common conditions:* Frequently presented conditions require educational reinforcement to help prevent repeated episodes and ensure that pertinent routine facts have not been overlooked.

Rare conditions

6 *Rare conditions:* Providing information about unusual conditions (e.g., genetic disorders, anorexia nervosa) helps to enhance the patient's understanding of etiology and prognosis.

Misinformation

7 *Myths, misconceptions, and controversies:* Pregnancy, sex education, infant care, cold remedies, and laxatives are among the topics about which many myths still exist in our society. In addition, the public may possess a lot of misinformation or controversial facts on mental health, cancer, heart disease, vitamin supplements, diets, and fitness techniques, to mention a few. People tend to lump illnesses together, often associating their condition with the negative experience of a relative or friend.

Chronic
diseases

8 *Chronic conditions:* Families involved in caring for the chronically ill, handicapped, or terminally ill require guidance in coping with the physical and emotional adjustment of ongoing responsibility over lengthy periods of time.

Aging

9 *Geriatrics:* Printed aids may help in the management of problems associated with the aging process (e.g., foot care, bowel routines, nutritional habits, and drug administration).

Lifestyle
changes

10 *Lifestyle habits and behavior:* Printed aids can be used effectively to provide statistics on self-imposed or environmental health risks. Subjects might include smoking or alcohol and drug abuse; highway, home, and recreational safety; nutrition, physical fitness, and mental health.

Read before
giving out

Most preprinted aids are prepared on a national-average basis with the "typical" patient in mind. Whether commercially designed, custom-produced, or self-prepared, printed materials should be carefully evaluated before being presented to patients. Otherwise, their beneficial effect will be lost. Several health educators are developing standardized, shortcut methods of evaluating printed materials used in family practice.[26]

CLASSIFICATION AND SOURCE OF MATERIALS

Pamphlets, Booklets, Flip Charts, and Graphic Illustrations

Voluntary
agencies

An abundance of printed materials is available from governmental departments or voluntary community agencies. Some of this material is free. Government publications cover a wide range of health and social topics of interest to the general population (e.g., immunization, safety, lifestyle risks). Private organizations try to create public awareness of a particular disease or other health topic through distribution of information at clinics, schools, community fairs, and so on (e.g., cystic fibrosis, arthritis, or family planning). Hospitals and community health centers, as well as health education centers, are additional sources of both general and specific health care information. Pertinent information on a subject of particular relevance to family medicine is often available through national or local chapters of medical associations (e.g., *Guide for Physicians in Determining Fitness to Drive a Motor Vehicle,* published by the Canadian Medical Association, and *Pride in Family Practice Kit,* published by the American Academy of Family Physicians).

Hospitals and health centers

Professional associations

Pharmaceutical firms, industrial manufacturers, and insurance companies are good sources of printed aids; however, be aware of the fact that a few of these are commercially rather than educationally oriented. One popular aid produced by drug companies is the personal health record notebook, or daily diary. These are commonly used by patients to record blood pressure and list diabetic food or medication routines. Food manufacturers produce some useful aids for nutrition counseling, insurance companies for safety programs. One comprehensive listing of printed materials from many sources is *The Guide to Health Information Resources in Print,* available from Health Information Library, PAS Publishing Co., Daly City, CA 94015.

Commercial suppliers

Daily diary

Annotated guides

Companies specializing in communications and education in the health care industry (e.g., Trainex, Professional Counselling Aids Inc.) market a variety of elaborately packaged learning systems for sale or rent. Resource catalogues list a choice of anatomic models, flip charts, filmstrips, and audiotapes for office use.

Education companies

Figure 40-4 shows a sample of colorful information booklets available from the Patient Information Library of Krames Communications at a minimal cost.

Patient booklets

Local hospital or university libraries receive current publications, and staff are most helpful in researching a health subject on request. Physicians could also encourage their patients to use public libraries to obtain printed aids. Although some physicians have established a lending library in their offices, the time required to run it efficiently gives such a system little appeal. One alternative to the lending system is to provide patients with a reading list appropriate for their individual needs. A concise list offering three or four carefully selected references will limit confusion and duplication. Recently paperbacks have become a recognized source of teaching aids, providing health care information at a price most people can afford. Consumer health guides and books on self-care algorithms are becoming very popular with the public.[27] *Consumer Health: A Guide to Intelligent Decisions* by H. J. Cornacchia and S.

Libraries

Selected reading list

Paperbacks

Self-care algorithms

Figure 40-4 Patient information booklets, Krames Communications, Daly City,
CA 94015.

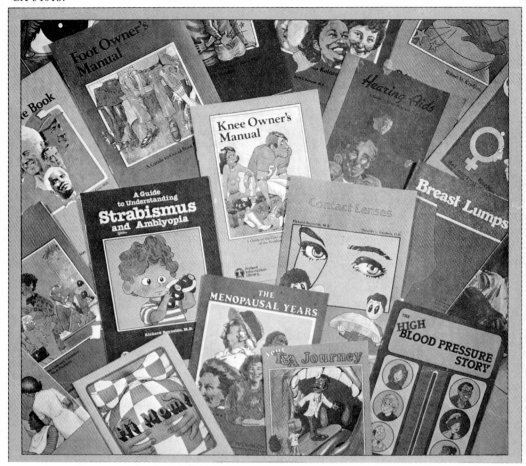

Barrett (1980) and *Take Care of Yourself—A Consumer's Guide to Medical Care* by J. Fries and D. Vickery (1976) have received wide distribution.

Simple
illustrations

Anatomical pictures and graphic illustrations should be kept simple when used for patient teaching, since extensive detail may cause more confusion than enlightenment. Plastic models with a

Models

three-dimensional effect usually provide a more realistic perspective of anatomy and physiology. Cartoon illustrations are another effective educational aid.

Handouts

The patient handout, a simple one- or two-page information sheet, is now commercially available from a variety of sources for patient teaching. Four instruction manuals consisting of a variety of handouts applicable to family medicine are listed below.

Patient Instruction Manuals

1 *Compendium of Patient Information* 1983–84, Biomedical Information Corporation, 800 2d Avenue, New York, NY 10017.

Hand-bound book containing multiple copies of each handout; perforated tear-out format.

2 *Instruction for Patients,* 3d ed., 1982, H. Winter Griffith; W. B. Saunders Co., West Washington Square, Philadelphia, PA 19105.

Multiple one-page sheets to be copied.

3 *Medication Guide for Patient Counselling,* 2d ed., 1982, Dorothy L. Smith; Lea & Febiger, Philadelphia, PA. 19106-4198.

Information sheets on the use and side effects of medications.

4 *Patient Education for the Family—Practical Patient Aids for Health Care Professionals,* 1979, David Brunworth and Scott Rigden; Harper & Row, Publishers, 2350 Virginia Avenue, Hagerstown, MD 21740.

A ring binder of multiple handouts to be copied.

Space has been provided for additional comments to individualize the handouts, making them more personalized. Some physicians prefer to develop their own information sheets using an instruction manual as a guide. Many hospitals and special clinics provide standardized information sheets for patients today. *Patient Care* is one journal which produces patient education handouts for distribution. More than 100 sheets on topics ranging from alcoholism to vasectomy are available. Upon written request, most scientific journals will allow reprinting of individual articles for teaching purposes.

Personalized handouts

Journal source

Reprints

Patient advisory leaflets (PALS) are another commercially produced counseling aid aimed at enhancing patient compliance with prescription medications. Individual leaflets can be purchased in bulk quantities on approximately 200 of the most popularly dispensed items. They are available from Pharmex Patient Counselling Aids, Automatic Business Products Co., Inc., Tuckie Rd., P.O. Box 57, Willimantic, CT 06226.

Drug leaflets

COMMUNITY RESOURCES

Resources available in patients' homes, neighborhoods, and communities extend the team concept far beyond the office of the family physician. To use community resources effectively, one needs a carefully organized referral process conducted by well-informed health care personnel. Table 40-6 suggests guidelines for effective use of community resources.

Know resources available

The physician and office staff should acquaint themselves with the resources in the community in order to promote good com-

Table 40-6   Effective Use of Community Resources

1 *Recognize* need for referral, explain reasoning to patient, and agree on possible goals for solution. Refer early, not as a last resort.
2 *Know* resources available, eligibility criteria, service parameters, and costs.
3 *Limit* the number of contacts; be selective.
4 *Motivate* patient to use referral resource as part of treatment plan; explain what to expect.
5 *Maintain continuity* of care by follow-up contact during resource's involvement.
6 *Evaluate* effectiveness through feedback from both patient and resource.

munication and ensure that the referral process will run as smoothly as possible when services are subsequently requested.

Personal encounters

Personal introductions provide more meaningful communication than form letters, telephone conversations, or chance meetings. Moreover, established community workers are often a source of new patients for the practice.

Reassess practice needs

Even a well-established physician may not be making optimal use of community services. One easy way to evaluate this is to review the charts of three patients chosen at random from your practice, asking yourself the following questions: How well are these patients' needs met? What specific health or social problems could be handled or reinforced by community resources? Would the utilization of community services improve the quality of care, patient satisfaction, or compliance?

Whom to Refer for Education

Acutely ill patients require considerable personal education from the physician, whereas chronically ill patients are ideal candidates for more formalized programs[28] (e.g., amputee clinics, pacemaker classes, diabetic day care). Physicians may have particular areas of interest for which they prefer to provide individual counseling initially, later making a referral for more detailed instruction (e.g., prenatal teaching, family planning, or psychotherapy). This practice is acceptable provided that consistency is maintained and the referral made *within a reasonable period of time*. Community agencies should not be used as a last resort to improve patient care, as a "dumping ground" for overwhelming social problems, or for intervention only in a time of crisis.

Resources for patients can be divided into two categories: informal (personal resources) and formal (agency resources).[29]

Informal Resources

Personal contacts

Personal resources include a patient's family, relatives, and friends. It is wise to involve family members or close associates in treatment whenever possible, since sick people appear to cope more readily if they remain in familiar surroundings. If family is nonexistent, uninterested, or mentally or physically handicapped, the availability of help from agency sources will have to be explored. Although formal community services may be limited in some rural areas, the personal care that is found in country areas is often envied by city dwellers. The physician must always ensure that personal resources in any setting do not become exploited or exhausted due to long-term involvement. All care givers, patients as well as staff, benefit from shared responsibility.

Formal Resources

The large number of government and private agencies may cause confusion for both patients and physicians. Public services offered vary with the size of the community and the health needs of the population. Since government services are regionally allocated, it behooves the physician to become familiar with the three major sources of health and social services available in North America: Departments of Public Health, Departments of Social Services, and Child Protection Services, or in rural areas, Agricultural Extension Services.

Organized services

Since government health agencies are designed to serve a large number of people, their programs focus on health maintenance, control of disease, and reduction of environmental health hazards to the community. Home nursing services, sexually transmitted disease clinics, immunization programs, and nutritional counseling are but a few of the services that a physician may use. Legal, social, and financial services, as well as employment and family counseling services, are also available through government sources.

Government

Volunteer or private agencies provide health or social services for the perceived needs of a particular segment of society. They may be categorized as follows:

Voluntary agencies

1 *Perceived-need organizations:* Associations organized at the national, regional, or local level to provide specialized services. Their focus is on public education and research (e.g., cancer, heart, and mental health organizations).

Specific need

2 *Sectarian agencies:* Many religious organizations provide support to families at times of crisis or emergency; also to those in financial or social need, such as hospitalized, isolated, or handicapped individuals (e.g., Catholic Charities, Salvation Army, and Jewish family service organizations).

Church activities

3 *Nonsectarian agencies* organized by the community and supported by fee-for-service or canvassed funds (e.g., Homemaker Services, Red Cross, YMCA): These are often organized collectively under the United Way.

Charitable organizations

Self-help

4 *Self-help organizations:* Persons with a particular condition or problem may form groups to share information and provide mutual support services (e.g., Alcoholics Anonymous, colostomy clubs, mastectomy visiting services, multiple sclerosis societies). Parent organizations for sudden infant death syndrome (SIDS), cystic fibrosis, and muscular dystrophy have contributed greatly to research and treatment for childhood diseases. Programs initiated by health action groups are steadily increasing.

Service clubs

5 *Service clubs:* Community fellowship groups finance special services for the underprivileged, such as summer camps, prosthetic equipment, ambulatory devices, or transportation services (e.g., Shriners, Rotarians, and fraternities).

Auxiliaries

Hospital and school auxiliaries, as well as volunteer bureaus and volunteer fire departments, are additional community resources that should not be overlooked.

Directory

A directory of community services is available in many metropolitan or regional areas. Copies should be strategically placed in the doctor's bag, physician's office, and the desk of the nurse-receptionist to provide a quick reference for required information. When in doubt about community services, contact the health educator at the local hospital or the staff of the department of health in your area.

If resources are inadequate or lacking, the physician should *initiate* community action to provide for unmet health needs.

REFERENCES

1 W. D. Squyres (ed.), *Patient Education: An Inquiry into the State of the Art,* Springer Publishing Co., New York, 1980.

2 *Patient Education: A Handbook for Teachers,* Report of the National Task Force on Training Family Physicians in Patient Education, Society of Teachers of Family Medicine, 1740 West 92d Street, Kansas City, MO 64114, 1979.

3 M. Ulrick and H. M. Kelly, "Patient Care Includes Teaching," *Hospitals,* **46:**59–65, April 1972.

4 A. R. Somers, "Consumer Health Education: Where Are We Going?" *Canadian Journal of Public Health,* **68:**362–368, September-October 1977.

5 E. Bartlett, "The Contributions of Consumer Health Education to Primary Care Practice: A Review," *Medical Care,* **18:**862–871, 1980.

6 L. Green and C. Kansler, *The Professional and Scientific Literature on Patient Education,* Gale Health Information Series, vol. 5, Gale Research Co., Detroit, 1980.

7 S. G. Rosenberg, "Patient Education Leads to Better Care for Heart Patients," *HSMA Health Reports,* **86:**793–802, 1971.

8 D. Sackett, R. Haynes, and D. Taylor (eds.), *Compliance in Health Care,* Johns Hopkins University Press, Baltimore, 1979, pp. 286–294.

9 B. Svarstad, "Physician-Patient Communication and Patient Conformity with

Medical Advice," in D. Mechanic (ed.), *The Growth of Bureaucratic Medicine*, Wiley, New York, 1976, pp. 220–238.

10 L. S. Levin, "Patient Education and Self-Care: How Do They Differ?" *Nursing Outlook*, **20:**170–175, March 1978.

11 A. Skiff, N. J. Goodwin, and M. F. Goldstein, "A Practical Approach to Assessing Patient Learning Needs," *Journal of the National Medical Association*, **73**(6):3, 1981.

12 J. Coope and D. H. Metcalfe, "How Much Do Patients Know? A Multiple Choice Question Paper for Patients in the Waiting Room," *Journal of the Royal College of General Practitioners*, **29:**482–487, August 1979.

13 W. L. Stewart, "Clinical Implications of the Virginia Study," *Journal of Family Practice*, **3**(1):15, 1976.

14 M. F. Fass, "Problem Oriented Patient Education: Defining and Assessing Educational Problems in Primary Care," in *Patient Education in the Primary Care Setting*, proceedings of a conference, Department of Family Medicine and Practice, University of Wisconsin, 77 South Mills Street, Madison, WI 23715, 1977.

15 L. Litwack, J. M. Litwack, and M. B. Ballow, *Health Counselling*, Appleton-Century-Crofts, New York, 1980.

16 D. Fireman, G. A. Friday, C. Gira, et al., "Teaching Self-Management Skills to Asthmatic Children and Their Parents in Ambulatory Care Settings," *Pediatrics*, **68:**341–348, 1981.

17 G. G. Stephens, "The Role of the Physician in Patient Education," in *Patient Education in the Primary Care Setting*, proceedings of a conference, Department of Family Medicine, University of Tennessee, Memphis, TN 38163, 1980.

18 Patient Education Advisory Board, "Making Your Patient a Partner in Care," *Patient Care*, **8**(18):108–124, September 15, 1974.

19 M. G. Landry, "Questions and Answers: Avoiding the Obvious with a Patient Information Booklet," *Canadian Medical Association Journal*, **118:**1130–1131, 1978.

20 D. McGinty and C. A. Kratz, *Tips on Publishing a Newsletter*, Muscatine Community Health Center, 1514 Mulberry Street, Muscatine, IA 52761.

21 C. F. Stirewalt, M. W. Linn, G. Goday, et al., "Effectiveness of an Ambulatory Care Telephone Service in Reducing Drop-In Visits and Improving Satisfaction with Care," *Medical Care*, **20:**739, 1982.

22 W. H. Bryant, "Patient Education in the Doctor's Office: A Trial of Audiovisual Cassettes," *Canadian Family Physician*, **26:**419–422, March 1980.

23 M. A. Chen, Jr., T. P. Houston, et al., "Microcomputer-Based Patient Education Programs for Family Medicine," *Journal of Family Practice*, **18**(1):149–150, 1984.

24 B. G. Valanis and C. S. Perlman, "Home Pregnancy Testing Kits: Prevalence of Use, False Negative Rates and Compliance with Instructions," *American Journal of Public Health*, **72**(9):1034, 1982.

25 Patient Education Advisory Board, "Written Aids: A Step towards Better Patient Education," *Patient Care*, **12**(9):88–224, May 15, 1978.

26 D. Bosshart and J. H. Rennear, "A Checklist for Evaluating Written Aids," in "Getting the Best out of Handouts," *Patient Care*, **12**(9):108–113, May 1978.

27 A. O. Berg and J. P. LoGerfo, "Potential Effect of Self-Care Algorithms on the Number of Physician Visits," *New England Journal of Medicine*, **300:**535–537, 1979.

28 M. D. Weller, H. Ruth, and R. Seller, "Effective Use of Patient Resources: A Training Guide for Family Physicians," *Journal of Family Practice*, **4**(3):515, 1977.

29 Patient Education Advisory Board, "Staff and Community Resources for Patient Teaching," *Patient Care*, **8**(18):126–145, September 15, 1974.

CONTACTS FOR ADDITIONAL PATIENT EDUCATION INFORMATION—PUBLICATIONS, DIRECTORIES, AND AUDIOVISUAL MEDIA

Local, state, or national offices of government health departments and voluntary agencies

American Academy of Family Physicians
1740 West 92d Street
Kansas City, MO 64114

Bureau of Health Education
U.S. Department of Health, Education and Welfare
Centers for Disease Control
Atlanta, GA 30333

Brady's Patient Education Series
Robert J. Brady Co.
A Prentice-Hall Company
Bowie, MD 20715

Canadian Medical Association
1867 Alta Vista Drive
Ottawa, Ontario, Canada K1G 0G8

Harvard Medical School Health Letter
Department of Continuing Education
Harvard Medical School
79 Garden Street, Cambridge, MA 02138

Health-Line Library
WARF Building, Room 465C
610 Walnut Street, Madison, WI 53706

Information Resource Unit
Health Promotion Directorate
Health and Welfare Canada
Tunney's Pasture
Ottawa, Ontario, Canada K1A 0S9

International Union for Health Education
North American Regional Office
c/o CHES, P.O. Box 2305, Station "D"
Ottawa, Ontario, Canada K1P 5K0

Krames Communications
Patient Information Library
312 90th Street
Daly City, CA 94015

Medfact
420 Lake Avenue, N.E.
Massillon, OH 04646

National Health Information Clearinghouse (NHIC)
P.O. Box 1133
Washington, D.C. 20013-1133

National Medical Audiovisual Center
Atlanta, GA 30333

Professional Counselling Aids, Inc.
90 Northline Road
Toronto, Ontario, Canada M4B 3E8

Trainex Corporation
P.O. Box 116
Garden Grove, CA 92642

Part Five

Team Function

Chapter 41

The Family Practice Nurse

S. Urquhart, R.N.
L. Muzzerall, B.N.

Most medical students, interns, and residents do not have the opportunity to appreciate fully the expertise of the nursing profession because they train separately from nursing students; there is no sharing of perceived roles and no development of a "co-professional relationship." Therefore, as family physicians, these former medical students will fail to recognize the scope of the knowledge a graduate nurse possesses. The purpose of this chapter is to outline the skills that nurses can contribute to a family practice.

"The Family Practice Nurse is one who provides continuing, comprehensive family-oriented nursing care in association with a family physician and in accordance with the professional guidelines for the conduct of medical-nursing activities."[1] Following is an outline of the qualifications and job description that a family physician may find helpful when hiring a nurse to fill this role in the practice. Depending upon education and experience, some nurses may not have acquired all of the suggested skills. Many nurses are trained on the job by the physician. The suggested outline is not intended to be all-inclusive, as the physician may wish to have the nurse develop other skills—and therefore should allow the nurse time for continuing educational courses.

NURSE QUALIFICATIONS

Educational background:

(1)   Bachelor of nursing
(2)   R.N. with diploma plus additional education

Helpful experience:

Background
training

Hospital ambulatory care (at least three years)
Emergency room experience
Community health
Palliative care
Crisis intervention
Teaching—community and/or nursing

Attributes:

sensitive, flexible, eager to learn

ROLE OF THE NURSE IN FAMILY PRACTICE

1   Patient care.

Job tasks

Provide continuity of care for patients.
Interview new patients.
Obtain basic personal and family history.
Take preliminary measurements and do investigations for basic
data record.
Encourage positive attitudes of health and self-management.
Certified in basic cardiac life support (BCLS)
Capable of providing care for epistaxis, hypoglycemic reac-
tions, foreign bodies, fractures, sprains and strains, bites and stings.

The health and best interest of the recipients of care are the
foremost considerations of the family practice nurse.

2   Patient education.

Teaching role

Teach patients (a) how to manage problems at home, (b) when
to ask for help, (c) how to make use of community resources.
Teach care and coping skills to patients with chronic illness,
e.g., diabetes, hypertension.
Provide prenatal care—advice on common disturbances, measurements (blood pressure, weight, fundal height, fetal position,
etc.), nutritional assessment and advice

Contraceptive counseling.

Encourage behavior change, e.g., smoking, home glucose monitoring.

Give nutritional advice, e.g., for obesity, patients with colostomies, the insulin-dependent, children.

3 Practice management.

Record and transmit clinical data.

Maintain supplies and stock equipment.

Organize tests and referrals and consultations.

Assist in interpreting physician's orders to patients and family.

Sterilization and maintenance of instruments.

Maintain doctor's bag.

Maintain narcotic control book.

Handle most medical phone calls (up to 90 percent).

Organizational tasks

Most often, the nurse's training, experience, and awareness of the doctor's preferences allow a response involving simple advice, support, and education so that direct physician involvement is unnecessary.

The management of the team is optimum when adequate time is allowed for communication. Regular team meetings including nurse, physician, and office staff facilitate continuity of care to patients. These meetings also provide a forum for review of general policies and sharing of ideas where all team members take an active role in discussion.

4 Nursing assessment–treatment.

Suture removal.

Immunizations.

Desensitization.

Venipuncture.

Wart treatment.

Check ears and throat.

Tonometries.

Breast examination.

Cervical smears—Pap—fit for diaphragms.

Ear syringing.

ECG—understand basic purpose and able to read 12-lead ECG.

Microscopic urinalysis.

Prepare trays for wound cleaning and repair.

Assist in biopsies, joint aspirations, and other procedures.

Procedures

5   Psychosocial support.

Provide sympathy, listening, and encouragement to improve the overall situation and state of mind.

Examples of problems amenable to support and reinforcement are anxiety, family dysfunction, loneliness, frustration, and lack of assertiveness.

ADVANTAGES OF NURSE-PHYSICIAN TEAM

Team approach

Complementary roles

To Physician	*To Nurse*	*To Patient*
Better-informed, satisfied patients	Application of acquired skills	Additional attention
Whole-person approach to health care	Intellectually and emotionally rewarding	Better informed
Deal with more challenging aspects of care	Complementary role with physician	Providing continuity when doctor absent or otherwise occupied
Fewer interruptions and telephone calls	Nursing opportunities to enrich patient care with education and support	
Flexibility within the team		

How Do We Make This Arrangement Work?

The physician must be committed to sharing the practice.

The physician should be comfortable delegating responsibility and enjoy a supportive supervisory role; discussion, planning and working together will be needed for two professionals to achieve trust, understanding, and appreciation for interwoven roles.

Openness in communication must be practiced.

Physician and nurse must behave in a mutually supportive way that helps patients understand roles.[2]

The following situation is presented as an example of the complementary roles of physician and nurse:

At 9 a.m. one Friday morning the practice receives a phone call from a 26-year-old mother with a 2-week-old baby. The mother and nurse identify two areas of concern, breast feeding and fussy baby. The nurse suggests that the mother bring in the baby at the time of feeding so that feeding technique may be observed.

Nursing assessment includes weighing the baby before and after feeding, observing breast feeding, and offering suggestions, reassurance, and praise where appropriate. The nurse should be aware of bonding in the mother-child relationship.

The physical condition of the baby is observed, and the mother's concerns are addressed. The nurse will discuss baby's different cries, sleep patterns, number of wet diapers, and stool consistency and will emphasize to the mother the importance of her own physical and mental well-being.

The situation can be described to the physician, who in turn can examine the infant, prescribe if necessary, and support the nurse's suggestions. Together the patient, nurse, and physician decide the best way to proceed with follow-up care.

CONCLUSION

The nurse in family practice is able to augment care given to patients. At a time when there is increasing public awareness and consumer interest in health issues, physicians are having less time to respond to patient education concerns. The majority of nurses employed in doctors' offices are functioning as receptionists, secretaries, and/or office managers. It is unfortunate that the value of a nurse in family practice is often measured only in financial terms. Perhaps the next generation of doctors will come close to developing a preventive attitude that will incorporate the full utilization of the nurse's skills and lead to more whole-person patient care.

Appropriateness of nurse's role

REFERENCES

1 D. Walters, "The Family Practice Nurse—Current Status," submission to Patterns of Practice and Health Care Delivery Committee for Canadian College of Family Physicians, Toronto, Ontario, Canada, November 1983.
2 L. I. Solberg and J. M. Johnson, *Physician and Nurse: A Manual for Collaboration*, University of Minnesota Medical School, Minneapolis, MN, 1981, pp. 3, 16.

ADDITIONAL READINGS

Brotten, D. A., L. Hayman, and M. Naylor, *Leadership for Change: A Guide for the Frustrated Nurse*, Lippincott, Philadelphia, 1978.
Chambers, L. W., and A. E. West, "The St. John's Randomized Trial of the Family Practice Nurse: Health Outcomes of Patients," *International Journal of Epidemiology*, Oxford University Press, 7(2):153–160, 1978.
Clarke, E. M., "The Primary Health Care Team. Working Together: The Team Concept," *Nursing Mirror Supplement*, 147(14):i–iii, 1978.
"Joint Practice Committee of the State Medical Association of Wisconsin and Wisconsin Nursing Association. Guidelines for Implementation of Joint Practice of Physicians and Nurses," *Wisconsin Medical Journal*, 80:38–40, June 1981.

MacDonald, H., and B. K. Hennen, "The Family Practice Nurse," in D. B. Shires and B. K. Hennen, *Family Medicine: A Guidebook for Practitioners of the Art,* 1st ed., McGraw-Hill, New York, 1980, chap. 16.

Mourin, K., "The Role of the Practice Nurse," *Journal of the Royal College of General Practitioners,* **30:**75–77, 1980.

Spano, L., "The Family Practice Nurse: Sense and Nonsense," *Canadian Family Physician,* **20:**93–99, 1974.

Chapter 42

Consulting Wisely

D. B. Shires, M.D.

Consultation is communication between two individuals with different areas of expertise. Although it is a common procedure in family practice, it sometimes produces unnecessary frustration. The purpose of this chapter is to clarify the process of consultation and to illustrate ways in which this communication can be made more effective for the family physician, the consultant, and—most important—the patient.

THE CONSULTATION PROCESS

As providers of primary care, family physicians often find that they need help with a particular condition (e.g., undefined neuropathy), procedure (e.g., gastroscopy), or manner of care (e.g., coronary care unit). Thus they will rely frequently on consultation.

To use consultation effectively, family physicians must realize that they will be consulting a number of individuals for varying reasons and in different ways. Who is consulted, how, and why will critically influence the information the family physician receives. In consultations, the physician asks for advice about a specific problem, not about the patient's total care, and the task is to obtain the information needed to make the most effective decision.

Table 42-1   Consultation Rates in England, the United States, and Canada

Location	Rate per 100 patient visits
Private practices* (Yorkshire, England)	1.3
Private practices† (Sheffield, England)	2.4
Rural practice‡ (United States)	2.4–5.9
Urban practices§ (London, Canada)	4.4

*Metcalfe and Sischy.[2]
†Pemberton.[3]
‡Penchansky and Fox.[4]
§Brock.[5]

Define the
question

    To consult wisely, family physicians must understand that consultation involves communication. Consulting family physicians seek specific information, and it is their responsibility to indicate clearly what they want to know. The family physician must become an expert in posing the question so that the information received is precisely the information requested. Neither the physician nor the patient should ever regard a request for consultation as an indication of failure on the part of the physician. Rather, such a request shows that the doctor perceives the seriousness or ambiguity of the situation, is aware of his or her limitations, or is sensitive to the concern of the patient.

    In the process of consultation, problems arise for both the consulting family physician and the consulted specialist (whether physician or nonphysician). One study reported that in over 30 percent of their referral letters to a large teaching hospital, general practitioners did not supply a relevant history of the problem that necessitated referral.[1] Another study showed that in over 40 percent of all consultations the family physician did not receive a report within 24 days of initiating the process.[2]

FREQUENCY OF CONSULTATIONS

The frequency of consultations for the average practitioner varies widely. Various authors have reported rates of consultation for different practice populations, as shown in Table 42-1.

    A physician can expect to have at least one or two consultations during a busy day. The frequency of consultations appears to vary with factors such as the age, sex, marital status and socioeconomic level of the patient. One study reported that patients under age 14 are seldom referred for consultation by family physicians, whereas for patients aged 15 to 34 the rate of referral can be as high as 4.6

Table 42-2   Patterns of Referral by Specialty according to Recent Reports

Specialty	Percent of referrals				
	United Kingdom		United States		Canada
	N = 673*	*N* = 178†	*N* = 126‡	*N* = 102§	*N* = 1883¶
Surgery	40.9	38.8	44.4	46.1	28.2
Medicine	14.1	8.4	19.8	15.6	24.9
Ophthalmology	4.1	13.5	11.1	5.9	12.1
Obstetrics and gynecology	7.0	12.3	11.9	10.8	10.9
Otolaryngology	12.1	15.2	2.4	9.8	9.2
Dermatology	4.4	4.5	0	6.9	6.1
Psychiatry	7.8	1.1	5.6	3.9	3.0
Pediatrics	1.0	1.7	0	1.0	1.1
Other (speech therapy, physiatry, podiatry)	8.6	4.5	4.8	0	4.5
Total	100.0	100.0	100.0	100.0	100.0

Source: Reproduced with the kind permission of Rodger M. Hines and D. J. Curry from their article, "The Consultation Process and Physician Satisfaction: Review of Referral Patterns in Three Urban Family Practice Units," *Canadian Medical Association Journal*, **118:**1071 (May 6, 1978).
·Pemberton.[3]
†Metcalfe and Sischy.[2]
‡Penchansky and Fox.[4]
§Brock.[5]
¶Hines and Curry.[6]

percent.[2] Table 42-2 illustrates the patterns of referral according to specialty in the United Kingdom, the United States and Canada.

The rates referred to in Table 42-2 are for family physicians consulting specialists. One can reasonably assume additional consultation of nonmedical consultants. Also, the number of consultations of family physicians by other family physicians and by specialist agencies is increasing. Consequently, consultation may be an even more common process than the published data indicate.

Family physicians as consultants

Factors Influencing Consultation Rates

The rates of referral are higher for women in the childbearing age, older men than younger men, and older unmarried patients of both sexes. (Older married patients are referred less frequently than older unmarried people.) Consultation rates appear to be lower among black patients and those of foreign origin, patients with limited education, patients in rural areas, and patients who are beneficiaries of medicare and Medicaid programs in the United States.[3−5]

Referral rates may be affected by individual physicians' awareness of their own limitations, their willingness to place themselves in a position in which they will be open to scrutiny, or their desire to make consultation a learning process.[6] In general, however, the patient who is able to demand extra or more complete service is the one who will be likely to receive a consultation.

SOME GENERAL DEFINITIONS

Expanded
definition

Our definition of a consultation is perhaps broader than would be generally accepted. According to the generally accepted definition, the patient's problem is referred to a medical consultant who sees and bills the patient for advice and refers the patient back to the family physician. However, we find that concept of consultation to be too narrow and have expanded our definition to include the seeking of advice from a variety of health professional consultants. Our definition primarily involves the concept of obtaining advice on a problem and does not necessarily require the presence of a patient. A consultation may take place on the telephone or at a social occasion.

It should be noted that in the United Kingdom the term *consultation* refers to a regular general practice visit; as used in this book, however, the term refers to a specialist consultation, according to North American usage. With this in mind, our definitions for the terms we shall use throughout the chapter follow.

Consultation

Consultation (physician retains responsibility) is the process in which advice is sought from a consultant regarding a particular patient problem either because of the complexity, obscurity, or seriousness of the care required or because another opinion is requested by the patient or an authorized person acting on the patient's behalf. The consultant responds by advising the referring physician on the specific problem but has no responsibility for the continuing care of the patient. (The exception to this is a consultation for advice on general care in which the total patient and his or her multiple problems are evaluated for a comprehensive opinion.)

> *Example:* A diagnosis of noncardiac chest pain, in which the consultant is positive that the pain is not myocardial but musculoskeletal in origin, and so advises the family physician.

Referral

Referral (physician transfers responsibility) is the process in which a patient with a specific disease is diagnosed and managed completely by the consultant for the duration of the illness. For example, in the case of a patient with diabetes in pregnancy, responsibility for the care of the patient is transferred, albeit temporarily in most cases. Some illnesses, for example, multiple sclerosis, may require a lifelong transfer of responsibility for the management of that specific illness. In such cases, the specialist consultant should keep the family physician informed of the patient's progress.

Transferral is the process whereby a patient transfers total care to another physician, for whatever reason.

Shared responsibility (concurrent care) is the process in which a particular problem is managed by the consultant, while the responsibility for general care is maintained by the referring physician.

> *Example:* A multiple-problem patient who is having surgery for an orthopedic malformation. The surgery and rehabilitation will be undertaken by a consultant orthopedic surgeon, but management of the other problems, e.g., diabetes, angina, hypertension, will remain the responsibility of the family physician.

Shared responsibility also refers to the style of care in which a variety of physicians (e.g., a gynecologist, a pediatrician, an internist, and the family physician) share the primary care responsibility for a family or an individual. This is a fairly common practice in the United States, but the general pattern in Canada and in most parts of the United Kingdom is to make the family physician the provider of family care.

Cross-referral is a commonly used term, although *cross-consultation* would be more accurate. This process occurs when a primary care physician sends a patient to a consultant for an opinion and the consultant recognizes additional problems and sends the patient to other consultants without discussing the situation with the referring physician. This kind of practice has been condemned by family physicians because it fragments care and does not allow coordination through a central focus—the family physician. It is also very discourteous to the referring physician, who is expecting an opinion on a particular problem for which he or she has sought advice. Finally, and perhaps most important, cross consultation is confusing to the patient. It is only fair to point out that some consultants who have cross-referred patients have done so because, in the past, the primary physician had done nothing to carry out the consultant's advice, resulting in neglect of the patient. This only reinforces our belief that consultation requires effective communication. To avoid cross-referral problems, you should clearly inform consultants when you first approach them that you wish to institute an effective method of communication and that cross-referral is not your style of practice.

Transferral

Sharing care

Cross-referral

Reasons for cross-referral

INDICATIONS FOR CONSULTATION

A physician may decide to use the consultation process on his or her own initiative or on that of the patient or family.

Whether a physician chooses to consult depends on his or her interests and abilities, the time available to perform the given procedure or task, the availability of the appropriate consultant, and the physician's personal knowledge of the patient.

A request for consultation from the patient may arise because of knowledge of a particular consultant (for example, an obstetrician who delivered her previous baby), because of a perceived need for more expertise, or simply to get a second opinion. Occasionally a patient requests a consultation because he or she is dissatisfied with the family physician. Some patients request a consultation as a result of their family's insistence.

Some reasons for referrals or consultations are outlined in Table 42-3.

WHOM TO CONSULT

Choosing consultants

One of the problems in setting up practice is to select a group of consultants to whom you will send your patients. How do you choose such a group? Initially, you may ask your colleagues' advice about who provides the best service to the community. Simply by talking to the community physicians about this problem, new practitioners will often gain valuable insights into the practices that are appropriate for that community. In addition, they will be able to evaluate the community physicians to whom they go for information. This is helpful because they will probably be using these physicians for consultative advice as well. Some considerations for choosing consultants are presented in Table 42-4.

Expanded list of consultants

Referral patterns in family practice are well documented.[2,7,8] From the studies made, it is obvious that surgeons are the consultants most frequently used by family physicians, accounting for

Table 42-3   Reasons for Consultation

1   Insufficient available resources (human or physical)
2   The need for more sophisticated diagnosis and therapy
3   Institutional policy
4   Patient or family request
5   Loss of rapport between patient or family and physician
6   The need for a team approach
7   Ethical conflicts in patient or family or physician
8   Reassurance for physician

Table 42-4 Considerations in Choosing Consultants

1	Potential for establishing mutual confidence
2	Convenience
3	Proximity to the practitioner's office and to patients
4	Prior knowledge of the consultant's ability
5	Unique expertise of a particular consultant

more than 40 percent of general practice consultations. However, one must not forget the referrals that are made to nonmedical specialists or agencies.[9] These include nursing services, adolescent behavior clinics, government liaison organizations (public health organizations, social workers, children's aid, welfare), therapists (physical, occupational, speech, etc.), mental health organizations, Alcoholics Anonymous, detoxification agencies, and community service organizations (cancer societies, arthritis societies, etc.). In addition, many family physicians find that they themselves are being used increasingly by their colleagues as consultants on problems of family dynamics, for multiple-problem patients, and for continuing care referred by tertiary care specialists.

Non-medical consultations

HOW TO CONSULT

The methods of consultation are as varied as the reasons for consultation. The family physician often consults with members of the primary health care team several times a day. For the purpose of this discussion, we will include only consultations outside the primary team.

The physician may request information on patients for diagnostic discussions, management decisions, or both. The purpose should be clearly outlined in the consulting request. It must be kept in mind that consultation is an *exchange* of information.

Consultation begins not with the patient's problem, but with the patient and his or her family.[10] The family should always remain the focus of attention for the family physician, even though this focus is sometimes lost in the consultation process. Figure 42-1 illustrates the series of steps along the consultation pathway.

Casual requests beget casual answers. The information required from consultation may be a simple "yes" or "no" answer to a "should I or shouldn't I?" question. In such a case, it must be *clearly* stated that this kind of answer is *expected*. Moreover, the family physician should not take the position that preliminary investigations are unnecessary since the consultant will repeat them anyway. It is frustrating for consultants when basic investigations

Writing the consultation request

Basic investigations

Figure 42-1   The consultation pathway.

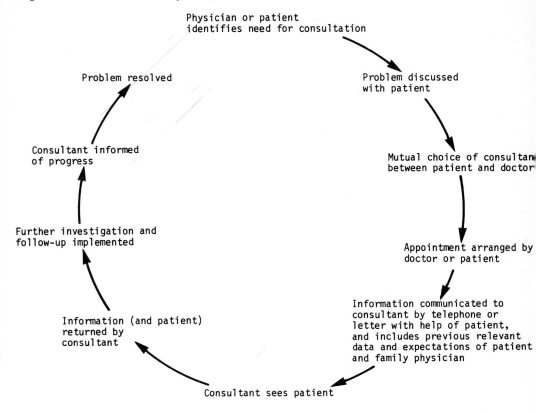

relevant to the patient's problem have not been completed, since this causes delay in defining and managing the problem.

Increasingly, family physicians are involving patients in the consulting process and encouraging them to make their own appointments with consultants. This approach increases patients' insights into their problems.[6]

In the past, a consultant often saw the patient only in the presence of the referring physician. Although this practice is now almost extinct, it represents the ideal to which all consultant communications should aspire. A letter or telephone communication should convey the same quality of communication that would exist if the referring physician were present.

Consulting letters must be carefully composed. A sample format for such a letter is given in Figure 42-2. Remember that consultation is an exchange of information, and use simple courtesies. It is *never* acceptable to send a consultation letter that states only "Please see and advise."[10]

Figure 42-2 Example of consultation request.

PLUMTREE MEDICAL CLINIC

TEL. 444-7729

Appointment date: *11 Sept. 1986*

Patient's Name: *Jean Smythe*
Patient's Address: *61 March Street*
Erie, Pa.
Telephone Number: *255-6472*
Health ID Number: *839-613-001*

TO: *Doctor R. Wilson*

ADDRESS: *Professional Building, Suite 1001*
Main Street
Erie, Pa.

Dear Doctor:

PROBLEM, as seen by patient: *Can't walk up more than one flight of stairs without stopping for breath; getting worse.*

PROBLEM, as seen by our staff: *Is this an increase in his emphysema or a new cardiovascular problem?*

OTHER SIGNIFICANT PROBLEMS: *Lives alone*
Smokes (++)

PREVIOUS CONSULTATIONS: *Respirology consultation (Dr. Jones, Nov., 1979) for lung function evaluation. Diagnosis of chronic bronchitis/emphysema.*

INVESTIGATION AND MANAGEMENT TO DATE:
Lung functions '84 and '85 (attached copies). ECG - possible ischemic changes (see attached).

REASON FOR CONSULTATION: *Assessment of cardiac function.*

Thank you for seeing this patient.

Yours sincerely,

Margaret Blough

Margaret Blough, M.D.

SUGGESTIONS FOR MORE EFFECTIVE
CONSULTATION COMMUNICATION

Effective
communi-
cations

The urgency of the problem should be stated when the appoint-ment is made. If the problem is really urgent, it should be discussed with the consultant over the telephone before he or she sees the patient. The problem should be defined as clearly as possible to-gether with any associated problems. Guesses, queries, and ruled-out diagnoses should *not* be included, but relevant investigations and results to date should be listed. The reasons for consultation, both general and specific, should be mentioned. If a "yes" or "no" answer to a "should I or shouldn't I?" question is being requested, this should be made clear. Any specific questions to which the re-ferring physician needs an answer must be clearly stated. The re-ferring physician should have a printed form with his or her name, address, and telephone number so that the reply from the consul-tant can be given in an appropriate time period. If the reply is slow in coming, the referring physician should not hesitate to request it.

Timeliness of
letter

It is important that the referral form be available to the consultant at the time of the patient's visit. Legible, handwritten (or block-printed) information on hand is preferable to a typewritten letter lost in the mail. Some physicians have the patients carry the form themselves.

Obviously, it is difficult to design a form that meets the needs of all consultants and referring physicians. New family physicians should consider the requirements presented above in designing a form to suit their particular needs.

There are many other methods of consultation in addition to the formal consultation process—for example, those conversations regarding patient care which take place over the operating table, in the hospital corridor or parking lot, or in the coffee room or doctors' lounge. Often, problems can be solved by discussing in-vestigations or management plans with a consultant over the tele-phone. Family physicians in group practice are used to this format and are apt to wander down the hall to their colleagues' offices to ask questions about a particular drug or symptom. This, too, can be regarded as a consultative process.

Use of
telephone

Consultations
to family
physicians

As can be seen from this brief review, the problems of consult-ing are many. The efficiency of health care delivery in terms of primary, secondary, and tertiary care depends very much on whether the referral and consultative process works smoothly. It is vital that the method of consultation involve two-way communica-tion. Primary care physicians must fully understand the process of consultation and evolve methods that are suitable for the commu-nity in which they work. Moreover, consultations between family physicians are becoming more and more common. These usually take the form of a referral to a family physician with specific expertise in family dynamics or to a family physician in another city or town.

SUMMARY

Consultation is widely used in organizing primary care, although its frequency varies with factors such as locality, physician's interests, and patient expectations. The indications for consultation are numerous and are a function of the qualifications and skills of the referring physician. The choice of specific consulting physicians depends on disease factors, previous experience, and the level of patient rapport.

Methods of consultation range from formal interviews to hallway coffee meetings, and each of these is a learning experience. Consultations are a two-way exchange of information and should include the problems of both the patient and the family. Anything the family physician or consultant can do to facilitate this exchange will improve the consultative process and the care given to the patient.

REFERENCES

1 D. C. Morrell, H. G. Gage, and N. A. Robinson, "Referral to Hospital by General Practitioners," *Journal of the Royal College of General Practitioners,* **21:**77, 1971,

2 D. M. Metcalfe and D. Sischy, "Patterns of Referral from Family Practice," *Journal of Family Practice,* **1**(2):34–38, 1974.

3 J. Pemberton, "Illness in General Practice," *British Medical Journal,* **1:** 306–308, 1969.

4 R. Penchansky and D. Fox, "Frequency of Referral and Patient Characteristics in Group Practice," *Medical Care,* **8:**368–385, 1970.

5 C. Brock, "Consultation and Referral Patterns of Family Physicians," *Journal of Family Practice,* **4:**1129–1134, 1977.

6 R. M. Hines and D. J. Curry, "The Consultation Process and Physician Satisfaction: Review of Referral Patterns in Three Urban Family Practice Units," *Canadian Medical Association Journal,* **118:**1065–1073, May 6, 1978.

7 C. Elliot and D. Backstram, "Referral Patterns in General Practice: Report of a Pilot Survey," *Australian Family Physician,* **1:**155–156, April–May 1972.

8 J. P. Geyman, T. C. Brown, and K. Ribers, "Referrals in Family Practice: A Comparative Study by Geographic Region and Practice Setting," *Journal of Family Practice,* **3:**163–167, 1976.

9 J. W. Villaveces, W. W. Welcher, and G. R. Evans, "A Family Practice Survey in Ventura County," *California Medicine,* **117:**85–89, November 1972.

10 B. L. Barnett and J. J. Collins, "A New Look at the Consultation Continuum," *Journal of Family Practice,* **5:**665–666, April 1977.

Part Six

Research and Teaching Skills

Chapter 43

Patient Care Appraisal: Evaluating Performance

R. W. Putnam, M.D.

The belief that physicians should try to improve the care they give through an awareness of their successes and failures is not at all new. However, those physicians who have wished to assess their care in any continuous and organized fashion have been largely left to their own resources, since, until recent years, medical schools and organized medicine have not promoted any formal programs of self-assessment. This chapter will explain how to do patient care appraisal (PCA) in your own practice.

Patient care appraisal is a systematic method of self-assessment, developed in the past decade, which is potentially highly useful. First, it can give physicians a clear idea of how their care compares with standards set by themselves or their peers, an important matter for any conscientious physician. More important, perhaps, PCA enables physicians to define deficiencies in their care precisely enough to allow a "prescription" for improvement. Such changes could, for example, include a better selection of educational material (e.g., reading, audiovisual materials, formal courses). Time is always valuable to the family physician, and one important feature of PCA is that the time needed for participating physicians is very low—half an hour to an hour for each separate review.

Rx for change

Medical audits

It is important to differentiate PCA from other forms of medical review that may be less acceptable to the practicing profession. PCA is, in effect, a review designed to yield information for educational purposes as opposed to reviews designed for punitive, administrative, fiscal, or other purposes (e.g., reviews done by hospital administrations to improve bed use or by third-party paying organizations to examine billing practices).

Bi-cycle
concept

PCA was developed on the principles of the "bi-cycle" concept, described by Brown.[1] The bi-cycle links a patient care cycle with an educational cycle so that the continuing education of the physician is directly correlated with clinical practice. (A simplified diagram is shown in Figure 43-1.) This concept was applied in the northwestern United States and in the Washington-Alaska-Montana-Idaho (WAMI) program of the University of Washington, and it is important to note that some of its earliest successes were in community hospital settings.[2] A detailed description of the bi-cycle concept and its application to quality assurance systems is contained in "The Quality Assurance System" in *Medical Peer Review*, a reference text on peer review in medical practice.[3]

PCA is essentially a simple method by which a physician or group of physicians establishes explicit standards (criteria) of care for diseases (or conditions, symptoms, etc.) being treated in the office or hospital. The criteria used will vary with time and place, and physicians measure themselves only against standards that are appropriate for a particular setting at a given time.

Flexibility of
PCA

The basic steps in PCA are outlined in Table 43-1. It is important to stress at the outset that PCA is highly flexible and can be applied to all members of the health care team. Nurses, physiotherapists, nutritionists, and other health professionals can participate in setting standards using the same expertise they provide as members of the health team. Their standards can be considered separately or integrated into a comprehensive "package." It is also important to note that standards can be set for treating not only specific diseases but also symptoms (headache or low back pain), conditions, injuries, physiological states, problems, etc.

EIGHT STEPS IN PATIENT CARE APPRAISAL

This section discusses the steps in PCA outlined in Table 43-1. Table 43-2 provides a sample set of criteria.

1 The first step in the PCA process is to select the health problem or diagnostic area to be considered. Only conditions that occur fairly frequently and have a substantial impact on the health of patients should be chosen. At the beginning of your PCA program, select only conditions that are fairly well defined and for

Figure 43-1 The Bi-Cycle concept—relating continuing education directly to patient care. (*Adapted from Brown and Fleisher.*[1])

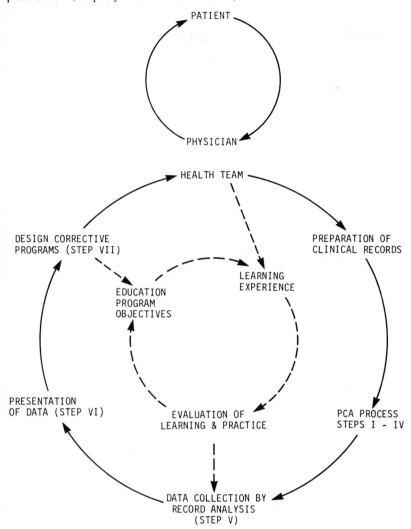

which there is a clearly established management regimen. Acute otitis media might be a good example for a family physician.

   2 Next, establish the specific criteria for optimal office management of the condition, beginning with points in the history or physical examination that you feel to be essential for validating the diagnosis. The criteria define the critical steps to be taken rather than indicate whether pathology was present (e.g., "inspection of tympanic membrane," not "normal t.m.," "inflamed t.m.," etc.). You should then list important steps in investigation, management,

Table 43-1   Steps in Patient Care Appraisal

1   Determine the health problem or diagnostic area of interest you wish to study.
2   Establish criteria for:
   a   Diagnosis.
   b   Investigation.
   c   Management.
   d   Follow-up.
3   Assure that criteria meet guidelines. They should:
   a   Reflect important aspects of patient care.
   b   Require *no* medical judgment by health record personnel (e.g., health record administrator).
   c   Be available in chart form.
4   Establish acceptable level of performance in relationship to criteria which reflect ideal level of care.
5   Have medical audit performed (preferably by health record personnel or similarly trained individuals).
6   Review data on actual performance using the criteria established for ideal performance (step 2).
7   Design corrective programs.
8   After appropriate interval, return to step 2 and begin again.

Clinical example

Practical criteria

and follow-up, taking care not to list every possible element of care but only elements essential to optimal care in a typical case.

3   The criteria must reflect only the most important aspects of patient care and, to be practical, those normally recorded in office records. If a physician records the elements of care necessary to make diagnostic or management decisions either at the present visit or in the future, this record should be "auditable." This means that evaluating the criteria should require no medical judgment on the part of the audit abstractor, and that they should be phrased in the clearest and most concrete terms. Table 43-2 contains a list of sample criteria generated by family physicians for treating acute suppurative otitis media. It is obvious that this is not a "cookbook" list or a protocol for care, but rather a list of measures that the physicians felt were absolutely necessary in the majority of cases.

4   An acceptable level of performance must be established based on the criteria that reflect the ideal level of care. In most cases, when criteria have been determined as suggested above, 100 percent performance level is required. However, there is an occasional exception for which a lower percentage may be acceptable. For example, in the treatment of otitis media, a physician may think it is appropriate to inspect the tympanic membrane in 100 percent of cases but realize that in practice this can be achieved in only 80 percent due to the presence of cerumen.

The physician may wish at this point to recheck his or her criteria against other standards, such as those set by peers or by other teams working in the area of quality of care investigations. This step is by no means necessary, however, since it has found that community physicians participating in PCA have set particularly stringent criteria and very little is to be gained by such validation except reassurance.

Mechanics of PCA audit

5   The next step is the audit itself, which, when possible, should be performed by trained health record abstractors. Health record abstractors perform this function in the hospital; in the office, a nurse or other health professional could be trained in this important task. A number of charts (the exact number is not important—15 to 30 should be adequate in the majority of instances) containing episodes of care of the selected condition are reviewed, and the physician's performance is compared with the criteria he or she has set.

Feedback

6   Next comes a review of the actual performance compared with the ideal standards and a definition of discrepancies. The discrepancies can be examined with a view to changing behavior for the better—an updating of factual knowledge may be necessary, a new skill may be required, or an old one may need improvement. In many cases, performance is less than ideal because of the lack of, or malfunction of, a necessary piece of equipment (e.g., an otoscope for examination of the tympanic membrane).

7   One may decide to deal with a deficit of knowledge or skills, to plan administrative changes, to buy new equipment, etc. In the example given in Table 43-2, use of inappropriate drugs might be corrected by a reading program for the physician. Poor patient

Table 43-2   Sample Criteria for Acute Suppurative Otitis Media

	Ideal, %	Acceptable, %	Actual, %
Diagnosis			
History			
1 Symptoms of ear discomfort	100	100	46
2 Prior URI	100	100	22
3 Past history of otitis media	100	100	38
4 Fever, chills, or sweats	100	100	13
Examination			
5 Inspection of tympanic membrane	100	80	66
Investigation			
6 Any lab tests (other than ear swab if tympanic membrane is perforated)	0	0	0
Treatment			
7 Was an antibiotic prescribed?	100	100	90
8 Was it an appropriate drug?	100	100	95
9 Was the appropriate duration (5 to 7 days) used?	100	100	*
10 Was a follow-up in 7 to 14 days ordered?	100	100	30
Follow-up			
11 Note stating otitis media cleared or referral to otolaryngologist	100	100	24

*Not recorded.

compliance with respect to return for follow-up might be improved by more patient education to be given by the practice nurse.

Effect of results

8 The appraisal process is not complete without a measurement of its effect on health care. After an appropriate interval has passed (to examine additional episodes of care similar to the ones used in the first study), the original criteria should be reviewed for their continuing relevance and another review done by the health record abstractors. Only when this step has been performed has the cycle been completed and high-quality care been assured.

It is obvious that the educational value of the appraisal process begins with the first step—the selection of the condition to be considered. If a physician looks closely at a list of the problems or diagnoses being managed, he or she will inevitably learn something about the care being provided to patients. Moreover, giving critical thought to the process of diagnosing and managing a specific condition may motivate the physician to return to tests or journals for further information about the condition.

Continuing medical education

Clearly documenting a physician's shortcomings can provide a motivation for change. Furthermore, if a physician is aware of deficiencies, he or she will be better equipped to choose the continuing medical education programs that will be of greatest value (see the next chapter, "Continuing Medical Education").

Relicensing

Looking to the future, it is conceivable that participation in evaluations of patient care (of which PCA is one example) might form the basis for recertification or relicensing, replacing the mandatory tabulation of study credit hours that became popular in the early 1970s. Quality assurance, achieved through patient care appraisal, is a more meaningful indicator of a physician's efforts to improve the care given to patients.

REFERENCES

1 C. R. Brown, Jr., and D. S. Fleisher, "The Bi-Cycle Concept—Relating Continuing Education Directly to Patient Care," in N. S. Stearns, M. E. Getchell, and R. A. Gold, *Continuing Medical Education in Community Hospitals: A Manual for Program Development*, Massachusetts Medical Society, Boston, 1971, pp. 88–97.
2 M. R. Schwartz, "WAMI, A Concept of Regionalized Medical Education," *Journal of Medical Education*, **48:**116, 1973.
3 C. R. Brown, Jr. and R. McConkey, "The Quality Assurance System," in *Medical Peer Review: Theory and Practice*, P. Y. Ertel and M. C. Aldridge (eds.), C. V. Mosby, St. Louis, 1977.

Chapter 44

Continuing Medical Education

M. Nixon, M.D.

The increase of information about health care delivery is so rapid that there is real danger of the recent graduate's knowledge quickly becoming obsolete. Moreover, new knowledge is retained in memory for relatively short periods of time. Consequently, continuing medical education is essential for the family practitioner if he or she is to maintain skills and keep up with new developments. This chapter outlines various methods of continuing education that are available to meet differing needs.

WHAT IS CONTINUING MEDICAL EDUCATION?

Continuing medical education (CME) is the education the physician acquires after entering practice. It is a lifelong process of acquiring knowledge, skills, and attitudes that can be applied in practice, and it is essential for maintaining competence. CME is self-education, not continuing instruction arranged or implemented by others.

Definition

Self-education

MOTIVATION FOR CONTINUING MEDICAL EDUCATION

One requirement for certification in family medicine by the College of Family Physicians of Canada reads, "The family physician

Table 44-1   Motivators for CME

Desire to be up to date (competence)

Individual patients' needs

Stimulation from students

Unusual medical problems

Requirement for membership in professional organizations

Desire to learn a new skill

Curiosity

Maintaining
professional
competence

shall understand and accept the responsibilities of a professional as he practices medicine."[1] In the United States, the Academy of Family Practice has similar requirements. Certainly, a part of the responsibilities of a professional is engaging in regular assessment of professional competence and needs and taking steps to increase effectiveness in weak areas.

Continuing medical education aims to improve the quality of patient care; consequently, it must be relevant. For the family physician, CME can be particularly useful in areas such as preventive medicine, counseling, and rehabilitation.

Desire to grow

Professional
society
requirements

Based on our own (unpublished) data we believe that the family physician's own standards and his or her desire to learn and grow are common motivators to continue medical education. Exposure to unusual medical problems is another stimulus. Involvement in learning that can be related directly to practice is a satisfying experience and one that promotes further involvement. Still another motivator comes from the requirements of certain professional family medicine societies, for example, the College of Family Physicians of Canada and the American Academy of Family Practice. The expectation is that exposure to the educational process will stimulate a further interest in learning. Table 44-1 lists a number of common motivators for CME.

WHAT TO LEARN AND HOW TO LEARN IT

Appropri-
ateness of CME

Clement Brown describes how the concept of CME conjures up the picture of a roomful of preoccupied but hopeful physicians anticipating a learned presentation by the medical school faculty. He depicts the members of the audience as being caught between the demands of their practices and the hope that the program will somehow be useful in the care of patients. Brown points out that such an approach is limited and may only incidentally or accidentally meet the needs of the learner.[2]

With constant and conflicting demands on their time, physicians should be able to choose the educational method most compatible with their own learning styles and practice needs, for the most effective and efficient learning. Properly designed, continuing medical education becomes an ongoing, individually focused process rather than a "potluck" selection of refresher courses.[3]

Making Time

Finding time is the worst problem in CME.[2] The wise family physician will incorporate time for organized CME into his or her work schedule. If CME is left for "when there's time," it will be low on the list of priorities and the time may never become available. Moreover, by building CME into the regular work schedule, a physician avoids losing personal and family time. Devoting relaxation time to CME may lead to resentment on the physician's part, and the effectiveness of learning will be impaired.

Organize yourself for CME

A significant part of a family physician's CME is informal and unstructured; it occurs during the day's practice from association with patients, other physicians, and health professionals and does not require extra time.

Unstructured learning

How to Learn

As George Miller stated, "The first step in learning is to identify educational needs and select learning experiences most likely to help meet these needs."[4] (See Tables 44-2 and 44-3.)

What to Learn

How do we determine what we need to know? One way is to keep our ears open. If a patient finds his or her medical care unsatisfac-

Patients' criticism

Table 44-2   Learning Experiences from Which to Choose

Reading

Small group discussions

Workshops

Lectures

Videotapes and movies

Consulting

Audiotapes

Journal clubs

Individualized programs

Intensive short courses

Table 44-3   Identifying Learning Needs

1 Feedback from patients
2 Inability to solve patient problems
3 Practice audit
4 Peer review
5 Consultants
6 Reading

tory, the physician will probably hear of it. Patient dissatisfaction offers a simple way of identifying possible areas of deficiency.

Peer review

Another way is through peer review. Opportunities exist, particularly in association with hospital privileges, for the family physician to participate in audits of medical performance. These often take the form of record reviews, which are discussed in Chap. 43. Patient care appraisal allows the physician to identify clinical areas and conditions in which the care he or she is giving is less than ideal. Such appraisals should lead us to take courses not only in what we like but also in what we need.

Self-assessment

Self-assessment is yet another way to determine what we need to know. Self-assessment programs are available to the family physician, particularly through professional societies. To use such a program effectively, you need specific data on the medical problems in your practice so that you know exactly what to assess. Practice profiles based on the data you supply can be obtained through third-party insurance agencies and can provide a statistical breakdown of the makeup of your practice. It may surprise you to see the frequency with which you deal with certain patient care problems, and this should influence the direction of your continuing medical education.

Practice profile

Lectures and seminars

Although the lecture is generally accepted as the most widely used instructional method in CME, many family physicians find listening to lectures too passive a learning method and search for small group seminars, which offer more active involvement.

Reading

A survey of all physicians licensed to practice in Canada's Maritime Provinces demonstrated an overwhelming preference for independent learning methods, particularly reading.[3]

LEARNING IN YOUR COMMUNITY

Building and Updating a Library

Individual's library

Both in training and in practice physicians are exposed to an enormous number of texts. These libraries should, however, be revised and expanded yearly after entering practice.

Family physicians practicing in clinic settings are often fortunate enough to have a library in their building, and even the smallest community hospital can develop a library of texts and journals suitable for its staff. Professional assistance, especially through national family medicine organizations, is available to family physicians, individually or in groups, who wish to develop libraries of core material. Many medical school libraries provide a regional loan service by mail.

Regional library services

The Role of Medical Journals

Journals provide the most up-to-date information, something even the newest text is often unable to do. But which journals are of most help to a busy physician? It is important to decide what we expect from a journal—updating, practicality, stimulating controversy, or relaxation—and be aware of the content and style of major journals in order to determine which can best meet our needs. As time goes on, needs and tastes change, and it is necessary to reevaluate journal subscriptions, keeping in mind the availability of journals from local clinics or hospitals. It is usually impossible to keep back copies of journals, but many physicians find it useful to remove and retain special articles, which can be kept in an indexed office file for handy reference during daily practice.

Which articles in what journals

Some physicians may benefit from a journal club. Getting together on a regular basis (weekly, every 2 weeks, or even every month) with a group of colleagues specifically to discuss recent journal articles of common interest in a relaxed setting—whether clinic or hospital, library or lounge, or private home—is a stimulating continuing education experience.

Journal clubs

Tapes and Television

Audiotapes are often used by family physicians to keep up to date; these can be obtained through various medical organizations. Television offers the opportunity for the most outstanding lectures to reach a national audience and for the physician to view a videotape at home or attend in his hometown a course that originates many miles away.

Audiotapes

Videotapes

Videodiscs and microprocessors now promote active learning by requiring the physician to solve problems and answer questions.[5] Within a few years physicians will be using terminals attached to their home television sets to research clinical problems.[3]

Computer-based learning

INFORMAL LEARNING

Informal learning goes on constantly. Few days pass without a discussion of a problem with a colleague in a hospital coffee room or

Discussions with colleagues

corridor. The colleague may have been faced with a similar problem recently, researched it, and found an article that helped. Sharing professional concerns and frustrations is not only a healthy aspect of medical practice but also an excellent learning opportunity.

The official consultation is also a learning experience for the family physician. Preparing a patient for a consultation and subsequent discussion with the consultant are active forms of CME.

Hospital rounds and conferences

Most family physicians participate in organized rounds, seminars, workshops, or clinical days in their hospital, often with a local or visiting expert as a resource person. Many feel they learn more effectively in their regular working environment than away from home as long as practice responsibilities do not interfere. Educational programs that are designed to meet the specific needs of the physician in the office or hospital, and include informed outsiders who understand the local family physicians' problems, can be very productive.

Learning Away from Home

Reasons for CME away from home

On occasion, despite the best intentions, learning in one's community is disrupted by the business of managing a practice. When a physician can obtain coverage for the practice and participate in CME away from home, he or she can give undivided attention to the course. Other reasons for participating at least once a year in a CME program away from home are (*a*) the availability of specific resources not found locally, (*b*) the stimulation of a different atmosphere, and (*c*) the opportunity to meet new people and discuss common interests.

Vacation/CME combinations

Although it is necessary to separate vacation time and CME time, under some circumstances a resort atmosphere may be conducive to learning provided the times for learning and for relaxation are carefully defined. A short course on sports injuries at a ski resort that schedules instruction from 7 to 10 a.m. and 5 to 8 p.m. and skiing from 10 to 4 p.m could be very effective—and might even provide some practical experience!

MANEUVERING THROUGH THE MAZE OF COURSES

Variety of offerings

The number and variety of CME courses is immense; the choice appears unlimited. Only the individual physician can decide which courses are valuable to him or to her. The department of continuing education in your regional medical school can provide information on locally available courses as well as those offered at other institutions.

Evaluating the Course Offerings

Read the descriptions of course programs carefully. Are the goals outlined so that you know what the course is designed to accomplish? Do these goals fit in with yours? Is the intended audience (e.g., family physicians) for the course specifically identified? Is it a refresher course with many topics presented, but possibly just touched upon, or is the course content limited to allow a more intense coverage of a single topic? What is the format of the course? Any mention of audiovisual aids? Are opportunities for audience participation built into the course? If not, how do you get your questions answered? Are there small group discussions? If skills are involved, will you have a chance to practice them? Is the course approved for study credits by specific professional societies? How will you be able to assess what you have learned? What expenses can you deduct from your income tax?

Selecting the right course

You should also investigate individualized learning opportunities in which participants identify a specific need and subsequently work with a tutor to develop the required knowledge and skills. Some centers offer this type of carefully planned one-to-one CME experience in the form of a clinical traineeship.

Clinical traineeships

LEARNING THROUGH TEACHING

In addition to the above, if a family physician wants to be an effective learner, he or she could consider teaching medical or health science students. The stimulation of being challenged by an inquiring student is constantly cited as one of the main rewards of teaching and may be a strong motivation for further continuing medical education.

Consider teaching

REFERENCES

1 The College of Family Physicians of Canada, Educational Objectives for Certification in Family Medicine.
2 C. F. Brown and H. S. M. Uhl, "Mandatory Continuing Education," *California Medicine*, **112**(5):69, 1970.
3 L. Curry and R. W. Putnam, "Continuing Medical Education in Maritime Canada, the Methods Physicians Use, Would Prefer and Find Most Effective," *Canadian Medical Association Journal*, 563–566, March 1, 1981.
4 G. E. Miller, "Continuing Education for What?" *Journal of Medical Education*, **42**:322–323, 1967.
5 P. R. Manning, "Continuing Medical Education—The Next Step," *Journal of the American Medical Association*, **249**:1042–1045, 1983.

Chapter 45

Teaching

B. K. Hennen, M.D.

Teaching is learning. Most family physicians who teach in their practices do so primarily because the presence of medical students is stimulating and rewarding. The stimulation comes from the challenge of having to recall and demonstrate to the student a rationale for the practice of medicine as well as a practical approach. The reward comes from acquiring the latest knowledge from the student and from the satisfaction of helping the student learn about family medicine through direct experience. To be asked to teach is a compliment. To agree to provide good learning opportunities for a medical student is an important responsibility.

PLANNING AHEAD

Define
expectations

In preparing to teach in one's practice, it is necessary to plan appropriately. First, establish or review the contract you have made with the medical school and find out what is expected of you by the education program coordinator. Insist on clear statements about objectives, expected teaching methods, evaluation, amount of time required, physical requirements in the office, accommodation and travel arrangements for the students, number of students to expect, and the need to change patient appointment schedules in the office. Find out also what you can expect from the

Table 45-1   Teacher's Expectations of Program

1   Clear statement of learning objectives for the student
2   Advance information regarding student
   a   Academic performance
   b   Class curriculum
3   Schedules and amount of notice expected
4   Workshops to improve teaching skills
5   Visits to practice by representative from program
6   Available resources
   a   Books, handouts
   b   Slide-tape shows
7   Financial arrangements

Table 45-2   Advance Planning Checklist

Review the contract with the medical school.

Prepare nurse, colleagues, and office staff so as to create an appropriate learning environment.

Alert hospital personnel, nursing homes, etc., of student's arrival and your expectations.

Prepare patients by means of a patient brochure and a sign in the waiting room and by talking to patients who will be visiting during the student's tenure.

Determine the consultants' willingness to take part.

Set aside space for the student.

Have objectives and evaluation forms available.

program in terms of resources, teaching materials, and written information about the students' previous curriculum. Ask how much notice you can expect about changes in schedules, whether teaching workshops are provided, whether there will be faculty visits to your practice, whether travel allowances will be provided, and about the extent of remuneration. Teachers' expectations are summarized in Table 45-1.

The introduction of the student to your practice and of the practice to your student should be carefully planned (see Table 45-2). A mention of your teaching activities in your patient brochure may be helpful, and a sign in the waiting room can introduce your patients to the idea of having a student at the practice.

Review with the office staff members their role in teaching the student and in introducing the student to patients. A negative comment by a receptionist ("You'll have to see a student today") can virtually destroy a learning opportunity, while a positive statement ("The student we have today comes from your old hometown, and

Inform patients

Office staff attitudes

I think you will like her") can help the student get off to a good start. Alerting the hospital administrator, the hospital nursing staff, and medical colleagues (especially the consultants likely to be involved with your patients) helps make the student aware that he or she is expected.

Other arrangements

Do accommodations have to be arranged for the student? In some cases the preceptor's office staff makes these arrangements, while in others the students make their own. We have our students phone the preceptors the week before they are due to arrive. This serves as an introduction and as a final reminder to the preceptor that it is time to get ready for the student.

WHEN THE STUDENT ARRIVES

Introduction

In the first day or two after the arrival, plan to spend a few quiet moments with the student to learn something about what he or she expects to get out of the time with you. Tell the student how likely it is that those expectations will be met in your practice.

Expectations of student

Be sure to clarify the ground rules and tell the student what you expect. How does the student wish to be introduced? (It is best to be direct—"This is John Wilson. He is a senior medical student working with me this week.") Have you decided how much autonomy the student should have? What do you expect of the student in reporting to you? How much time is it reasonable for the student to spend with a patient? Do you expect the student to be on call at night, to meet you at the hospital in the morning, to accompany you on house calls? What does the student expect? A sample of a typical student schedule can be found in Table 45-3.

LEARNING OPPORTUNITIES IN FAMILY PRACTICE

Clarify objectives

The principal learning opportunities for medical students in family practice settings are identified in Table 45-4. Each objective should be considered according to your ability to provide opportunities for the student to achieve it, keeping in mind the student's expectations and the overall program goals.

THE LEARNING-TEACHING PROCESS: A THREE-STEP APPROACH

Simply stated, the three steps in the learning program correspond to the answers to three questions which can be directed toward the student and indirectly apply also to the teacher. These questions are: Where are you headed? How are you going to get there? How will you know when you have arrived?

Table 45-3 Sample of a Typical Week's Schedule for a Student in a Family Physician's Office

Sunday	Monday	Tuesday	Wednesday	Thursday	Friday	Saturday
			Morning			
Meet for a half hour to discuss personal expectations	Hospital rounds	Early arrival to practice endotracheal intubation	Credentials Committee hospital	Hospital rounds	Minor procedures in OPD	Hospital rounds
Give schedule	Coffee—meet administrative superintendent		Hospital rounds	OR assist for gallbladder	Hospital rounds	Patients in office
	Introduction to office staff, office patients	OR assist for mastectomy, hernia	Visit nursing home	Marital counseling session	Review of financial management	Sign out to on-call associate
		Hospital rounds	Patients in office		Feedback session	
		Student to go over appointment system with receptionist				
			Lunch hour			
	Rotary lunch	Student on own for lunch	Student on own for lunch	Lunch meeting with office staff	Student on own for lunch	
			Afternoon			
	Patients	Patients	Student has afternoon off	Patients	Patients	
			Evening			
	Off call	Evening office hours	School board meeting			
	Student on own	After 9:30 p.m.—on call				

Table 45-4   Possible Learning Opportunities in Family Practice

Patient contact activities
  In office
  In hospital
  In nursing home
  House calls
  Special procedures, for example, minor surgery, confinements, assisting with major surgery

Office management activities
  Interpersonal relationships
  Appointment system
  Roles of receptionist, family practice nurse
  Answering service
  Bookkeeping, billing, and supplies
  Financial management

Professional responsibilities
  Medical staff rounds
  Hospital committee responsibilities
  Service club attendance

Personal
  Family life
  Outside interests
  Financial status

Where Are You Headed?

Office teaching routine

This first question should be answered in the context of stated objectives. The general objectives provided by the program should identify what the student can expect to learn from the experience. However, it is necessary to set up more specific objectives based on the situation at hand. In the case of a particular patient with a particular problem, it is important that both student and teacher not try to accomplish all the objectives at once. The student and teacher should jointly decide to focus on a defined problem or area of interest. The patient facing the student may be very cooperative, may have a highly interesting disease or a fascinating family history, or may be following a complex management regime. No matter how interesting the patient's case, it is nevertheless necessary to focus on a single realistic objective. You may decide to focus on the opening and closing gambits of the interview with the patient. This does not mean that the student will not learn anything else during the interview or that you may not address yourself to other things that come up.

How Are You Going to Get There?

This second question relates to the learning-teaching process. It concerns the activities that will make it possible for the objective to be achieved. Table 4 outlines four general areas of learning, all of which can be approached in many ways. We will focus only on models which might be used in dealing with patient contact activities.

Continuing with the previous example, how to open and close an interview with a patient, how can we teach the student what we want to communicate?

The procedure may simply involve observation of the teacher   **Observing**
by the student. This approach is useful for certain kinds of teaching and in our example may provide a model, with the teacher demonstrating how to handle the opening and closing gambits. By and large, however, passive learning is less desirable than learning that actively involves the student.

In an active approach, the student may do part of the interview   **Direct**
under the direct supervision of the teacher; that is, the teacher ob-   **supervision**
serves directly what happens either by being in the room throughout the interview or, given our sample objective, by being present only at the beginning and end of the interview in order to observe the opening and closing gambits.

If finances allow, a one-way mirror can be built into any teaching practice with a microphone and amplifier for less than $500. This allows direct observation without the interference of the supervisor in the room. A video camera and recorder provide an even more sophisticated, more expensive method of direct observation. It has the distinct advantage of playback.[1] These methods require the patient's informed consent and generally are well accepted.

A third model is one in which the student talks directly to the   **Indirect**
patient with indirect supervision by the teacher. Indirect supervi-   **supervision**
sion may involve discussing the interview and the patient's problems after the interview has taken place; after their discussion the teacher and the student together may discuss management with the patient. Or the student may come out from seeing the patient, discuss the problem with the supervisor, and then go back in alone to give the patient an explanation of the management. At some point in the process, the teacher-supervisor makes a personal contact with the patient to indicate that he or she knows what is going on and has assessed the student's ability to handle the situation. In this way, one ensures that the patient's needs are satisfied.

Another method of indirect supervision, while not usually ac-   **Record review**
ceptable for medical students, may be used with qualified resident   **with resident**
physicians. This is the record review, in which the patient's problem   **learners**
and its management are checked at the end of the day through a chart review by both the learning physician and the supervising physician.

In our own practice, we have found it most useful to allow stu-

Dialogue with
the student

dents to describe and comment on what they felt was happening during an interview, what their findings were, and what management they suggested. We then take the diaglogue from there, challenging points put forth by the student and raising questions and alternatives. Here, one important point should be emphasized. Even if what the student reported sounds feasible, what he or she found on examination sounds reasonable, and the management proposed is satisfactory, it is not enough to say, "Well, that sounds good to me. Why don't you go and see the next patient?" It is important to check by means of a few careful questions that what the student perceived actually did happen, that the rationale for the proposed management plan was valid and was based on an understanding of the patient and the illness. The student may have the right answer, but may not have arrived at it through the correct or the most efficient route.

In a short chapter such as this, we cannot elaborate further on the actual process that takes place between the teacher and student, but we refer you to books that have been written on this topic.[2,3]

How Will You Know When You Have Arrived?

Evaluation with
constructive
feedback

This third question is one of evaluation. Constructive criticism is the basis for successful evaluation. The teacher who fails to criticize at all is performing as poorly as the one who destroys his student's self-confidence. The solution to both problems is to refer to the behavior that was observed and not to the person who performed the behavior. The feedback should be both specific and detailed. "That was a terrible review" is a destructive comment. It implies total failure and suggests no hope for remedy. We have found that letting the student assess his or her own behavior first almost invariably leads to a focus on the main points that need to be addressed. "How did you feel about that interview?" may lead to the student's making the general comment, "I thought it was terrible." That can be followed by a facilitating question such as "When did you feel for the first time that the interview was not going well?" that in turn leads to a specific learning point. One can nearly always find some positive things to say, and although there is always a tendency to bring them out first in order to soften the criticism, it is sometimes more useful to save them until the end of the discussion. They can then be used as a building block for remedying some of the negative behaviors.

Formal
evaluations

Most programs have formal evaluations, and these are usually done through written assessment forms. We think that there should be two-way assessments, with forms to be completed by both learner and teacher. These should be filled out with both student and teacher present, and both should ultimately sign them. A two-way evaluation in a milieu in which feedback is expected is usually less threatening and results in more constructive comments.

Evaluation can come from sources other than the student and the teacher. Patients often make very useful comments about students. If the patient agrees, these should be shared with the student. A family practice nurse is often in a position to observe a student for long periods of time, as are other members of the office staff. Consultant colleagues who have been involved in the teaching of the student can also be asked for their comments.

Patient and office staff comments

Finally, the people who plan the program appreciate feedback. As a member teacher in a department of family medicine, you have a responsibility to keep the program planners informed about the adequacy of the arrangements, the preparation that has been possible, the student's knowledge of the general curriculum, and the degree to which you as a practicing physician in the community think the medical school is fulfilling its mandate in preparing its graduates.

REMUNERATION FOR TEACHING

It is our belief that no teacher who is in practice should lose income because a student has been assigned to the practice.[4] If the teacher is expected to reduce patient volume, put in extra hours, travel long distances, or give up practice time for workshops, the medical school should offer some financial recompense. Many medical societies now give study credits for teaching activities. But the ultimate satisfaction for the physician comes from the stimulation of having young tyros asking questions and raising new concepts, and from having contributed to the education of a future physician.

REFERENCES

1 B. S. Cole "Teaching Medical Interviewing in Vocational Training," *Journal of the Royal College of General Practitioners,* **32:**665–672, 1982.
2 W. E. Fabb, M. W. Heffernan, W. A. Phillips, and P. Stone, *Focus on Learning,* Royal Australian College of General Practitioners, Melbourne, 1976.
3 P. S. Byrne and P. E. L. Long, *Learning to Care,* Churchill-Livingstone, Edinburgh and London, 1973.
4 G. L. Pawlson, R. Watkins, and M. Donaldson, "The Cost of Medical Student Instruction in the Practice Setting," *Journal of Family Practice,* **10**(5):847–852, 1980.

Chapter 46

Research

D. B. Shires, M.D.

Before the advent of specialization and the orientation of medicine toward technology, the family doctor contributed greatly to the description of the natural history of disease and to the unveiling of what were then medical mysteries. This process is now commonly described as "research." In the last 50 years, however, the family doctor has taken a back seat. It is only recently that the opportunity for research in primary care is once again presenting itself and the potential is being generated for young family practitioners to organize their practice so as to conduct research that can be useful to the doctor, the patient, and the scientific community. This chapter will explore methods of organization and the development of a research concept, following its progression through the collection and analysis of data to the final publication of the research study.

History

"The seeds of great discoveries are constantly floating around us, but they only take root in minds well prepared to receive them." So said Joseph Henry, a nineteenth-century American physicist. In no field of endeavor is this more true than in family practice. The roots of family practice research are strong, going back to the contributions of Edward Jenner, who discovered the smallpox vaccination, Wilfred Pickles, who described the natural history of disease in his book *Epidemiology in Country Practice*,[1] and James

MacKenzie, who is regarded as the father of cardiology in the United Kingdom. These men were all country doctors with a strong, natural curiosity who pursued ideas and made their discoveries available to their scientific colleagues.

Many family doctors are intimidated by the word "research" possibly because of a misconception, acquired in medical school, that research requires huge funding, elaborate facilities, and familiarity with areas not generally within the scope of an average family practitioner. In reality, the family physician has much to offer in terms of research—for example, an available patient base and a knowledge of early and undifferentiated illness and of the social and behavioral aspects of clinical medicine. In addition, many opportunities exist for collaborative studies with research-based institutes and specialty groups. The research community appears to be renewing its interest in primary care, and Kerr White[2] has recently forecast a renaissance in clinical research based on the "new epidemiology, involving ambulatory patients at the earliest stages . . . in the natural history of illness."[3]

Research potential

OFFICE ORGANIZATION FOR RESEARCH ACTIVITY

In order to carry out a research project successfully in family practice, certain organizational steps must be taken. They include the development of an age and sex register and possibly even a disease register. If an *E-Book* is used in the practice, this can provide a defined practice base, sometimes called the *practice denominator.*[4] However, with the advent of *computer-based accounting systems* that record the diagnosis and the reason for each visit, a far more powerful tool has now become available. In practices that have their own microcomputer system, the opportunity to pursue research activities is greatly enhanced. The *written medical record,* which contains essential information for providing exemplary clinical care, can be another important source of clinical research data. *Risk registers* are useful in any practice for patient recall, and can serve as another source of data. The register might include data on patients who need to have Pap smears done at appropriate intervals, those who need immunizations, those who are on certain medications, those with diseases requiring periodic recall, and people who are at high risk for certain diseases such as cardiovascular disease.

How to get going

Use of computer

Registries

TYPES OF RESEARCH STUDY

Most research studies in family medicine are applied epidemiology, and novice researchers should acquaint themselves with basic epi-

Figure 46-1

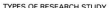

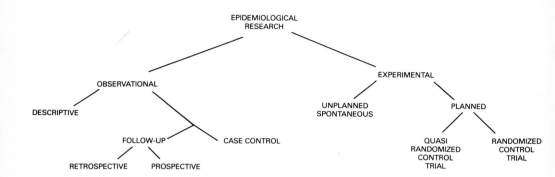

demiological texts to gain an understanding of the principles involved in this type of research. In summary, epidemiological studies can be subdivided as illustrated in Figure 46-1.

A brief description of the types of epidemiological study will assist the potential researcher in focussing on his or her scientific interests and the resources available in the practice setting.

Descriptive   This type of study is a description of the circumstances pertinent to a rare or highly unusual event (e.g., the first description of the unusual circumstances of an illness involving American Legionnaires attending a Philadelphia convention).

Follow-Up Study   This is a study in which a group of patients are subject to a specific intervention (test/therapy) and are followed up for a period of time to measure the occurrence of a defined outcome (e.g., patients given ASA followed up for possible future occurrence of Reye's syndrome). A follow-up study may also be retrospective where both the intervention and the outcome have already occurred (e.g., radiology treatment for benign thymoma of the neck given to children 30 years ago followed up for occurrence of thyroid cancer).

Case Control Study   In a case control study, the outcome event has already occurred and the cases are matched with controls except for the factor of investigation (e.g., patients with myocardial infarction [outcome event] matched with noncardiac patients for all variables except smoking to determine possible relationship of smoking to myocardial infarction).

Spontaneous Experiment An unplanned event is investigated for specific consequences (e.g., the Bhopal tragedy in India and the resulting effects on vision, in comparison with a nonexposed population).

Quasi-Randomized Control Trial (QRCT) This is a planned experiment involving a *test* and a *control* group where the randomization of the two groups has been suboptimal usually due to factors beyond the control of the researcher (e.g., randomization of centers in a multicenter trial rather than randomization of patients in each center).

Randomized Control Trial (RCT) This is a planned experiment involving a test and control group where there is true randomization of patients; i.e., each patient stands an equal chance of being included in either the test or the control group by use of a random number generator (e.g., in a double-blind controlled drug trial). The "blind" is usually implicit in an RCT, referring to the fact that the researcher does not know to which group a patient has been assigned (single-blind) and neither does the patient (double-blind).

Most powerful epidemiological evidence

It would be wise for novice researchers to gain more understanding of the advantages and disadvantages of each of the above techniques as it related to the family physician's research idea. Several excellent publications are available, including the monograph *Critical Skills of Medical Literature* published by McMaster University.[6]

It would be appropriate at this point to introduce another type of research being undertaken with increasing frequency by family doctors, namely, drug trials funded and administered by research divisions of drug companies.

Drug trials

These can be trials of efficacy and human safety or trials related to marketing of a new product. The family physician is usually approached by the company research division to be part of a multicenter trial and asked to contribute a certain number of patients from the practice to the pooled results from other like practices.

Contract research

Although these types of studies raise issues of social responsibility, ethics, and scientific credibility, they can be of research value to the family practitioner if they follow the following guidelines:

1 In most cases (if not all) the drug company offers to pay the direct costs, overhead, and due compensation for the family physician involved in the study. This may be in the form of a negotiated budget or a flat fee per evaluatable patient submitted to the study pool. Whatever the payment method, in no case should money be

Underestimated costs

the dictating reason for undertaking the study. As a further point of advice, whatever the predicted costs calculated prior to the start of the trial, the time involvement and costs are almost always at least a third higher than estimated.

Involvement
with protocol

2 The family physician should insist on being involved in an investigators' meeting called to review the protocol. The drug company must be flexible enough to alter the protocol according to reasonably expressed needs. Problems that frequently occur are overrestrictive entry and exclusion criteria, lack of adequate controls, wrong frequency of testing, and drug supply/administration. If reasonable alterations are not acceptable to the drug company, the family physician would be advised not to participate in that particular trial.

Ethics

3 An ethical review of the patient consent form and research protocol is mandatory. This should be done by the university, hospital, or medical society independent of the family physician investigator. Legal opinion should be sought as to protection of the family physician from liabilities should a harmful effect of the tested new drug arise.

Publication
rights

4 Publication rights of the family physician should be documented so that the physician has the right to publish what are considered valid results and to refuse publication of data for what are considered invalid conclusions.

5 Marketing studies are rarely of scientific interest to the practitioner unless he or she has special interest in investigating, in a scientifically credible manner, the efficacy of a newly packaged aerosol, transdermal, or implant technique. In this instance, it is the method, not the drug, that should be evaluated.

The above remarks should not be interpreted as being negative to requests from drug companies for participation in trials. There are many highly ethical drug companies that will gladly fulfill all the above criteria, and it is appropriate that family physicians involve themselves in ethical studies so that the true value of new therapies in family practice can be evaluated.

STEPS IN THE SUCCESSFUL COMPLETION OF AN ORIGINAL RESEARCH PROJECT

The first and most important step in establishing a research project is to develop a hypothesis, or concept. This concept may be investigated through one of four general types of study:

1 A clinical study, e.g., the management of hypertension with a new drug

2 An epidemiological study, e.g., the prevalence of influenza in a community

3 An organizational study, e.g., the development of a medical record system

4 An educational study, e.g., an analysis of residents' learning techniques

Once the family practitioner decides what type of study is most appropriate, it would be wise to seek expert advice on its planning and execution. Whatever advice is received, the procedure usually falls into the following stages:

Step 1 Define the idea. Establish the primary question you wish to answer. Think about it for a short period of time before writing an outline of what it is you wish to achieve.

Define the idea

Step 2 Read around the subject. Obtain relevant literature through local health library services or colleagues' reference files. Contact people with knowledge of the field. Follow through on other people's ideas that may provide insights for dealing with your own. Ask yourself whether what you are doing has been done before; review all the available literature you can find on the subject. This may be done by using your own journals, books, clippings, etc., a local medical library service, or bibliographies of family medicine from your college or academy of family medicine. You might also make a specific research request to a medical school library, or use a national computerized library service such as *Medlars* or *Index Medicus*. Further information on these services is available through your local health services librarian.

Read all you can

Library assistance

Step 3 Draw up an outline of how you wish to obtain an answer to your question. Do not forget the primary question you asked yourself in step 1—it is amazing how often it appears to be forgotten.

Primary question

Step 4 Whatever answers you expect to get, list the available mechanisms for collecting data and discuss these with your colleagues, asking for their support and possibly their assistance.

Obtain colleagues' support

Step 5 The next step is to refine your question. Break up the problem into realistic, workable units, trying not to answer too many questions in one project. By delineating the problem carefully and rigorously, you will make the primary question self-evident and the answer you are looking for will be honed down to something pure, simple, and clear. Be aware of the danger of answering other questions and neglecting the primary question.

Keep question simple

Step 6 It is essential to define all the terms and provide clear meanings and descriptions. If you cannot define a term, put the project aside until such time as you can.

Define terms

Step 7 Once you have phrased the question in realistic terms, it is not too early to think in terms of final publication. The publication should almost be written prior to the project, with the details filled in when the project is completed. Although this sounds strange, it is often done. It should be emphasized that early advice

Write up your project prospectively

Table 46-1   Suggestions for Completing a Successful Research Project

1   Follow through on your bright ideas.
2   Seek advice early in defining the question and all the variables.
3   Estimate your requirements carefully; avoid underestimation.
4   Consider advantages of a prospective vs. a retrospective study.
5   Define the denominator of the group to be studied.
6   Consider the value of a pilot study to eliminate operational problems.
7   Identify and eliminate all biases in the study.
8   Review all measurement techniques for accuracy.
9   Write up your results as soon as possible after the project data are collected
     and analyzed.

from an expert is essential. Too often epidemiologists complain that a researcher arrives at their office with a pile of data and the request to "feed this to your computer and see what you come up with."

Data collection

Step 8   Begin to collect your data, possibly at first as a pilot study, to work out the operational problems. In many cases, this is the most frustrating phase as it often has to be fitted into an already overloaded schedule.

Step 9   Write up your results as soon as possible. It is common to see piles of data on researchers' shelves waiting to be written up.

Publish

Step 10   Decide in what journal you would like to publish your paper, and write it according to the editorial instructions for that journal. Circulate copies of your paper for your colleagues' comments before you submit it for publication. Often this results in clarifying obscure concepts or bringing up points which you have overlooked.

In working through to completion of a research project, the points made in Table 46-1 need to be borne in mind.

Writing skills

Although physicians spend considerable time writing medical records, charts, letters, etc., they often lack the skill of scientific writing. This may prevent family physicians from undertaking a

Editorial assistance

research project. However, this skill can be acquired or improved in many ways. Courses in scientific writing are available and are sometimes connected with medical meetings of national associations. There are also publications available to assist the novice scientific writer.[5] Other opportunities for research writing present themselves in terms of grand rounds, community activities, hospital conferences, and continuing medical education activities. It is always wise to present your research findings to your colleagues prior to submission for publication, since their advice and receptivity often alter the way certain ideas are expressed. A number of journals publish their editorial requirements and offer assistance to authors. A letter to the editor of any family physician journal will usually be answered with helpful advice at least. Do not be put off by rejections. A rejection slip with the reviewer's comments is often very helpful in making the article more readable and bringing out the real value of your work. Use rejection slips with review comments as a tool to help improve your writing.

Research is an activity often neglected by the family physician but one in which a renaissance is taking place. Family physicians should make every effort to organize their practice so that research activities become a part of their routine.

REFERENCES

1 W. Pickles, *Epidemiology in Country Practice,* 2d ed., Devonshire Press, Devon, England, 1972.
2 K. White, "Primary Care Research and the New Epidemiology," *Journal of Family Practice,* **3:**579, 1976.
3 J. Geyman, *Research in Family Practice,* special edition of *Journal of Family Practice,* **7:**49–160, July 1978.
4 Journal of the Royal College of General Practitioners (1977). Age-sex registers. Editorial, **27;** 515–517.
5 *Research Manual for Family Physicians,* College of Family Physicians of Canada, Willowdale, Ontario, Canada.
6 McMaster University, *Critical Skills of Medical Literature,* 1985, available from Department of Family Medicine, McMaster University Medical Center, Main Street, Hamilton, Ontario, Canada.

Part Seven

Office Management

Chapter 47

Setting Up Practice: Staffing

G. C. du Bois

Industry has long recognized that success depends largely on the loyalty, skill, and effectiveness of company employees. The management of personnel is therefore a very important part of a successful business, and many years of training are needed to learn this skill. The physician, who has no such training or experience, is at a serious disadvantage in selecting, training, and motivating staff. If you are to acquire and keep the right staff, you must pay attention to providing the atmosphere and conditions that will give your employees continuing job satisfaction. This chapter offers guidelines for selecting the best personnel for your practice. The average physician has little difficulty attracting job applicants; the problem is to find the right type of person for the job.

Family physicians can neither train nor personally supervise all of the training and introduction of new staff (with the possible exception of the family practice nurse). Nevertheless, their receptionists and secretarial and accounting staff must be reliable, be able to work with little or no supervision, and be "self-starters." Some physicians seem to believe that the selection process simply involves finding a person who has the training to do the job and is willing to work for a given salary. Needless to say, there is much more than this to finding the right employee. The two main rules the physician should bear in mind when selecting staff are:

General
definition

1 Find the person who has the most suitable background as well as the proper mental, physical, and emotional qualities to give satisfactory performance.

2 Ensure that the employee has the necessary skills to perform the job properly.

WORKLOAD ANALYSIS

An analysis of the workload of your office is the first step in hiring staff. Before writing individual job descriptions, you should record all the tasks to be performed by all your personnel. You will then be able to divide up the workload and write up the job description and required skills for each job, according to the task analysis and delegation scheme shown in Figure 47-1.

JOB DESCRIPTIONS

List all duties

A job description is a list of the duties and responsibilities of each employee. To ensure that these are completely understood, the list should be as detailed as possible. In preparing such a list, state in an unambiguous way *all* the duties that you expect an employee to be able to perform.

When interviewing an applicant, use the job description to ensure that the individual's declared skills are adequate to meet the requirements. Suggested job descriptions for a receptionist-secretary, a receptionist–nurse's aide, and a family practice nurse are included in Table 47-1.

JOB SKILLS

Once you have written the job description, you should prepare a second list of job skills. This list should set out in detail the accomplishments needed to carry out the job described. The job description may state, "Maintain routine correspondence of Dr. Blough," whereas the job skills list may state that a minimum typing speed of 60 wpm is required. Table 47-2 indicates the skills required for the job description of receptionist-secretary.

Testing the Skills

Telephone
answering

Be sure to satisfy yourself (through a testing program if necessary) that applicants actually possess the skills they claim to have and can carry out the required work efficiently. Shorthand, typing, and dictaphone transcribing can be tested readily during the selection process. Other skills can be acquired by special training or experience. Be sure not to overlook or dismiss as unimportant a routine part

Figure 47-1 Task analysis and delegation of medical office tasks.

	RECPT	NURSE	DOCTOR
Answer the telephone			
Schedule patient appointments			
Maintain listing of telephone call-backs			
Determine the nature of patient incoming calls			
Check for messages with answering service			
Telephone pharmacists			
Return non-emergency patient calls for doctors			
Maintain chart filing system			
File all reports, X-ray, laboratory, etc.			
Receive patients			
Register patient's arrival			
Communicate with "no show" patients			
Schedule appointments with accountant			
Maintain doctor's personal appointment log			
Prepare a daily work schedule (patient appointments)			
Conduct daily work schedule staff meeting			
Maintain laundry supply records			
Maintain equipment maintenance schedule			
Maintain patient annual physical reminder file			
Maintain "periodic" task reminder file			
Open the office			
Open, sort and distribute mail			
Order needed janitor services			
Do office housekeeping chores			
Quiet noisy children			
Renew magazine subscriptions			
Check doctor's bag and refill			
Inventory and order medical supplies			
Review & authorize medical supplies purchase orders			
Inventory & order office supplies			
Review & authorize office supplies purchase orders			
Inventory and originate drug orders			
Review & authorize drug purchase orders			
Make arrangements for hospital admissions			
Pull medical records for all of today's appointments			
Complete Medicare claim, except for diagnosis & fee			
Prepare workmen's compensation form (patient information)			
Prepare attending physician's statement (patient information)			

	RECPT	NURSE	DOCTOR
File claim forms in suspense file until payment is received			
Follow up control procedure on old claims			
Telephone insurance company about unpaid claims			
Prepare letters to insurance company about unpaid claims			
Post payments from medicare, insurance company & patients to accounts receivable ledger			
Dispose of any difference between patient bill and reimbursement			
Endorse checks received			
Handle disposition of patient "rubber checks"			
Determine what correcting entries are needed in the patient ledger			
Prepare patient ledger adjustment forms			
Maintain petty cash fund			
Balance and replenish petty cash fund			
Check invoices from suppliers for discounts			
Prepare checks for doctor's signature			
Review and sign expense checks			
Record cash disbursement in daily journal			
Record all cash received in daily journal			
Prepare bank deposit slip			
Make bank deposit and obtain receipt			
Reconcile bank balance			
Run a trial balance of accounts			
Prepare payroll checks			
Sign payroll checks			
Record payroll disbursements in ledger			
Remit income tax, Unemployment Insurance, Canada Pension, etc.			
Issue T4 slips			
Maintain a list of office problems			
Schedule and assign unusual tasks			
Take corrective action on employee problems			
Conduct a salary review			
Compose correspondence (business and personal)			
Compose patient medical correspondence			
Edit draft of outgoing correspondence			
Type and prepare correspondence for mailing			
Determine fee reduction or adjustments			
Communicate fee adjustment to patients			
Conduct office staff training in new procedures			

Table 47-1 Job Descriptions

Receptionist-secretary

Screens phone calls

Prepares medical care insurance forms

Files patients' charts and reports

Maintains charts in filing system

Bills patient for uninsured services

Records professional income and expenses in account books

Pays expenses following physician's approval

Handles bank deposits and reconciliation of account

Orders stationery supplies

Opens and sorts mail

Delivers mail to post office

Types correspondence

Family practice nurse

Screens phone calls

Gives injections for immunization

Gives prenatal physical

Gives well-baby checks

Gives skin tests

Gives venopunctures

Takes history

Takes throat swabs

Changes dressings

Removes sutures

Does urinalysis and pregnancy test

Initiates proper blood work

Reviews test reports and refers to physician

Checks patients' charts

Additional tasks for either receptionist–nurse's aide or nurse

---

Urinalysis—dipstick only

Sterilizes instruments

Stocks examining room with instruments and supplies

Calls patients for further investigation following test results

Escorts patient to examining room and instructs on preparation for examination

Makes appointments and arranges for patients' tests

Records weight, height, and blood pressure of patients

Table 47-2   Job Skills—Receptionist-Secretary

Primary skills
1   Telephone manners: Can handle calls efficiently, avoids lengthy calls, and displays an interest over the phone instead of acting as an answering service.
2   Bookkeeping: If this is your first receptionist, have your accountant go over account book procedure. If a replacement, have departing employee go over procedure.
3   Good typing speed: Minimum 60 wpm.
4   Knowledge of dictation equipment. (Dictate on *your* time—shorthand dictation takes up prime office time.)
5   Knowledge of medical terminology.
6   Ability to file and retrieve records.

Secondary skills
1   Previous experience in physician's, dentist's, or hospital office.
2   Neat appearance.
3   Well spoken.
4   Expresses a genuine interest in people.
5   Bright and cheerful.
6   No commitments to preclude meeting job hours.
7   Willing to make a job commitment for at least 2 years.

of the job that seems to require no particular skill, for example, answering the office telephone. The idea that anyone can answer a telephone, receive messages, and record a physician's office appointments is simply not true. *How* your employee answers the phone is of great importance, since he or she is your first contact with the patient. The impression left by an abrupt, uninterested, or uncooperative receptionist can destroy the good public relations every physician strives to maintain. A poor impression may cause patients to question the efficacy of all the doctor's staff as well as the quality of medical care provided.

FINDING APPLICANTS

Suitable applicants can come from a number of sources:

> Advertising in local newspapers
> Business schools
> Commercial employment agencies
> Hospitals or other medical offices

Advertising in Local Newspapers

Advertising in newspapers is usually the most productive method, but it takes some skill to write an advertisement that will attract replies from the most suitable people. The advertisement should include a descriptive title, location of the job, and general duties. Do *not* provide your name or telephone number or you will be deluged with phone calls. Merely state that the employer is a physician and use a box number for replies.

The following example shows a sufficiently specific advertisement for a receptionist-secretary.

```
                    SECRETARY RECEPTIONIST

       Required for medical practice in west end of
       town.Should possess good working knowledge
       of typing, bookkeeping,accounts receivable
       and appointment systems, medical terminology.
       Previous experience in a medical office an
       asset.  Send application indicating
       experience, education, and salary require-
       ments to Box 310, Daily News and Herald.
```

Hopefully, if specific qualifications are listed, those who lack them will not bother to reply. Most likely, you will receive a large number of applications and can reject those who do not have the necessary skills and retain for possible interview those who have either some or all of the skills listed. During the initial review of applications you should use a checklist to score each applicant on a predetermined scale.

Business Schools

Need for experience

Business schools will provide a list of graduating students and are usually willing to advertise a job to their prospective graduates. When considering an applicant from this source, the physician should remember that skills acquired through attendance at a business school have not yet been applied and the applicant will have little, if any, related business experience. This type of applicant might be suitable for a clinic in which there is staff to provide training, but not for the solo physician who would not be able to afford the considerable time needed for supervising and for teaching basic skills.

Commercial Employment Agencies

Advantage

Disadvantage

The advantage of a commercial employment agency is that it usually has knowledge of the applicant's skills and abilities. As the prospective employer, you can be assured that the agency has done the preliminary screening and will only refer applicants who have the necessary education, experience, and background. An agency will usually bill the employer for a fee which is a percentage of the employee's annual salary. These fees range anywhere from 7 to 10 percent of the salary paid to the employee during the year. Since this is a substantial amount of money, hiring through an agency should be carefully weighed. However, an agency will usually provide a replacement for employees who prove unsatisfactory within an indicated probationary period.

Recruiting from Hospitals or Other Medical Offices

A physician may know of competent staff in local hospitals or other doctors' offices. Although a doctor may not actively hire away a member of a hospital staff or of a colleague's staff, he or she may indirectly create some interest in the vacancy. The physician may find it useful to use the grapevine to publicize the opening and trust that someone suitable will apply. The employee whom the physician has in mind may recommend the job opening to someone else who is as competent. Since the physician, the local hospital, and the other doctors are likely to work closely together, it is never a good idea to offer a position *directly* to employees of the hospital or the other doctors. Such an action would certainly cause resentment from the hospital administration or the physician involved.

Other doctors' offices

THE HIRING PROCESS

The staff selection process need not be difficult if it is approached with common sense. The objective is to select competent, well-trained, interested staff who will provide excellent support. This will allow the physician to concentrate on providing good medical care, secure in the knowledge that all other aspects of the practice are being handled well. The teamwork required to achieve these objectives depends, to a great extent, on a feeling of mutual respect between employer and staff.

Respect must be earned. The employer gains the staff's respect by providing them with the proper tools and a pleasant atmosphere in which to work, and by adopting good personnel and salary policies and intelligent supervisory attitudes. The staff, on the other hand, earn their employer's respect by displaying an interest in their jobs, showing good work habits, and being efficient and effective. Above all, staff must be aware of the employer's objectives and work toward realizing them.

Good office milieu

Both employer and staff must have an interest in the community and must develop and maintain a medical practice which satisfies patients, staff, and the physician.

Selecting from Applicants

Application
letters

Applicants should in all cases be asked to submit written applications. In their letters of application, suitable candidates will indicate their knowledge of the job requirements and state their qualifications. It is, however, unlikely that everything the employer wishes to know will be in the letter of application. It is therefore appropriate to send each applicant a formal application form for completion before arranging interviews (Figure 47-2). Applications from those who are unsuitable can be discarded at this point.

The formal application form should be detailed and should permit a comparative evaluation of candidates based on a common standard. A further weeding out is then possible so that a manageable number of applicants can be more thoroughly investigated.

References

Uses of
references

Obviously, candidates will list only friendly references, so that there is little likelihood of obtaining an unbiased opinion from them. The best sources of information are the candidate's immediate supervisors in previous jobs. Always telephone; verbal answers are likely to be more frank than written ones. It takes some skill to question previous supervisors. It is not sufficient merely to ask for an opinion of the capabilities of the applicant, since this will elicit rather general and incomplete answers. Instead, list the exact duties the employee will be expected to perform, as well as the specific skills needed, and ask whether the applicant fulfills these requirements. Remember to use a reference check form to record the results of the telephone conversation (Figure 47-3).

Consider as an example the following situation. Mary Smith has applied for a position as a receptionist-secretary. She has had several years experience as a receptionist at Central Hospital, where her immediate supervisor was Jane Simpson. If you telephone Ms. Simpson and simply ask what she can tell you about Mary Smith, the reply may be that Mary worked there for four years and that she was a good worker and got on well with other staff members. Is that what you want to know? Not entirely.

Be specific

You should ask Ms. Simpson more specific questions. First tell her that you are looking for someone who can work effectively *without supervision* and who must type medical reports, answer the telephone, make appointments, record income and expenses, bill for medicare, etc. Then ask Ms. Simpson how effective Mary Smith might be for this job.

Ms. Simpson can now give definite opinions. She tells you that Mary is a good typist, knows medical terminology, gets on well with others, and handles phone inquiries well. Mary has not been good at billing, and bookkeeping was not part of her job at the hospital.

Figure 47-2 Employment application form.

```
                        EMPLOYMENT APPLICATION
                    (Please write - do not print or type)

        DATE:_____      POSITION APPLIED FOR: _____

A. GENERAL HISTORY

   NAME: _____      MAIDEN NAME: _____

   ADDRESS: _____

            _____ How long at address _____

   PREVIOUS ADDRESS: _____

                     _____

   TELEPHONE #: _____     SOCIAL SECURITY #: _____


   ----------------------------------------------------------------------

B. EDUCATION

   School (list most recent first)    Dates attended    Courses or Special Training

   _____

   _____

   _____  _____

   _____  _____

   ----------------------------------------------------------------------

C. EMPLOYMENT HISTORY (list most recent employment first)

   Name & Address of Employer _____

                              _____

   Dates of Employment:_____ to _____   Position held: _____

   Supervisor: _____      Phone #: _____

   Starting Salary _____     Salary at end _____

   Reason for leaving _____
   ----------------------------------------------------------------------
   Name & Address of Employer _____

                              _____

   Dates of Employment: _____ to _____    Position held: _____

   Supervisor: _____      Phone #: _____

   Starting Salary _____     Salary at end _____

   Reason for leaving _____
   ----------------------------------------------------------------------
```

- 2 -

D. REFERENCES (do not list relatives)

Personal: Name _____ Phone #: _____

        Address _____

        Name _____ Phone #: _____

        Address _____

E. EXPERIENCE AND SKILLS

Please enter a check mark by any of the following activities in which you are
qualified by reason of previous experience or training:

Technical:

__ Dental Assistant	__ Lab Procedures, Dental	__ Dental Terminology
__ Dental Hygienist	__ Lab Procedures, Medical	__ Medical Transcription
__ Injections	__ Insurance Forms	__ Nursing, General
__ Instrument Sterilization	__ Medical Terminology	__ X-Ray Exposure
__ Other, specify _____		

Administrative:

__ Accounts Receivable	__ Collection Procedures	__ Stenography
Control	__ Filing	__ Switchboard
__ Billing	__ Reception	__ Typing
__ Bookkeeping	__ Posting	__ Appointment Scheduling
__ Other, specify _____		

Office Equipment:

__ Adding Machine	__ Dictation Equipment	__ Typewriter
__ Bookkeeping Machine	__ Duplicating Machine	— Word Processing
	__ Minicomputer	
__ Other, specify _____		

F. EMPLOYMENT CONDITIONS

Indicate Salary Expected: _____/yr   Date you could begin work:_____

Any limitations on Working Hours? Explain _____

How would you get to work? _____ How long would it take _____

G. GENERAL INFORMATION

	YES	NO
Would you prefer to work alone, rather than with others?	__	__
Do you enjoy meeting new people?	__	__
Do you dislike talking on the telephone?	__	__
Are you good at remembering names and faces?	__	__
Would you appreciate an opportunity to learn new skills and techniques?	__	__
Is it important to you to be punctual?	__	__
Are you active in community, church, political or similar activities?	__	__
Do you smoke?	__	__
Would a restriction on smoking make you uncomfortable?	__	__
Would you object to being bonded?	__	__
During the last three years, has illness prevented you from engaging in normal activities more than 5 days a year?	__	__

What did you like best about your last job? _____

What did you dislike most about your last job? _____

What are your favorite recreational activities? _____

What is your primary purpose in applying for this position? _____

Figure 47-3 Preemployment telephone reference check.

Applicant's Name	Date of Application	Position for which Applicant is applying

Name of firm where Applicant worked   Address   Phone

Former Supervisor   Title

When did Applicant work for you? What kind of attendance record did Applicant Have?

FROM: TO:

What was Applicant's job when (he)(she) started to work? When (he)(she) left?

Applicant states (his)(her) earnings were $ per   Was Applicant bonded?

YES   NO $_____

Did Applicant supervise others at any time? What kind of supervisor was (he)(she)?

How did Applicant get along with superior and associates?

 Was Applicant a competent and conscientious worker?

What was the biggest problem you had with the applicant, on the job?   personally?

Why did the employee leave your employ?

Would you rehire (him)(her)? YES   NO   If No, why not?

What else can you tell us about this applicant that will help us make a decision?

Comments

Reference Checked by   Date:

If you still have an interest in Mary Smith (and you might not if she is poor at billing), you should ask why she left the hospital. She may have had good personal reasons, or she may have been asked to leave.

Now that you know Mary's capabilities and her strengths and weaknesses, you may decide to hire her and overlook, or provide training to correct, her deficiencies. The decision will depend largely on the strengths of the other applicants.

PREINTERVIEW EVALUATION

Since your time is valuable, you cannot spend countless hours interviewing job candidates. Interview only those who have the necessary qualifications, understand the job requirements, and are interested and challenged by the position.

Before interviewing, review the letter and application form of each applicant. Have the applicants meet other members of the staff and discuss working conditions, inspect the working place, and examine the equipment. Candidates should have the opportunity to find out what kind of employer you are and decide whether they want to work for you.

Involving current staff members in the selection process helps

How to select
interviewees

Figure 47-4 Checklist for review of interview candidates.

```
                              POSTINTERVIEW
                               CHECKLIST

APPLICANT:                 Mary Smith

DATE AND TIME INTERVIEWED: June 15 - 2 p.m. to 2:45 p.m.

APPEARANCE:                Neat.  Brown-Eyed.  Short Brown Hair.

HOBBIES:                   Interests:  Music, composes songs, plays
                                       piano, plays on softball team.

CAREER PLANS:              Wants to work three years to save money
                           to return to college - music career.

FAMILY:                    No marriage plans.  Boyfriend in law
                           school, finishes in 2 years.

PREVIOUS JOBS:             Enjoys - meeting public, typing.
                           Dislikes - Heavy supervision, shift work.

SKILLS:                    Good typing test, misspelled some medical
                           words, good diction.

STAFF EVALUATION:          Liked her very much.  Felt comfortable talking
                           to her.  No experience in medical office but
                           they will help her get started.

COMMENTS:                  A good candidate - attractive, seems interested
                           in the job.  Can use the dictionary for
                           medical terminology.  Pleasant outgoing
                           personality.  Should fit in well here.
```

to ensure that the candidate will be accepted. Staff opinion is valuable and may save you the unpleasant job of dismissing an employee who later proves to be incompatible with existing personnel.

THE INTERVIEW

Conducting the interview

Many job applicants are apprehensive, ill at ease, and perhaps a little overawed when they appear for an interview. For these reasons, start the interview informally. Talk about the weather, or local news of interest. If you have some unusual decorative articles in the office, describe what they are and where you got them. Use any means possible to break the ice. A relaxed applicant will be more inclined to be talkative, and that is a prime objective.

Before commencing interviews prepare a checklist of items to question or discuss, and later fill it in. (See Figure 47-4.) It is surprising how quickly one forgets which applicant was which after interviewing several people over a period of a week or two. This is why the sample checklist identifies Mary Smith as being "brown-eyed" and having "short brown hair."

Interviewing is both an art and a science. The objective is to learn as much as possible about the candidate. A good interviewer will talk about 25 percent of the time and encourage the candidate to take the initiative during the interview. Doctors are usually skilled interviewers, since they must often elicit as much information as possible from patients. Interviewing job candidates is similar to interviewing patients. Asking leading questions that require an explanatory answer gives the best results. It should always be remembered that interviewing is a two-way street: you are evaluating the candidate and the candidate is evaluating you.

How to obtain information

A good leadoff is "Why do you want to work here?" A good answer, among many others, is "I like to be able to use my own initiative, work without close supervision, and be part of a medical care team," or words to that effect. Candidates who have the fanciful idea that "working with doctors is fun" or say "I always wanted to help the sick" may not realize that working in a doctor's office is sometimes hectic, occasionally boring but never routine. Candidates should be asked what they think the job requirements are and should also be questioned about their long-range career objectives. You may find plans include returning to school or university in the foreseeable future, which would make the appointment a temporary one. If the change in career is planned for a long time in the future, it may not deter you from offering the position. You may ask general questions about the applicant's outside interests. A candidate's hobbies may not seem relevant to the job, but people with interesting hobbies are usually interesting people.

What to listen for

Your application form may provide you with more questions—for example, "What did you like and dislike about your last job?" The likes may be an indicator of job interest, the dislikes an indicator of personality clashes, dissatisfaction with routine work, or an aversion to close supervision.

Ask questions about past employment. What were the applicant's duties? Why did he or she leave the job? What was the best and most satisfying job ever held? Find out if any personal commitments will prevent the applicant from giving full attention to the job. For example, responsibility for small children at home may cause difficulties if any overtime work is needed. Such commitments should not necessarily deter you from selecting a candidate, but you should know about them.

Past employment

The occupation of the spouse, if there is one, is also of interest to the employer. What are the career objectives of the spouse? Will any problems arise if, for example, the vacation period most convenient for your business does not coincide with that of the spouse?

Figure 47-5   Sample letter for confirmation of employment.

June 20, _____

Ms. Mary Smith
Anytown
North America

Dear Ms. Smith:

I am pleased to confirm your appointment as receptionist.

Your qualifications and interest in the post impressed me and I trust this
is the beginning of a long and mutually satisfactory working relationship.

As we discussed on June 15, the starting salary is $_____ per year with a
review at the end of the 3 month probationary period. The salary will then
be increased to $_____ and the position made permanent if we both are in
agreement. You may terminate employment without notice or giving cause
during the probation period and I reserve the right to this same privilege.

The starting date is July 2, _____.   Please report to me at 9 a.m.   I will
have my accountant, Mr. Jones, instruct you on our bookkeeping practices
on July 3.

On your last visit we reviewed the personnel manual and I enclose a copy
for your records. All the details respecting sick leave, vacation, overtime, etc., are in the book. Rather than repeat the rules here I am asking
you to confirm your familiarity with the manual by signing one copy of
this letter.

I sincerely hope you will find your work interesting and satisfying.

Yours truly,

Elizabeth Trask, M.D.

Dr. Trask:

I accept the appointment under the terms and conditions stated in this
letter. I have read the personnel manual and understand and accept the
practices and procedures contained therein.

_____

Mary Smith

June ___, _____

HIRING FRIENDS AND RELATIVES

Finally a word of caution. Try to avoid selecting a friend, a friend of a friend, a relative, a relative of an employee, or even a friend of an employee. A physician's office is a place of business and should be run on a businesslike basis. The injection of personal attachments between employer and employee or between employees creates problems. Other employees may suspect that friends and relatives of the employer enjoy special consideration and privileges. Although there may be no evidence to support the suspicions, they are difficult to dispel. It is best to avoid problems, which may include the need to dismiss an incompetent friend or relative—a most difficult task.

The Final Choice

The applicants have all been interviewed and the decision made to offer the position to Mary Smith. What now? Mary Smith should be recalled for a second interview, if for no other reason than to confirm that she was the applicant who impressed you. People have been known to confuse applicants; perhaps Mary was not the person you really meant to hire. Another good reason to call her is so that you may be able to assess her *telephone* personality.

Once you are sure that Mary is the best candidate, make her a verbal offer of employment. Decide on the starting date, tell Mary of the induction procedure, and confirm the starting salary and other details of employment. Having reached agreement with Mary on the terms and conditions of employment, provide her with a written confirmation (Figure 47-5). The confirmation letter need not be detailed; it should simply confirm the appointment, salary, and starting date. It should also refer to your personnel manual, and ask the new employee to certify that she has read and understood the manual and agrees to work under its terms and conditions. If you do not have a personnel manual, the letter of confirmation must be more precise about the terms of employment.

Letter of confirmation

Staff manual

GETTING THE NEW EMPLOYEE STARTED

No employee will give satisfactory performance without being told how the job is to be carried out. The fact that an employee has the skills and experience to do the job does not guarantee superior performance. Instruct the employee yourself in the areas in which you are competent to do so, e.g., appointment scheduling, telephone message disposition, telephone screening, chart filing, handling test reports. In the areas in which you are not competent to

Starting up

Use a checklist

provide instruction, involve people who are. For example, your accountant can show how to keep the books, the hospital laboratory can provide instruction on the proper handling of laboratory materials, and the hospital can provide information on proper admitting procedures. Encourage the employee to join associations relevant to his or her employment. The employee will be exposed to ideas that may be valuable in your office organization. You may want to use a checklist to remind yourself of information to be passed on to the new employee (Figure 47-6).

PROVIDING MOTIVATION

There are many ways to motivate people, but unfortunately, none is universal; different things motivate different people. It is only by careful observation of employees that appropriate motivations

Figure 47-6 Checklist for teaching new employees.

Be prepared:
    Do you know anything about the employee's past training and experience?
    Is the desk and equipment ready?
    Do you have something relatively simple for the employee to start on so that he or she can begin to feel part of your operation immediately?

Be human:
    Have you asked about personal interests?
    Do you know how the employee is going to get to work?
    Has the interval between jobs left the employee short of funds? (Tactfully offer a salary advance.)

State the facts:
    Have you stated your policies on office procedures, lunch hours, breaks, sick leave, and vacations?
    Have you told the employee what he or she must or must not do?
    Have you explained your overall philosophy of patient care?

Explain the job:
    Have you given a clear explanation of what the employee's responsibilities are?
    Have you given the employee a job description?
    Have you provided any guidelines that may help the employee to learn the job?

Show interest in the employee's progress:
    Do you check often to see how the employee is getting along or if there is something he or she does not understand?
    Have you encouraged questions?
    Have you provided encouragement by giving compliments when they are deserved rather than confining yourself to pointing out errors?
    Have you advised that you are available for help beyond the probationary period?

can be identified. For example, Mary Smith may be motivated by being given tasks and left to her own devices. John Jones, on the other hand, may by nature be a procrastinator and perform best when given a deadline. What motivates Mary and John can be determined by results.

A title is a motivation for some employees. The duties of a receptionist-secretary may include bookkeeping, billing, purchasing supplies, etc., as well as routine reception duties. Changing the job title from receptionist-secretary to office manager, or from billing clerk to accounts receivable supervisor, may make the job more attractive.

The greatest motivator is the recognition of the employee as an important member of a team. People tend to lose interest if they work in a vacuum. If there is no recognition of their efforts and no apparent importance to the job they do, their attitude is often "Why do anything at all?"

Recognize employee's efforts

Management experts once denied that money motivated people to give superior performance. "Provide the atmosphere for job satisfaction," they said, "and you have provided motivation." More recently, opinions have changed and money is once again considered a motivation. Spiraling inflation and high taxes have made money important to everyone; consequently, monetary rewards do stimulate more conscientious work. The key is to pay a salary as good as or slightly better than what is paid elsewhere for similar jobs and to give salary increases on schedule. Pay close attention to salary scales, job titles, and all conditions required to create job satisfaction for employees.

The money motivator

EVALUATING EMPLOYEES

During the probationary period, evaluation of the employee should be an ongoing process. The tool for evaluation is the job description. When an employee is aware of the job requirements and the employer is satisfied at the time of hiring that the employee has the needed skills, evaluation is used to check performance. The process, which is simple and effective, involves keeping a record of performance. To illustrate, we will continue with the example of Mary Smith. Mary's principal duties are typing, making appointments, ordering supplies, billing medicare, and filing charts and test reports. A record of Mary's performance might read as follows:

Typing	Neatly done, no spelling errors, prompt (evaluation good).
Appointments	No problems, booked patients properly (evaluation good).

Supplies	July 10—ran out of swabs (otherwise okay).
Billing	August 15—got medicare payment. Several accounts not paid, wrong identification numbers (not so good).
Filing	Okay, no problems.
General observations	Pleasant on phone, always on time for work, no reluctance when asked to work overtime. Appears interested in the job.
Final evaluation	Acceptable if the problems of billing can be sorted out. Must see accountant to get an opinion. Jane Simpson, her previous supervisor, warned me about the billing problem.

It appears that Mary is competent except at billing, which was apparent at the outset. If you are satisfied that the problem can be resolved, retain Mary on a permanent basis; if not, she should be dismissed during the probationary period.

A periodic evaluation form for all employees is a good idea. A sample is shown in Figure 47-7. The physician should also provide an opportunity for staff to evaluate his or her performance as an employer. An example of an employee checklist is shown in Figure 47-8.

DISMISSING EMPLOYEES

It is always distressing to decide that the only solution to a problem is dismissal of an employee. There is a tendency to delay taking action, but putting it off does not help the situation.

Document valid reasons   There must always be valid reasons for dismissal; it is not good enough to fire someone on "general principles." Carefully document daily all inappropriate actions by the employee, recording them in your diary. An accumulation of evidence will make the task of dismissal easier. Present the data item by item to the employee; such evidence will prevent repercussions. In other words, make certain the reasons for firing are valid and the employee is aware of them. Although it is usual to give notice of dismissal, you may prefer to tell the employee to cease work at once and supply the appropriate amount of pay in lieu of notice. Have the check ready

Figure 47-7 Evaluation of employee by employer.

1. ON TIME FOR WORK: a) Always	10
b) Usually	5
c) Seldom	0
2. COFFEE BREAKS: a) Always observes allotted time	10
b) Seldom takes coffee breaks	10
c) Sometimes absent on break longer than should be	5
d) Often absent on break longer than should be	0
3. WASTES TIME BY PERSONAL TELEPHONE CALLS: a) Never	10
b) Sometimes	5
c) Frequently	0
4. TIME LOST: a) Seldom off work	10
b) Usually loses a few days a month for illness	5
c) Requests time off: i) Seldom	10
ii) Occasionally	5
iii) Often	0
5. TELEPHONE MANNERS: a) Trys to answer the phone promptly	10
b) Lets it ring awhile i) sometimes	5
ii) habitually	0
c) Trys to be pleasant: i) always	10
ii) most of time	5
6. ATTITUDE TOWARD PATIENTS/VISITORS IN THE OFFICE:	
a) Always pleasant	10
b) Usually pleasant	5
c) Patients annoy	0
7. WORK HABITS: 1) a) Always up to date	10
b) A few days behind	5
c) Usually well behind	0
2) a) Doesn't leave work at usual quitting time if there is work that must be done at once.	10
b) Always must leave because of personal commitments, but gets everything ready before leaving	10
c) When quitting time comes, leaves regardless of work to be done.	0
8. APPEARANCE IS NEAT AND APPROPRIATE: a) Always	10
b) Most of the time	5
c) No interest	0

Figure 47-8 Evaluation of employer by employee.

NAME: DATE:	POSITION: DATE OF LAST REVIEW:
QUALITY	COMMENT on each quality
AVAILABILITY Lets me know where he/she is.	
COMMUNICATES clearly when assigning tasks; makes priorities clear depending on workload.	
Maintains CONFIDENCES.	
RESPECT.	
Lets me organize him/her properly.	
DICTATION reasonable.	
Understands clearly what I think my job is.	
Encourages creativity.	
Facilitates interpersonal communication.	
SIGNATURE: _____ DATE: _____	

and make the final separation as quickly as possible. (Check appropriate regulations in labor laws applicable to state or province.)

The Gentle Art of Firing: An Example

Susan Billings has been on staff for a year. During her probation period, you had some misgivings but waited, hoping her performance would improve. It didn't. Susan is a nice person and has a lot of good qualities even though it seems she cannot handle the workload. You want to make the likely separation as painless as possible. How do you handle the situation?

Document mistakes

Explain the consequences

First, carefully document all relevant incidents. A simple note in your diary will suffice. The incidents may involve mistakes in making appointments for patients, giving garbled phone messages, sometimes with incorrect numbers, allowing necessary supplies to run out, or misfiling charts and test reports—none of them very serious but nevertheless frustrating. The first step is to discuss the problems with Susan and then offer a second chance. Set a time limit of perhaps a month. Susan should be quoted the dates of the incidents with an explanation of the consequences of her actions or mistakes. She will probably be grateful for the second chance and, if her capabilities allow, will be careful not to repeat the errors.

Suppose, however, that at the end of the probationary month, her work has *not* improved. Be firm at the end of the period and do not procrastinate. Interview Susan again, give firm evidence of her areas of incompetence, and tell her you are ending her employment immediately. Have the final check ready including appropriate salary in lieu of notice. Susan should also be told that if she seeks another position, you will be pleased to give a good report in the areas in which she is competent. Advise her to seek a job that requires the skills in which she excels. Although Susan may not be equipped for the position in your office, she may do better in a more suitable job. Do not destroy a person by giving prospective employers a blanket report of incompetence.

The act of firing

The practices and procedures for hiring, induction, evaluation, and dismissal discussed in this chapter are suggestions only. People develop individual methods ranging from simply saying "that's for me" about the first strong applicant to an abrupt dismissal note in the pay envelope. Induction may simply be, "There's your desk, you've done this type of job before, away you go." Regardless of the method, the objective is to recruit a contented, competent staff who are interested in their jobs and strive to meet the employer's goals. The likelihood of achieving these objectives is greatly increased by logical, sensible selection practices.

SUGGESTED READING

Medical Practice—Business Practice, M.D. Management Limited, C.M.A. House, Ottawa K1G 0G8 Canada.
Personnel Administration Handbook, Center for Research in Ambulatory Health Care Administration, Denver, Colo.
Redden, Charles S., monthly articles 1971–1975, *Canadian Family Physician.*

Chapter 48

Office Organization

D. B. Shires, M.D.

Before entering practice, the new family physician must make a number of decisions regarding the how, where, and what of family practice. The realities of practice are not generally taught in medical schools, and it is the purpose of this chapter to give the new family physician some guidance in specific areas and direction as to further sources of information according to individualized needs.

Because of the complex nature of practice management, we have found it necessary to restrict ourselves to a few important topics that are of greatest relevance to the new family physician: time management, office procedures, appropriate practice organization, clinical record management, patient's registry, appointment scheduling, billing procedures, and preventive law. Personnel selection has been dealt with in the preceding chapter, and computer usage is discussed in the next.

SOLO OR GROUP?

Selecting a
practice

Probably the most important decision for the graduate is whether to "go it alone," start out with a group of novices, or join an established group or institution. Often this decision is dictated by factors beyond the immediate control of the physician. These include personality, the ability to live with the other people's decisions, specific opportunities created by relatives, colleagues, or friends, available funds, community needs, and family adaptability.

Each decision creates the need for specific management skills. Should you choose to join a group practice, the problem will be to find the right job opportunity in the right location to meet your needs as well as those of your spouse.

EVALUATING A GROUP

In seeking a group position through medical journal advertisements, medical society secretariats, departments of family medicine, or social contacts, the big problem is finding out what you need to know about the group to decide whether it suits you. Charles Redden,[1] a noted clinic management consultant in Canada, has devised the following series of questions that should be answered at the interview.

Getting information

General Questions

1 What is the reputation of the group in the community?
2 How stable is the group?
3 How many doctors have joined or left the group in the past 3 years?
4 If any left, why did they go?
5 What is the earnings record of the group?
6 What percentage of cash income goes to overhead expenses?
7 How does the group divide income? Is there a formula?
8 What are the future plans—to remain static or to expand?
9 If expansion is planned, how is it to be financed and how will that affect partnership income?

Present Commitments of the Group

10 Are there any partners near retirement age?
11 What commitment has been made to them about retirement income?

Partnership

12 What is the partnership agreement? (Obtain a copy for legal opinion.)
13 Who administers the partnership?
14 Are there junior and senior partners, or is everyone equal?
15 How long must a new member be on staff to become eligible to join the partnership?

16 Is there an investment required, and how is it paid?

17 How is the investment calculated? Is there a formula, or is it based on book value?

18 If you leave later, how do you get your investment back?

19 Does the partnership provide all the equipment and instruments?

20 Who owns the furnishings and equipment, the partnership or a holding company?

21 If a holding company, can you buy shares in that company?

22 Does the partnership agreement provide for dissolution?

23 How would the assets be divided on dissolution?

Conditions and Benefits of Employment in the Group

24 What specifically are the required duties (office hours, on call)?

25 What is the workload? Is there a ready-made practice?

26 To what extent will the new member have to build his own practice?

27 Is support staff pooled, or does each practitioner have his or her own?

28 Will the new member be encouraged to help formulate clinic policy?

29 How are new ideas received and action taken?

30 Is the new member eligible for committee membership?

31 Is salary fixed or reviewed depending on volume, etc.?

32 If there is a fixed-period contract, are there provisions for automatic increase?

33 Does salary continue during absences for vacation or study?

34 Is a travel allowance provided for CME?

35 Is there an automobile allowance? If so, how much?

36 Are registration fees and memberships in professional societies paid?

37 What benefits are provided—health insurance, sick leave, pension plan, disability insurance, life insurance?

38 Is there a compulsory retirement age, and if so, what is it?

39 Is there any restrictive covenant in the agreement which could penalize a staff member who decides to set up another practice in the same community?

Weighing advantages and disadvantages

Job opportunities from which positive responses are obtained to all these questions are extremely rare. If you find one, grab it quickly! Usually you have to evaluate how far you are prepared to compromise or negotiate other terms to counteract deficiencies in the contract. Consider the possibility of doing locums (filling in for other doctors) in several communities to evaluate their strengths and weaknesses so that your choice of practice location can be based on firsthand experience.

CHANGES IN FAMILY PRACTICE

Evolutionary changes have taken place in family practice over the past two decades. In economic terms, rising overhead expenses, inflation, and restricted inefficient billing procedures have all narrowed the gap between gross and net income. The end of the first baby boom, the potential of the second baby boom, and the rising age of the population are further factors contributing to changes in practice patterns. The cost of ancillary office personnel and the expanded nature of practice have worked to the financial detriment of the fee-for-service practitioner. In addition, the public, particularly in North America, has become more aware of basic health principles and is demanding to be told "the facts,"[2] necessitating a more collaborative relationship between patient and practitioner. Many physicians find the changes difficult to deal with, but a competent family physician should try to be comfortable with them and to encourage new directions.

Changing practice norms

Finally, the technological advances of the past decade hold both the threat and the promise of having a major impact on family practice. Consider, for example, a physician's office computer system.[3] This should be seen not as an invasion of the doctor-patient relationship, but rather as a vital tool that, when used appropriately, will facilitate correlation of data, recall of patients at risk, bookkeeping, health hazard appraisal[4] and so on. (See the next chapter.)

TIME MANAGEMENT

The family physician is certain to be faced with a shortage of time, since time and money are the biggest managerial problems in any practice. Consequently, the efficient management of time is the distinguishing mark of the financially successful and content family physician, who will also probably be active in the community.

Principles for Organizing Time

1 Do not allow yourself to be interrupted by the telephone except in emergencies. Have your receptionist collect telephone messages, and reserve some time during your workday for dealing with them. Do not have telephones in your examining rooms.

Use time wisely

2 Have your receptionist call patients if you are running late or are delayed.

3 Try to schedule patients for counseling at the beginning or end of a workday and fix a time limit. Or you may want to use the last hour of your day for patients who can drop in to your office and be seen on an "available time" basis.

4 Learn to delegate, particularly mechanical tasks (billing, for

Delegate tasks

example). In clinical areas, if you provide clear instructions regarding level of authority, the nurse can easily handle upper respiratory infections, diarrhea and vomiting, and immunizations as well as more complicated situations, especially when guidelines are provided. (See for example, the problem algorithms in Chapter 11-30).

House calls   **5** Think out your policy regarding house calls and inform your patients about your availability. Although the science of medicine can probably be better practiced in the well-equipped office environment, the art of medicine is often better applied at home.

6 Use more than one examining room so that a patient can undress or dress in one room while you are seeing someone else in another. Each examining room should be completely self-contained.

7 Write your notes with clear *plan* directions for the next visit.

8 Establish your own method of achieving rapport with patients. Personal notes about patients are often useful, especially when a patient has not been in the office for some time. To keep such notes confidential, one physician adopted the habit of writing a brief phrase backwards; e.g., "likes golf" would be "flog sekil."[5]

Patient questionnaires   **9** Use preprinted questionnaires for new patients to reduce the time needed for detailed history taking.[6-8] Schedule any routine, noncrisis physical examination for these patients on another day.

10 Use rubber stamps for recording data on particular conditions (e.g., hypertension) or investigations (e.g., urinalysis).

Family time   **Reserve Time for Self and Family**   By employing some or all of these simple aids, you should have sufficient time at the end of your day to consider your own needs and those of your family. Perhaps a further word about family needs is appropriate. We all know at least one "excellent" doctor who is seen visiting his patients at all hours of the night and who never leaves the practice or hospital until 11 p.m. Little thought is given to the spouse, or to children who grow up with a father who is a stranger. Family time is important, as more and more family physicians are beginning to realize; many older physicians who adopted the "dedicated" role are beginning to regret it as they see the best years of their family life escaping from them. Make it a point to set aside a block of time, preferably daily but at least at regular times during the week, for your family. Your patients will be better off if your own home life is a happy one.

Time to think   **Time for Oneself**   Apart from family time, you need time for yourself. Such time has to be planned, or it will never be available. Some people appear to have an innate ability to find time for reflection while attending meetings, driving their cars, or "listening" at meetings. Others must deliberately set aside time for themselves, since procrastination may lead to frustration and a feeling that nothing has been accomplished.

Time must also be found for an activity for which the need has always existed but which is now becoming more formalized—continuing medical education (CME). This may involve reading journals, listening to tapes, participating in rounds, or attending courses. Whatever method you choose, let nothing interfere with your CME time. (For further advice, see the chapter on CME.)

CME time

OFFICE PROCEDURES

Space does not allow a comprehensive discussion of office procedures for family practice. Consequently, we urge the novice practitioner to acquire an office procedures manual[9-11] and adopt the recommendations that seem relevant. After you have read one of these manuals, you will have a general idea about how you want to run your office. The next and perhaps most important step is to make the community aware of your presence, your need for patients, and your office location and hours. For a small community (less than 2000) this will probably be unnecessary, since word will be around before you arrive on the scene. For a medium-sized community (2000 to 10,000) and especially for a larger community, it is advisable to place an advertisement in a local newspaper. The ad should conform to the ethical requirements of your local medical society. It will usually include your name and degrees, whether you are joining or associating with other doctors, what type of practice you are setting up, the office location and telephone number, and sometimes the office hours. Consider the advice of the newspaper on what items should be included. (See Figure 48-1.)

Office manual

Advertising

If you are moving to a small community as the only physician or into an "underdoctored" community, you will not be in competition for patients. If you decide not to advertise, you should nevertheless have a practice information brochure printed detailing your name and degrees, address and telephone number, limits of practice (e.g., no obstetrics) or special interest (e.g., geriatrics), office hours, names of physicians who will be covering your practice when you are not available, and billing procedures. Such a brochure will be useful to new patients for several years to come. (See Figure 48-2.)

Practice information brochure

In addition to providing information to patients, you need to make yourself known to other health personnel in the community who may be sending patients to you. The local public health department, social agencies, hospital staff, school supervisors, and police all need to meet with you at some time after you start practice. You might consider having an open house at your office.

Community agencies

Figure 48-1   New practice announcement.

PLUMTREE MEDICAL CLINIC
64 Plumtree Avenue, Thorndale

is pleased to announce that

DR. JOSEPH DWIGHT BLOUGH, M.D.

will be joining them in the

practice of Family Medicine.

For patient appointments,

please phone: 444-7729

Figure 48-2   Patient information brochure.

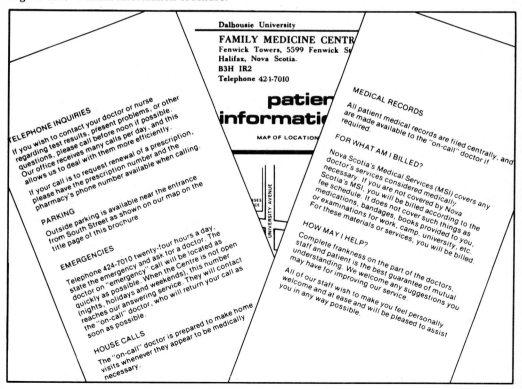

Social contacts with other physicians in the community must be worked at. The coffee break at the hospital lounge is an ideal place to do this. Not only will you be aware of the consultants available, but you will also have an opportunity to evaluate them.

In the past, emergency rooms provided excellent opportunities for establishing and increasing a practice; some still do. A surprising number of patients who come to emergency rooms have no family physician, and if they have been satisfactorily treated by you, such patients may decide to continue their care in your office practice.

Emergency rooms

During the first year or two of practice do not hesitate to make it known that you are available to fill in for other community physicians who are on holiday or on emergency room duty; the more rapidly you build your practice, the more leisure time you will be able to afford in the future. Try to attend medical society branch meetings and College or Academy meetings, and volunteer for jobs, especially those that involve contact with other physicians and health professionals, e.g., membership benefits, liaison work, work in CME. Your industry will be rewarded in time, and you will probably be more rapidly accepted in the community.

Contact local physicians

Entertaining at home is another way to develop better social relationships with your colleagues. It will also allow your spouse an opportunity to meet people with similar interests and problems in the community. If you have an open house at your office, make sure your spouse and those of your colleagues are invited.

Home entertaining

IMPROVING PATIENT COMFORT IN THE OFFICE

1   Try to avoid keeping people waiting. If you are running late or are delayed, ask your receptionist to call patients and explain. Patients will appreciate this courtesy.

Promptness and courtesy

2   Consider how accessible your office location is. If necessary, provide a map for new patients and possibly add a carefully marked "patients only" parking area if you are in a busy downtown area.

Accessibility aids

3   Choose office and waiting room furniture carefully, providing soft chairs and using muted colors. Avoid furnishings with sharp corners; supply rounded coffee tables if these are necessary. Lighting should be soft and carpet of the durable commercial variety, color-coordinated with furnishings and drapes. The whole effect should put patients at ease. Remember that a considerable percentage of your patients will be children and the elderly; provide toys and small chairs for children and firm seats with arms that are easy to get in and out of for the elderly.

Furnishings

4   Select your magazines or patient reading materials carefully and keep them current. Do not include journals intended for physician consumption.

Magazines

5 Adopt specific ideas for your practice that suit your individual style. Some examples are providing a large corkboard for displaying the artwork of child patients, a lending library of patient education books, or a convenience center with coffee and juice. (See also the chapter on patient education.)

RECORD SYSTEMS

Choosing
medical records

By the time your first patient enters the waiting room, you should have made decisions about several key organizational elements. One of the most important is choosing a clinical record system. In a group practice the choice is often dictated by the past decisions of the clinical management. Or, if you have taken over a practice, you may have inherited a record system from your predecessor. In either of these situations your options may be severely restricted. However, if you are dissatisfied with the clinical records and the opportunity arises, you should give serious consideration to an organized record system based on the flowchart system, the problem-oriented system[7,8] or a combination of the two. If you have started out with no clinical record system, you will have an ideal opportunity to choose wisely during the slow initial period. In years to come you will be glad that you took the time to build a system suited to your own style of practice. The three basic types of manual record system are as follows.

Traditional
records

1 *Content-oriented records* - the traditional way of filing patient notes, lab reports, x-ray reports, consultation notes, etc., separately without any linkage of related problems

POMR

2 *Problem-oriented records* - linkage of notes, investigations, and treatments to a numbered problem index so that any problem can be assessed at any time by searching in one place which can be located from the index

Flowcharts

3 *Flowcharts* - time-sequenced records in which lab data, investigations, consultations, and prescriptions are recorded on a flowchart for rapid identification of information or gaps in information

Starting Your Own Record System

If you are starting from scratch, the best compromise might be to use firm manila folders and have them printed locally with your name and office address on the front, leaving space for the patient's name (family name and family members if you wish to file by family), address, telephone number (including business number), medical insurance number, and anything else that is important in your community. It may be important to note religion if there are two strong religious groups in your community, each with its own hospital. If you have this information, you may save your-self the embarrassment of booking the patient into the "wrong" hospital. On the inside front cover of the folder you should have printed a list of patient and family problems and a therapy list. If these lists are kept up-to-date, they will serve as a rapid index of the patient's or family's problems and save valuable minutes going through the chart on each visit to ensure that nothing important has been missed. (See Figure 48-3.) If you do not wish to go to the trouble of having folders specially printed, charts are available commercially from various sources.

Included in the manila folder may be a variety of data collection forms, clinical notes, flow sheets, consultant reports, and laboratory and x-ray results. The note on the last office visit should be on the top; it should be the first page visible on the right-hand

Problem-oriented records

Figure 48-3 Problem-oriented record.

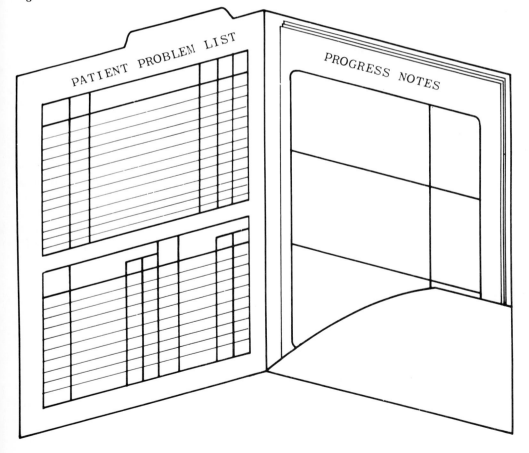

Flow sheets

Alert file

Data collection files

side when the folder is opened. The progress note and problem and therapeutic index inside the front cover can be considered as the *alert file* of the clinical record and the remaining forms as *data collection*. (Be sure to collect a supply of any available blank laboratory investigation, physiotherapy, or x-ray order forms, as well as social service requisitions, from your community facilities.) The data collection forms may include a health questionnaire, a health risk appraisal form, a past history and prenatal record for females, immunization records, and birth and preschool records. Flow sheets should be considered for particular patients' problems such as diabetes, hypertension, arthritis, or anticoagulant control.

A general-purpose front sheet which fits any 8½ × 11 in (20 × 80 cm) folder is the FACMIS sheet[12] (see Figure 48-4). This includes a problem and medication list and much of the flow sheet data. It provides an excellent compromise between the flow sheet and problem-oriented approaches.

Another useful device is peel-off labels to identify specific illnesses (e.g., hypertension) or "reminder" conditions (e.g., immunization needs). (Such labels are available from Anatomy with A-PEEL, Dave-son Medical Enterprises Ltd., 257 Arnold Avenue, Thornhill, Ontario, L4J 1B9, Canada.)

Dictating Notes

Dictation

Some doctors use a dictating machine and have all their notes typed. This ensures legibility and may save time. However, it has several disadvantages, which are that (*a*) dictating is relatively expensive, (*b*) doctors tend to be more verbose when using a dictaphone, (*c*) the records are usually not immediately available to the doctor on call, who may need to check a note for diagnosis or to identify a drug prescribed, and (*d*) the typed notes need to be edited to correct errors. Consequently, unless the doctor's handwriting is absolutely illegible and he or she (as well as colleagues) is prepared to accept the disadvantages, we do not recommend dictating notes in family practice.

Telephone Consultations

Notes on phone consultations

It is controversial whether notes should be made on telephone consultations. Certainly this makes clinical sense, and for legal purposes it is absolutely necessary if any diagnosis or management advice is given to the patient over the telephone.

Filing Systems

Filing systems for office records need not be elaborate; simple shelving will suffice. Always ensure that the office is securely locked in your absence.

Figure 48-4 Cumulative patient profile.

1. PATIENT IDENTIFICATION (Plate)	Codes /Nos.	6. ONGOING HEALTH CONDITIONS (e.g. problems, diagnoses, dates of onset)	Date Recorded	Date Resolved /Controlled

Mr Mrs Miss Other

Address

Home Phone

I.D. # or File #

OHIP Number   Sub. In.

Present Marital Status   Sex   Date of Birth
S M Sep. D W   Other   M F   D   M   Y

2. PERSONAL AND FAMILY DATA (e.g. occupation, life events, habits)	Dates

3. PAST HISTORY (e.g. past serious illnesses, operations) RISK FACTORS (e.g. genetic/familial diseases)	Dates	Codes /Nos.	7. LONG-TERM TREATMENT REGIMEN (e.g. medications, dosage/frequency)	Date Started	Date Discontinued

4. ALLERGIES/DRUG REACTIONS	Dates

5. DATES OF:	General Assessment	
Initial Visit	Summarized Record on CPP	

8. CONSULTANTS

Family and Community Medicine Information Systems (FACMIS)
UNIVERSITY OF TORONTO
© 1977

9.   M.D.

APPOINTMENT SCHEDULING

Appointment
systems

It is convenient for the patient, physician, and office staff to have a patient appointment system. However, an appointment system that cannot be maintained within reasonable limits is useless, as well as frustrating to patients. In urban communities, the appointment system is the accepted mode of practice, whereas in rural areas many practitioners have given up appointment systems because of the high percentage of "drop-in" patients. In some parts of the world the appointment schedule depends largely on local transportation systems. If an appointment system is to be efficient, careful thought must be given to it by the physician and also by the receptionist, who will be making the appointments and receiving the criticism from patients when the doctor isn't on time.

Time units

The appointment system should be as flexible as possible. A preprinted format should be used for each session and for each health professional, and a time unit should be decided upon. A basic unit of 10 minutes seems practical. Instructions should be given to the receptionist as to how many units to book for each type of visit. A new patient or a counseling visit may require three units (30 minutes), a regular visit two units (20 minutes) and a recheck visit one unit (10 minutes). An example of a patient appointment system designed along these lines is given in Figure 48-5.

PATIENT REGISTERS AND RECALL

Keeping track
of patients

A list of who your patients are can be very valuable in your practice. Various kinds of lists can be used, which may include any or a combination of the following:

A simple Kardex, which is verified and if necessary updated by the receptionist each time the patient comes to the office. This can be color-coded to allow simple age-sex retrievals. (See Figure 48-6).

An edge-punch card system such as the BJS system,[13] which allows for retrieval of patients in selected groups by age, sex, investigation, therapy, or disease.

An E-Book system,[14] which, like an edge-punch card system, provides both an age-sex search and disease- or prescription-indexed searches. (See Figure 48-7).

A computer listing, which allows for more complicated retrievals and statistical analysis. (Figure 48-8 shows a listing from our own practice.)

Recall methods

Any or all of these methods allow the physician to describe the practice so that decisions can be made on practice needs, trends,

Figure 48-5 Patient appointments.

PHYSICIAN ___

TIME	TEL.NO.	NAME
10:00	1	
10:15	2	
10:30	3	
10:45	4	
11:00	5	
11:15	6	
11:30	7	
11:45	8	
12:00	9	
1:30	1	
1:45	2	
2:00	3	
2:15	4	
2:30	5	
2:45	6	
3:00	7	
3:15	8	
3:30	9	
3:45	10	
4:00	11	
4:15	12	
4:30	13	

PHYSICIAN ___

TIME	TEL.NO.	NAME
10:00	1	
10:15	2	
10:30	3	
10:45	4	
11:00	5	
11:15	6	
11:30	7	
11:45	8	
12:00	9	
1:30	1	
1:45	2	
2:00	3	
2:15	4	
2:30	5	
2:45	6	
3:00	7	
3:15	8	
3:30	9	
3:45	10	
4:00	11	
4:15	12	
4:30	13	

PHYSICIAN ___

TIME	TEL.NO.	NAME
10:00	1	
10:15	2	
10:30	3	
10:45	4	
11:00	5	
11:15	6	
11:30	7	
11:45	8	
12:00	9	
1:30	1	
1:45	2	
2:00	3	
2:15	4	
2:30	5	
2:45	6	
3:00	7	
3:15	8	
3:30	9	
3:45	10	
4:00	11	
4:15	12	
4:30	13	

TEAM: ___
DATE: ___

SUMMARY

No. of physicians ___
No. of clinic hours ___
No. of patients seen ___
No. of new patients ___
No. of appointment cancellations ___
No. of "no-show" patients ___
No. of patient M.S.I. cards prepared ___
No. of patient statements prepared ___

Figure 48-6   Patient kardex.

```
JOHN ALEXANDER SMITH            yob: '40
100 High Street
Anytown, North America

Phone: business - 444-1000
                  444-5121

MSI #: 121-682-111-01
```

Figure 48-7   Sample page from E-book.

DATE			E.I.	SURNAME		INITIALS	DATE OF BIRTH			M.S.S.	S.S.	REF	A	B	C	D	E	F	G	H	I	J
12-13	14-15	16-17	18	19 20 21		22	23-24	25-26	27-28	29	30	31	32	33	34	35	36	37	38	39	40	41
28	10	78		MACKAY		J A	1968															

RCGP B-4

DIAG. CODE NO. 1-3: [0] [5] [3]   SEX 4: [0] (MALE)   DR'S. CODE NO. 5-11: [2]

and continuing education gaps. They also permit recall of particular patient groups. For example:

1 Children under 1 year of age for well-baby care
2 Children in immunization age groups according to protocol
3 Female children aged 11 years for rubella immunization
4 Females for well-woman care
5 All patients over 60 annually
6 Patients with high-risk conditions, e.g., hypertension
7 Patients with identified chronic diseases
8 Patients on medications requiring monitoring

Simple card systems

The first five groups above are classified simply by age and sex, so that a simple age-sex register would suffice for them. Alterna-

Figure 48-8 Computer-generated patient registration listing.

D A L H O U S I E   F A M I L Y   M E D I C I N E   C E N T R E   15 SEPT. 78

PATIENT DIRECTORY BY SURNAME, TEAM

SURNAME	FIRST NAME	PATIENT ID	OFFICE NO.	SEX	BIRTHDATE	STREET	CITY	PHONE	DOCTOR	TEAM DOCTOR
	Kanthi T.	359.814.01	000-0000	MALE	1946		Halifax	-4175	6787	Dr. Still
	Lorna	029.833.02	101-0293	FEMALE	1943		Halifax	-0368	4697	Dr. Still
	Alvina	840.659.02	100-8406	FEMALE	1907		Sackville	-5367	6387	Dr. Brown
	Robert	488.137.01	423-6321	MALE	1960		Dartmouth	-1285	5367	Dr. Hansen
	Lillian	595.580.01	107-0955	FEMALE	1886		Halifax	-0295	6387	Dr. Brown
	Brenda	513.416.02	429-2773	FEMALE	1956		Sackville	-8065	6697	Dr. Still
	Terence	400.111.01	106-0359	MALE	1950		Halifax	-1295	6387	Dr. Phillips
	John	850.677.01	429-2776	MALE	1913		Halifax	-6159	6787	Dr. Still
	Margarite	840.677.02	000-0000	FEMALE	1916		Halifax	-6159	6787	Dr. Still
	Ruth	034.184.02	423-8331	FEMALE	1924		Dartmouth	-0224	6787	Dr. Still
	Maureen	400.115.01	424-6700	FEMALE	1954		Halifax	-0005	5697	Dr. Brown
	Elizabeth	488.139.02	103-6152	FEMALE	1925		Sackville	-0219	6787	Dr. Still
	Anny	001.989.02	000-000	FEMALE	1929		Halifax	-2292	4697	Dr. Phillips
	Peter	809.612.01	715-8065	MALE	1050		Sackville	-5601	5387	Dr. Brown
	Michael	013.765.01	107-0137	MALE	1917		Dartmouth	-2224	4697	Dr. Brown

Figure 48-9   Patient folder.

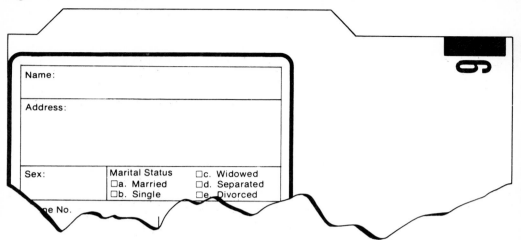

tively, a 12-file card box labeled with each month of the year could be used. In this system, a card with the patient's name and condition for recall is placed in the appropriate month slot. As each patient returns for a visit, the card is removed from the box. At the end of the month, the cards remaining in the box indicate which patients have not returned and need to be recalled. Another recall method is to edge-code the patient's records where they project from the file for easy identification and retrieval (see Figure 48-9). It is suggested that the receptionist place a number corresponding to the last digit of the year on the outer edge of the chart. Thus for a patient's first visit in 1986, the number 6 will be stuck to the outer edge of his or her chart. A quick glance at the files in 1988 will identify the patients who have not been into the office for 2 years and who need to be checked. A color code for diseases and therapies used in addition to this one-digit year code allows for rapid retrieval according to disease. One can search by color for those with a particular disease who have not been in the office for a given period (e.g., a blue sticker might indicate hypertensive patients).

Not only will these patient registry and recall systems help you in your daily practice, if you should become curious about particular aspects of your practice, they will also provide a built-in system for research and patient care appraisal. (See the chapters on research and patient care appraisal.)

OFFICE SUPPLIES

Maintaining office supplies, both clerical and medical, can be a problem unless some organizational rules are established. You should set these up with the nurse or receptionist and make sure that they are kept. We have summarized in tabular form three lists of rules which may be of use to you:

   1 Suggested contents of the doctor's bag (Table 48-1)
   2 Office rules to ensure that the doctor's bag is always "at the ready" (Table 48-2)
   3 A guide for maintaining adequate office supplies (Table 48-3)

COMMUNICATION

The family physician must ensure that there is effective communication among patients, office staff, and physician during regular hours and also in the evenings and on weekends.

Communication problems may start with the answering of the telephone when a patient requests an appointment. There is a world of difference between the response "Dr. Joan Williams' office—can we help you?" and the response "Plumtree Clinic." You will be judged by the impression given by the receptionist's initial opener! Decide on the format that suits you and your receptionist and make sure the established procedure is followed. Every practice should have at least two telephone lines and possibly an additional private line for the physician.

In telephone answering, particularly in a multiple-line system, a call should not be placed on hold before determining whether the call is an emergency call or not. This seems like an obvious precaution, but unfortunately emergency calls are put on hold every day—a potentially disastrous action. The receptionist should, of course, be trained to quickly ascertain the urgency of the call before requesting the patient to hold.

Another problem is communicating with the doctor when he or she is out of the office. Several mechanisms exist to accomplish this, some of which may be more suited to your practice community than others. In urban areas the most common method may be the telephone answering service with a "beeper" system. This is expensive but very convenient. Two types of beeper service are commonly available; the first has a buzzer that alerts you to call the answering service to receive a message, the second a small loudspeaker for the answering service to communicate a message. The disadvantage of the latter is that the answering service has no way of knowing if the doctor has received the message. Whichever beeper system is used, the physician should periodically telephone the answering service to ensure that no messages have been lost. In choosing an answering service, comparisons should be made of reliability (find out and call names of satisfied customers), battery life

Answering the phone

Instructions to receptionist

Answering service

Table 48-1   Suggested Contents of the Doctor's Bag

Drugs

Oral—tablets or solutions

Antibiotic of your choice—to be used for priming dose on emergency call until prescription filled
Antiemetic—dymenhydrinate oral and suppositories
Analgesic—aspirin or codeine (222, 292, buffered aspirin)
Minor tranquilizer—diazepam (Valium)
Antiangina medication—nitroglycerin
Narcotic—meperidine (Demerol)
Antihistamine—diphenhydramine (Benadryl)

Injectable—intramuscular and intravenous

Furosemide (Lasix)	Chlorpromazine (Thorazine)
Dymenhydrinate	Promethazine (Phenergan)
Diphenhydramine	Diazepam
Epinephrine (adrenalin)	Digoxin (Lanoxin)
Meperidine	Lidocaine (Xylocaine 2%—no
Morphine	adrenalin)

Utilities

Rectal as well as oral thermometers

Airway—pediatric and adult size

Tourniquet, vacuum tube, needles (disposable), and a variety of labeled blood tubes (with and without anticoagulant)

Tongue depressor, flashlight, and labeled culture tubes

Disposable gloves and lubricant

Dextrostix and Labstix

Gauze, elastic bandages, and alcohol swabs (disposable)

Prescription pad, note pad, pen, and billing material

Note: If you do not have spares in your bag, don't forget to take along your stethoscope, ophthalmoscope–otoscope set, sphygmomanometer, and reflex hammer from your office.

Table 48-2   Office Rules to Ensure That Doctor's Bag Is Always at the Ready

1   Don't leave the bag in your car unless you lock it in your trunk. Preferably take it with you.
2   Besides using the note pad in your bag to make diagnostic, therapeutic, and billing notes about the patients you see, underline the medications you use *at the time of the visit.* Give these notes to your nurse each day for patient follow-up, filing with respective patient's chart, and billing, as well as for replacing medications in bag.
3   Once a week make sure that your nurse does a general housekeeping of the bag to replace materials and medications used, as well as date-expired drugs, and to ensure an adequate supply of dressings and clean thermometers.

Table 48-3   Guide for Maintaining Adequate Office Supplies

1   Ensure adequate storage space where supplies are readily accessible to the office staff but *not* to the patients, in particular children. Make sure that certain drugs (e.g., narcotics) are locked up.
2   A fireproof office safe for keeping receipts, accounts, and legal documents is a worthwhile investment. It can also be used to store narcotics. Make sure only you and the nurse have a key. (There is a high incidence of addiction among health professionals.)
3   All supplies should be checked at monthly intervals against a stock list and reordered whenever necessary. The nurse may also keep a running list of low supplies. Don't forget stationery supplies.
4   If you have adequate storage space, stock supplies can be ordered in bulk to lessen cost. Drugs and solutions that can become outdated must be ordered on a short-term basis. Your use of these over an initial 6-month period will provide a guide to the quantity you will need to order.
5   Supplies of vaccines (MMR, DPT, etc.) may be obtained free of charge from local health departments, and this should be investigated.
6   An accumulation of drug samples will be left in your office by drug company representatives. Try to avoid accepting drugs you don't intend to use, or else you will simply clutter up valuable storage space.

and home recharge capability, one-way beep, voice, or two-way voice capability, effective range, and, of course, cost.

Home telephone

Probably the most common after-hours method of communication is using the physician's home telephone and relying on the spouse to redirect messages. The disadvantage is obvious: someone has to stay home to answer the telephone, and this may not be convenient or even acceptable to your spouse, particularly if he or she is acting as an unpaid office assistant. (Your accountant may be able to advise you on whether your spouse can be remunerated.)

Mobile telephones

Another method of communication involves the use of mobile telephones, citizens band (CB) car radios, and, more recently, cellular telephones.

However, since these mobile telephones and CB radios are expensive, unless you are the only physician in the area and therefore have a moral obligation to be in contact at all times for emergencies, you might find a better way to use your time in the car, for example, playing back self-learning CME audiotapes.

Finally, in a small town, the network in which everyone knows the doctor's car and thereby his or her location, often works as effectively in an emergency as the telephone.

Staff problem solving

A different aspect of communication involves the relations between staff in the office. The wise family physician will block out time for two-way discussions with the staff about communications problems and try to arrive at solutions acceptable to all. The doctor should be open to suggestions from staff, who usually bear the brunt of patient complaints.

PROTOCOLS AND OFFICE ETHICS

Office Staff Protocols

Instructions on office procedures should be worked out and clearly communicated to all your office staff. Office staff protocols should cover the following areas:

Called-away
protocol

1 *Telephone procedures, including canceling office appointments when the doctor is out on a call:* Emergencies should be directed to another physician or to an emergency room; other patients should be given new appointments. Unless procedures are clear, the receptionist will take action on your behalf, as the following short story shows.

A colleague of ours was called out of a busy afternoon office session to a difficult obstetrical case. On her way out she called to her eager new receptionist to take care of things while she was gone. After 3 hours of a tiring and difficult touch-and-go delivery, she returned to the office, physically and mentally exhausted. As she opened the office door, she heard music and was astonished to find the waiting room full of patients all singing together, conducted by her receptionist, who had kept them there for the 3 hours of her absence. She didn't get home that night until 10 p.m. Her receptionist (a gem) is still with her but doesn't conduct choir practice for her patients anymore.

Nonsmoking
areas

2 *Restriction of smoking to specific areas indicated by placement of suitably worded signs:* If you do restrict smoking, be sure that staff do not smoke in front of patients.
3 *Instructions about dealing with physically unruly, abusive, or intoxicated patients, and with fire and theft.*

Emergencies

4 *Acute medical emergencies:* These should not cause hysteria in your staff if you have planned for them by discussing and demonstrating cardiopulmonary resuscitation (CPR) methods, providing emergency telephone numbers, and having a resuscitation bag and oxygen cylinder located where all staff can find them quickly.

Drug company
representatives

5 *Handling visits by drug company representatives:* Make clear to your receptionist whether you wish to accord drug company representatives the courtesy of a visit. If you do and you are in a solo practice, you may wish to arrange for 10-minute visits between patient appointments. If you are in a group of physicians, you and the drug company representatives may find it more convenient to meet for a refreshment break during your workday. Although you may question the educational value of drug representative visits, they have several advantages. You can obtain information on new packaging, patient education materials, and free samples for indigent patients.
6 *Billing procedures:* If these differ from general patient expectations based on the community norm, they should be promi-

nently displayed and written in nonauthoritarian language; e.g., avoid "Pay here."

7 *Drop-in patients:* A clear policy should be established for dealing with patients who drop in without appointments.

8 *Staff addressing one another:* Staff should be informed of how you wish them to address one another in front of patients.

The above list represents only some of the areas in which decisions must be made in advance by the physician and the staff to avoid awkward, embarrassing situations or even disastrous outcomes.

PATIENT PROTOCOLS

Much of the information you wish to convey to patients about your practice can be transmitted through a clearly written patient information brochure, preferably illustrated. However, each new patient deserves a few minutes of your time to establish the working rules of the relationship. This time may be used to discuss special requirements or unique family situations or to explain how you wish to be addressed and find out how the patient wishes to be addressed.

Patient Educational Materials

Generalized patient protocols either distributed as patient educational materials or displayed as wall posters in examining rooms illustrating your schedule for immunization or listing items covered by the well-baby or well-woman check, cardiovascular risk charts, and illustrated instructions about breast self-examination can be very helpful to patients. Such materials serve to remind patients to initiate requests for special examinations or to ask questions about preventive care. Drug company handouts can also be useful, particularly those dealing with contraceptive methods, pregnancy problems, or the management of particular conditions. In addition, the physician's office should purchase copies of patient-oriented books that can be lent to patients. (See chapter 40 on patient education.)

Patient education

Billing Problems and Procedures

Billing is always a difficult problem, especially when doctors leave this chore to a secretary-receptionist to whom they have given insufficient direction. These doctors should not be surprised when the secretary-receptionist makes billing or procurement decisions that are not to their liking. Be sure that you have a clear under-

Patient accounts

standing with your receptionist regarding standard billings, exception billings, nonpayment, bad debts, etc. Be prepared to discuss the matters frankly with the patient and include your secretary-receptionist if you feel a problem in communication has occurred or if the situation otherwise warrants it.

Informing patients

Before you see your first patient, you must decide on your billing procedures in consultation with community colleagues and with your receptionist, particularly if he or she has had previous billing experience with another physician in the community. You may decide to bill according to the local medical society's recommended schedule or the third-party payer's schedule, or to bill directly to the patient (either the total amount or the balance from another paying agency). You must ensure that your procedure is conveyed to the patient by word of mouth or notice. This is especially important if you bill differently from other community practitioners.

Using an accountant wisely

You should also obtain advice from your accountant to ensure that the income you receive is adequate for the number of patients seen. (Most doctors have appallingly poor accounting systems.) You may wish to use voucher checks, which are larger than standard checks and have voucher space for recording details of the transaction. These have the advantage of being serially numbered, enabling you to keep track of missing checks and facilitating accounting procedures.

Your accountant, who will be involved in your tax calculations, can also advise you on purchasing or leasing equipment and on management services. The practice management books referred to earlier can also be of help.

PRACTICE MANAGEMENT CONSULTANTS

When to use a consultant

In the past decade, full-time professional managers have been increasingly used in group practice. In smaller group practices (less than eight practitioners), serious consideration should be given to retaining the services of a practice management consultant. These individuals, experienced in the business problems of practice, are better equipped to advise on the totality of practice than accountants, lawyers, or bank managers. A practice management consultant should be called (*a*) before setting up practice, (*b*) when the practice situation changes, e.g., because of a new partnership agreement or a change in locality, (*c*) periodically to review practice policies and advise on increasing efficiency (this is analogous to the periodic health examination we emphasize with our patients), and (*d*) when things *start* to go wrong (the earlier the better). Unfortunately, this last piece of advice is seldom heeded.

Efficient practice organization is vital to the success of your career. Think about it very carefully and seek help *early*.

LEGAL PROBLEMS AND THEIR PREVENTION

There are two major causes of patient lawsuits against a doctor. The first is a breakdown of the doctor-patient relationship, which affects consent to treatment. Such a situation can produce injury by default. The physician should always ask him- or herself two questions: "Am I misleading the patient?" and "Am I creating a false sense of security by promising or implying a cure?"

Avoid lawsuits

The second is patient injury either as a result of poor communication (e.g., failure to inform a patient of side effects or hiding something from the patient) or because of professional or technical error. Again, the physician should constantly ask, "Have I done everything within reason to avoid the risk of injury or damage?"

It is clearly impossible to prescribe a method of practicing medicine which will guarantee that a physician never faces legal action. Certainly all physicians should be protected by malpractice insurance and in addition, when starting practice, should retain a lawyer and consult that lawyer on all matters that could lead to a suit. It is nevertheless possible to organize a practice so as to minimize the possibility of a suit. Measures that might be adopted include:

Malpractice insurance

1 Carefully and immediately document clinical contacts including telephone contacts, particularly where explanations and warnings have been given regarding side effects and complications of drugs or the birth control pill and the side effects of hypertensive drugs.

Documentation

2 Be sure records are at least as secure as those of your fellow practitioners in the community.

Security

3 Transfer records, when this is requested by other practitioners, by copy only, after a signed authority has been obtained from the patient, retaining the originals in your files.

Retain originals

4 Give clear, legible, and concise written instructions to nurses and to physicians who will be covering your practice. Avoid telephone and other oral instructions except in cases of emergency. In those cases, make certain the recipient has recorded the instructions correctly—have them read back and put them in writing at the earliest opportunity. In some jurisdictions, this is required by law, and in many hospitals it is required by bylaws.

Clear instructions

5 Carefully consider actions (such as therapeutic abortions and the withholding of prescriptions) that may not be against the law but may contravene the code of medical ethics in the local jurisdiction.

While we cannot deal with all the situations with potential legal implications that may confront the family physician, we list below some of the more common situations and discuss them one by one, resisting the temptation to provide legal advice. Legal advice should be obtained from legal counsel in your own state because the law on these matters varies widely from one jurisdiction to another. The situations to be discussed are as follows:

1 Consent to treat a minor
2 Confidentiality and privacy
3 Security procedures for office records
4 Retention of records
5 Transfer of records
6 Disclosure of information
7 Use of patient information
8 Employment of a locum physician, a salaried employee, or a medical student
9 Ethical and social obligations
10 Computer record legality

Consent to Treat a Minor

This is a controversial problem that may occur during the first days of practice. In many jurisdictions, there is a difference between the age of majority and the age of consent. In others, there may be no statutory age of consent. This problem has particular relevance for providing birth control pills, abortion, physical examination, surgery, and other forms of therapy. In some jurisdictions, birth control pills can be provided for a 12-year-old at the discretion of the individual practitioner, while in others the College or Board code of ethics or the law may oppose such action.

Confidentiality and Privacy

Confidentiality and privacy are everyone's concern. They are the subject of congressional inquiries, royal commissions, and study groups of national societies and government administrations. Clearly, the physician must make every attempt to preserve confidentiality between the patient and the physician. When it comes to disclosure within a court of law, the advice of legal counsel should be sought.

Security Procedures for Office Records

Lock up records

The physician should ensure that there are adequate security procedures for the records in his or her possession. The theft of medical information has been widely reported, and the potential of medical information being used in attempted blackmail must be remembered. Consequently, the family physician should ensure that records are kept in a locked room or closet. Patient's records should never be left lying on desks or countertops.

Retention of Records

Records should be retained for the period of time advised by your lawyer. The time limit will depend on local legislation and in particular the period in which a lawsuit can be brought against the physician and in which the records could be required for defense purposes. The office should be arranged so that inactive files can be stored outside premium space but within the office. Such files should be available if patients return after several years of absence. Do not microfilm and destroy records without obtaining prior legal advice.

Inactive records

Transfer of Records

As has been previously mentioned, the original records should never be transferred to another physician; send only copies, preferably abstracted copies, which will be more valuable to the physician requesting them. In addition, the physician should obtain written permission from the patient to send a copy of the records to the other physician, and the permission should be stored with the record in question.

Retention of original records

Disclosure of Information

The physician will often be requested by a parent, an insurance agency, or other third-party group to disclose information. Great care must be taken in dealing with such requests. As regards insurance agencies, there is no question that prior written permission from the patient must be obtained, no matter how persuasive the agency may be. As regards parents, the physician should use discretion, ensuring that the confidentiality of a minor patient is not breached. The physician should also use caution in disclosing information to a spouse, and should consider documenting what is said by both parties regarding the issues.

Use of Patient Information

Using information for purposes other than that for which it was originally intended, namely, patient care, is a matter for concern. When physicians use their records for research, education, and other purposes, they must be sure to obtain permission from the patients concerned. Physicians can avoid this problem by not identifying the patients when using the data.

Employment of Locum Physician, Salaried Employee, or Medical Student

Arranging with another physician to cover your practice when you are not available must be carefully discussed with your lawyer and the legal implications verified. Where a medical student or resident is assigned to a physician, the student's actions may lead to a malpractice suit. In this situation, the preceptor-physician is directly responsible for the student; he or she should therefore be absolutely certain that the student is adequately supervised so as to prevent a malpractice suit.

Ethical and Social Obligations

Social responsibility

Conflicts between ethical and social obligations cause the doctor great concern. (They are further discussed in the chapter "Ethics and Issues.") Such situations occur when the clinical obligations of the physician conflict with the law. Examples are reporting an alcoholic patient to the driving authority, reporting venereal disease (particularly when the spouse is unaware of such disease), and reporting trauma that involves obvious criminal activity. In some cases, the social obligations may supercede the ethical. In some jurisdictions, physicians are legally protected when they report possible child abuse; similarly, legal protection is often afforded physicians who report drug or alcohol abuse or a disease condition which leads to a restriction of the patient's driving or flying license.

Computer Record Legality

Abuses of computer-based records

Many microcomputer suppliers state that their computer equipment is self-contained and, therefore, confidentiality is kept. However, in the case of time-sharing computers, information is sent over a telephone line to a central facility where it is processed and stored; consequently, the risk of loss of confidentiality exists. Again, the law varies in its definition of what is accepted as a legal record in a computer-stored format. An advantage and at the same time a potential danger of computers is their capacity to link a variety of records. Computers can lead to many patient benefits but also to a great deal of harm. (See chapter 49.)

All of the issues outlined above may confront the family physician shortly after the beginning of practice. Legal action cannot always be avoided, but a knowledge of the kind of situations that may lead to a malpractice suit will forewarn the physician and hopefully reduce the possibility of this unfortunate occurrence.

REFERENCES

1 C. Redden, "Joining a Group Practice," *Canadian Family Physician*, **117**: 67–78, May 1971.

2 A. P. Somers, "Consumer Health Education: Where Are We? Where Are We Going?" *Canadian Journal of Public Health*, **68**:362–368, September and October 1977.

3 D. B. Shires, "Physician's Office Computers Are Here to Stay," *Modern Medicine of Canada*, **33**(10):1412–1415, October 1978.

4 J. Milsum, C. Laszlo, and P. Prince, "A Pilot Evaluation of Introducing Health Hazard Appraisal in a Community Health Centre Environment," *Proceedings of the Twelfth Annual Meeting of the Society of Prospective Medicine*, 1977, pp. 92–102.

5 *Physician's Management Manuals*, Physician's Management Publications, 315 Victoria Avenue, Westmount, Quebec H3Z 2N1, Canada, Fall 1978.

6 A. Cameron, W. Gillis, and D. Shires, "A Message from MARS," *Nova Scotia Medical Bulletin*, **52**(6):253–254, December 1973.

7 Systemics Inc., Princeton Air Research Park, P.O. Box 2000, Princeton, N.J. 08540.

8 Available from COR—College Office Record System, College of Family Physicians of Canada, 4000 Leslie Street, Toronto, Ontario, Canada.

9 *Financial Planning for Physicians*, M.D. Management Ltd., Ottawa, Ontario, Canada, 1980.

10 *Organization and Management of Family Practice*, American Academy of Family Practice, 1740 West 92d Street, Kansas City, MO, 1984.

11 G. Korneluk and R. McKnight, "Writing an Office Procedure Manual," *Canadian Doctor*, **43**(4):44–47, April 1977.

12 *FACMIS: Family and Ambulatory Care Medical Informatics System*, Department of Community and Family Medicine, University of Toronto, Toronto, Ontario, Canada, 1975.

13 M. Brennan and L. Spano, "The B.J.S. System: Recording and Retrieving Data for Family Medicine," *Canadian Family Physician*, **22**:1064–1074, 1976.

14 *E-Book*, College of Family Physicians of Canada, Toronto, Ontario, Canada, 1960.

Chapter 49

Computers in Practice

R. MacLachlan, M.D.

Many factors lead family physicians to consider computerizing some of their office functions. These factors have complex interrelationships, and they must be carefully analyzed to ensure that the physician has the desired benefits at an acceptable cost.

The successful practice of medicine depends to a great degree on one's ability to manage information.[1] The family physician must integrate core medical knowledge with the medical life histories of 2000 patients and then synthesize appropriate management plans which consider current therapeutic recommendations. All of this must be done quickly and in a manner that involves patients in their own care, allows for proper recording of the decision-making process for future reference, and includes adequate documentation for billing purposes. This data management task leads many family physicians to consider using a computer in their practice.[2]

FACILITATION

A number of developments in the past few decades have greatly facilitated the introduction of computers into practices. These include:

1   The standard codification of diseases and morbidity in primary care, e.g., ICD-9, RCGP, ICHPPC-2, OXMIS (see the glossary at the end of this chapter)
2   The problem-oriented medical record with its problem and medication lists
3   The evolution of medical and social insurance schemes with unique identifier numbers for identification of each individual
4   Fee-for-service medical insurance schemes which require the physician to provide patient's identification, demographic characteristics, diagnosis, and a summary of the type of care provided
5   The standard codification of drugs and other aspects of the process of care, e.g., AAHP, ICPC - Process

WHERE TO START?

Assess Current Data Handling

Perhaps the best way to start thinking about using a computer in practice is to review how data are being handled at present. Table 49-1 lists many of the types of data handling encountered in family practice. Consider each task:

1   Is it being done? By whom?
2   How long does it take? What would be the benefits of increased speed?
3   How repetitive is the task?
4   How accurate is the data handling? What are the consequences of an error?
5   If the task is not being done at present, how would it augment care or efficiency if it were done?

Office data tasks

Two points are worth remembering at this stage:

1   If a manual system works well, be cautious about replacement. ("If it works, don't fix it.") The appointment book is an example.
2   A computer cannot correct for faulty or missing information. ("Garbage in, garbage out.")

Set Priorities

At this stage, the physician or group needs to look at this analysis and set priorities. What benefits would accrue from improving or

Importance of benefits

Table 49-1   Data Management Tasks

1	Patient register	
2	Appointments	Scheduling care-givers Booking patients Lists
3	Accounting	Insurance liaison Third party Payroll, expenses, accounts receivable
4	Word processing	
5	Medical record	Problem and medication lists Summaries Accurate demographic information
6	Chronic problems	Age-sex and morbidity register
7	Recall system	
8	Access to data banks	Medline, Toxline
9	Morbidity analysis	Listing and rank ordering
10	Screening and periodic health assessment	Ability to interact with patient record and prompt care-giver at time of interview
11	Medication analysis	Including interactions and contraindications
12	Algorithms or flowcharts for patients	

initiating these tasks? How important are these benefits? If one result being sought is increased efficiency in seeing patients, would the time saved be productive for the physician? If a recall system produced a listing of those overdue for cervical smears, is it ethically acceptable in your jurisdiction to contact the patient? It is vital to include staff in this process. They may have different perceptions of the level of efficiency in the current data-handling processes, as well as estimates of the consequences of change.

LOOKING AT THE OPTIONS

Types of Systems

Investigating systems

Once you agree on the tasks to be considered for computerization and their relative importance, start investigating possible systems. There are essentially three types of systems to consider—"off-the-shelf" packages, commercial packages designed for medical practices, and custom-designed systems—although there is some overlap between these groupings. Each has specific advantages and disadvantages, some of which are listed in Table 49-2.

Table 49-2 Types of Systems

Advantages	Disadvantages
Off-the-shelf	
1 Readily available in computer and general stores.	1 Software rarely designed for medical purposes.
2 Least expensive.	2 Hardware may have limited memory; expansion may be expensive.
3 Wide variety of software available.	
4 Allows some self-programming.	3 Service may be poor or from a distance.
5 Familiarity for home computer users.	4 The computer language and operating system may restrict number of users and speed of the system.
	5 May require accreditation by insurance schemes.
Commercial medical package	
1 Designed specifically for medical practice.	1 Restrictions on individual modifications or expanded functions.
2 Probably meets the standards of third-party payers.	2 More expensive than off-the-shelf.
3 Staff training and full maintenance available.	3 Commits one to certain suppliers; makes user dependent on their commercial viability.
4 Allows collaboration with other users.	
Custom-designed system	
1 System will be limited only by group's ability to define tasks and finances.	1 The most expensive.
	2 Collaboration is more difficult.
2 Allows tailoring to the group's particular characteristics.	3 May require accreditation by insurance schemes.
	4 Long lead time.
	5 Dependent on programmer for ongoing support.

Suppliers of Systems

Several sources of information on specific systems should be available in your area. Start with your local medical society or organization—they frequently have working committees looking at computer applications in practice and may have evaluated and possibly accredited systems. Talk to colleagues, in particular those whose practice is most like yours and who have no vested interest in any particular system. National or regional bodies such as the Canadian College of Family Physicians or the American Academy of Family Physicians frequently publish reviews of system applications, and may list appropriate suppliers.[3] Computer shops should be ap-

Obtaining unbiased advice

Table 49-3   Sample Questions to Ask Potential Suppliers

1   How do we add a new physician to the system?
2   If the diagnostic or therapeutic coding schemes must be modified, how is this done?
3   How are changes in the fee schedule incorporated into the system?
4   If an insurance company (private or governmental) changes the format of its forms, how is the system modified to respond?
5   If a dependent is living with one parent but is covered under health insurance of the other parent, how does the system handle this?
6   How does the system distinguish between active and inactive patients, and how can the latter be deleted if desired?

proached with caution, since their prime motivation is usually the sale of hardware, whereas review of available software first, should be your top priority.

First the Software . . .

Software most important

Programs are critical. They determine what tasks can be computerized, how they are handled, how quickly they are carried out, and how many people can work on them at any one time. Before you approach any supplier, have a listing of the current and future tasks that you want done, an estimate of the number of users of the system (present and projected), and an estimate of the number of patient files to be stored. You should also have decided on a ceiling for net expenditure on any system over the next 3 to 5 years. Arrange for a demonstration of the prospective system with ample time allotted for you (and your office manager, if appropriate) to inspect the system. Prepare a list of questions in advance;[4] some suggested ones are in Table 49-3.

Input methods

In evaluating different systems, consider carefully who enters what information. In most cases, demographic and billing information is entered by reception staff, but the entry of diagnostic and therapeutic information varies, both in the way it is entered and by whom. Many systems are designed for the record to be reviewed after the patient's visit. Information is then extracted and entered into the computer, often with the help of an encounter sheet completed by the physician and attached to the chart. This does not require the physician to make the entries at the terminal, but may lead to duplication or triplication of recording and the chance of attendant errors.

Other systems allow for direct entry of data by the physician at the time of the patient's visit; this type of system plays an active role in patient care with screening and computer-aided diagnosis packages. It does, however, mean that a terminal must be in the consulting room, with resultant ramifications relating to confidentiality vs. information disclosure.

There is also considerable variation in the way data are entered. In order to get maximum benefit from the computer, it is best to incorporate standard classifications—e.g., of diagnoses, drugs, laboratory tests, recall intervals, and similar categories. This means that these must be coded, at least within the computer. If other colleagues will be using the system, the codes should be widely accepted. For example, viral upper respiratory infection, coryza, and cold should be stored as a single entity in the system. Some systems accept only the code (e.g., 460); others will accept the free text (e.g., "viral upper respiratory infection") and will then respond by displaying the corresponding code (460). A refinement of the latter system is a prompter; when only a few letters of the free text are entered (e.g., "upp"), all diagnoses beginning with these letters are displayed, and the physician can choose from the list. This can apply to the patients' names, addresses, diagnoses, drugs, or any of the lists stored in the computer.

Coding

No software is perfect; inevitably there will be bugs in the system. You should determine how many physicians currently use this particular package, how long they have been using it, and in what type of practices. The supplier should be prepared to explain software maintenance: Whom does one call if trouble arises? How quickly can one get help? What are the costs? Also, maintenance contracts should include provision for periodic upgrading of the programs to include new functions and improvements.

Correcting software errors

If the system is to be used for direct billing of health insurance plans (private or governmental), then you should determine whether your system is acceptable to them. They may also be able to provide information about the reliability of the system and confirm or deny the supplier's claims of increased efficiency in billing.

Billing software

. . . Then the Hardware

Once you know what data you have to manage, how you will manage it, and what software package (program and operating system) best suits your needs, start considering your hardware options. Specific considerations depend on the particular piece of equipment, but some general considerations apply in all cases:

1 Who supplies the equipment? Who services it, and how long does service take?
2 How stable and well known is the manufacturing company?
3 What warranty applies, and what maintenance contract is available?
4 What provision is there to expand or upgrade the equipment as needs or use increases?

VDU

Terminals   While there are a variety of means of entering the data, the most common by far is the video display unit (VDU), with its televisionlike screen and a keyboard or touch screen for data entry. Some things to consider are:

1   Size
2   Noisiness
3   Adjustable screen angle
4   Availability of color screen (green or amber to relieve eyestrain)
5   Programmable function keys for common tasks (these relieve repetitious keystrokes)
6   Graphics capability if desired

Requirements for storage

Computers as Storage Devices   Computers have undergone great technical advances in the last 5 years, and progress will continue to be rapid. Knowing some of the computer jargon is of some help (see glossary at end of chapter). The requirements for computer memory will vary widely with the size of the practice and the number of users, as well as the amount of storage required. The minimum memory for any but a single user system should be 256K bytes (1K byte = 1024 bytes), and storage should allow for 2000 to 4000 bytes per patient at the outset, as well as storage for the programs themselves, word-processing files, and the like. Storage devices include floppy disks, hard disks, and magnetic tape; for any practice with more than one doctor, storage on hard disk is at present the most popular option. For a five-doctor, 10,000-patient practice, the minimum storage is probably 20 to 25 megabytes (1 million bytes = 1 megabyte).[5] Some practices may need 5 to 10 times this amount,[6] depending on the size of the patient file stored. Be certain to consider:

Desirable characteristics

1   How fast is the system? For common functions, a 2- to 3-second delay in response should be the maximum allowed under full usage.
2   How is the system "backed up"? All systems have problems and stop working ("crash") at some time, and the information stored in a computer needs to be duplicated on a separate memory device; these are usually floppy disks or magnetic tape machines. How long does the backup take? Does it involve inserting a new floppy disk into the machine every few minutes?
3   How many terminals will the system support?
4   Can the terminals switch from one task (word processing) to another (checking in a patient) without signing off the first task?
5   What other operating system and software will run on the system?
6   How much noise does the computer produce?

Printers   There are two general types of printers, which are beginning to overlap each other. Dot-matrix printers print characters by putting a series of dots on the page. Depending on the number of dots per character, these can approximate the appearance of a typewritten character, particularly if the letters with tails go below the line (*descenders*). They have the advantage of being relatively inexpensive and extremely fast, and are frequently used for lists, reports, and prescriptions.

Letter-quality printers produce type, like a carbon-ribbon typewriter, with well-defined characters. They are slower and significantly more expensive than dot-matrix printers and are best suited to producing letters, formal reports, and articles for publication.

Types of printers

Recently introduced laser-jet printers are very fast but probably out of the price range of the average doctor's office system.

Some pointers in reviewing printers:

1   How noisy are they, and what silencing devices are available?

2   How easily is the ribbon changed?

3   What graphics capabilities are there (if desired)?

4   How easily is the paper changed? This is of vital importance if one is doing multiple functions with the printer, such as insurance forms, letters, appointment list, and prescriptions.

What to look for

5   How is the paper fed? Unless the printer has the small cogs on either side of the paper roll (*tractor feed*), it is very difficult to keep the paper aligned for more than one sheet.

6   Does the printer have print buffers?

Modems   You will need a modem if you communicate with other computers over telephone lines. Most computers allow for the type of modem which lets a telephone handset be connected easily; the key specification here is an RS 232 port. This allows for connecting with large data banks such as Medline (the medical literature research service), Toxline (a drug information data base), and other service bureaus. If you are communicating with a central computer over dedicated phone lines, you will need a high-speed modem; your hardware supplier should be able to provide specifications.

Communicating with information data banks

Before any final decisions are made, it is wise to visit a practice of similar size using the same hardware and software that you think you may buy. This can be one of the most useful parts of the decision-making process.

COSTS

These will vary directly with your decisions made about tasks to be performed, number of users, and number of patient files. Be cautious about any claims that the computer will actually make money for the practice. It may indeed do so, but the profit will be small. Computers can save you money by:

Advantages

1   Increasing efficiency of billing, both insurance and private
2   Reducing time before reimbursement from third-party payers
3   Increasing returns from services based on recall system (where allowed)
4   Increasing efficiency in appointment booking and patient flow
5   Increasing staff efficiency

Note that for the last two to save money, the time saved must be put into financially productive activity or result in reduced staff costs. There are, of course, many nonfinancial benefits of office computers.[7] It is difficult or impossible to assign fixed values to these, but it is these benefits that will be the deciding factor for most family physicians.

Some general principles apply when reviewing proposed costs:

Considerations in estimating costs

1   Accept from the outset the eventual obsolescence of the hardware; a 3- to 5-year life span is common.
2   Include estimates of annual hardware and software maintenance; 15 to 20 percent of purchase price is normal.
3   Once the computer is installed, other uses and users will come forward. Consider expansion possibilities and costs at the outset.
4   Computers are fussy about their electrical source. Be certain that installation costs include both electrical and communication wiring, and consider a device that protects against voltage surges.
5   Installation may necessitate new desks, chairs, and even lighting (see "Installation" below).
6   Include full insurance of the hardware in annual ongoing costs.
7   The cheapest buy is rarely the best buy; purchase in circumstances that assure ready service.
8   Consider leasing, and investigate tax allowances and depreciation carefully; these frequently differ for hardware and software. Corroborate claims of suppliers with advice from your accountant.
9   Be certain to determine who pays for staff training.

It is prudent to put a ceiling on costs before getting into discussions with suppliers. A figure of 10 percent of annual gross earnings of the group might be a reasonable starting point, although significantly higher levels have been advocated.[4]

INTRODUCTION OF SYSTEMS TO THE OFFICE

It is wrong to believe that once the system is ordered the work is nearly over. In reality, successful introduction of the system requires careful planning and close monitoring.

Staff Training

Seasoned users invariably say that investing time and money in training all users to use the system pays the greatest dividends. If you have purchased a system from a medical supplier, these expenses may be included in purchase or lease costs; in other cases they must be paid out of your own budget.

Staff training is good investment

1 If at all possible, have the training sessions away from the office to ensure that participants are not disturbed.

2 Organize a schedule to ensure that office functions are maintained during training sessions.

Points to keep in mind

3 After familiarization sessions, have staff use actual office sources of information (records, invoices, insurance claims forms) even if these are fictitious.

4 If possible, include refresher sessions after several weeks of use in the office.

5 There are eight ways to insert a floppy disk; only one is correct.

A complete manual, written in plain language, is mandatory. A telephone contact procedure ("hot line") to the supplier is ideal.

Installation

Give detailed consideration to the work environment long before putting a terminal on a desk and plugging it in. There are now specific guidelines for VDU usage[8] and these are summarized in Table 49-4. Adjustable seating, lighting, and desk height are vital for any but infrequent users.

Ergonomics important

Consider carefully the flow of people and paper within the office. This particularly applies to the terminals and the printer. Injudicious decisions here can lead to miles of extra walking for staff each week in a busy office.

Computers are particular about their environment. At all costs,

Table 49-4   Recommendations For Users of Video Display Units

1   The workstation and devices should allow flexible adjustment of:
   a   Keyboard and screen height.
   b   Screen brightness and contrast.
   c   Leg room and viewing distance.
   d   Workstation illumination.
   e   Chair height, backrest support and height, and armrests.
2   Screen glare should be controlled by:
   a   Drapes or blinds to limit direct sunlight.
   b   Proper positioning in relation to lighting fixtures.
   c   Nonglare screen or screen shield.
   d   Amber or green screens may assist in reducing eyestrain.
3   There should be mandatory rest periods of 15 minutes every 2 hours under moderate visual demands and 10 minutes every hour under high visual demands.
4   Initial complete visual testing of frequent users, and yearly rechecks.

avoid installation in a carpeted room, as static electricity is a common cause of systems' "crashing." Stable ambient temperature, little dust, and no movement are also vital for problem-free operations. Have a fireproof storage container nearby for the backup disks or tapes, but do not have the computer directly under a fire-protection sprinkler outlet.

Start-Up

Careful planning

Various approaches to the actual start-up of operations have been used, and all have been successful when properly planned. The most critical factor is likely to be the type of demographic filing system already in operation; if there is a good existing patient or age-sex register, one can then enter information and create the patient file efficiently. Essentially the two options are:

Options for data entry

1   Enter each patient's registration information as he or she comes in for an appointment. This has the advantage of entering current (and more accurate) information and reduces or diffuses demand on staff.
OR—
2   Enter patient data in batches before or at the start-up of the system. This gives you a full register more quickly but costs staff time and may increase errors. The latter can be eliminated by checking demographic data when a patient comes in for an appointment.

Step-wise installation

Regardless of the type of system chosen, it may be wise to implement the various functions of the system at different times over the first year of operation. Creating the individual files with demographic information only can take several months for a large practice,[9] and only after they are in place can appointment scheduling, morbidity coding, and some forms of billing function efficiently. The corollary of this is to keep manual systems in operation until you are *entirely* satisfied with the function of the system *and* the security of its backup.

THE HUMAN ASPECTS OF COMPUTING

Several issues are frequently overlooked by practices planning computer installations. These relate to the real or perceived effects of the computer on the physician and patient involved.

The Patient

1 Confidentiality: Patients are naturally apprehensive about who has access to their information. A computer not connected to a phone line is much more confidential than a medical record legibly written, on a shelf, but patients may not be aware of this.

2 Who is making the decisions? The computer represents an intrusion into the doctor-patient relationship, and patients need to understand its role.

Make an information sheet on the computer system available for patients to read in the waiting room; this may greatly alleviate these concerns. | Information sheet for patients

The Office Staff

1 Radiation hazards: Current terminals have been declared to pose negligible radiation hazards.[8] It is vital to have a contingency plan available when a staff member becomes pregnant and is understandably concerned. | Radiation from VDU

2 Overuse syndrome: A growing body of research links prolonged work at a VDU with specific consequences.[8,10] These include eyestrain and painful and/or stiff neck, shoulders, forearms, or wrists. Prevent or reduce these by attention to the guidelines in Table 49-4.

The Physician

The impact of the system on the physician's modus operandi will vary greatly with the type of system chosen.

1 Behavioral change: The presence of the computer will demand organizational concessions within the practice.[11] The physician will be reminded to do things, and this represents a shift in locus of control. | Organizational concessions

Patient-doctor
relationship

2 Alteration of patient-doctor relationship: The medical interview represents a delicate balance of the art and science of medicine, constantly testing the physician's interpersonal skills. The intrusion of a bulky VDU and interruptions to enter data may affect this relationship.

PROSPECTS FOR THE FUTURE

The increasing involvement of computers in the practice of family medicine in the future is not in question. Metcalfe describes three phases through which computers are likely to evolve:[12]

1 The cross-indexing system: This is the level of operation of most current systems; it allows for selection of specified demographic and diagnostic characteristics, while maintaining the traditional medical record in its current forms. The system can facilitate administration, preventive medicine, medical audit, and research.

2 The narrative record: Systems will only effectively manage the complete contents of the record if their contents are standardized and organized, and if the physician allows the system to participate actively in patient care through prompts and cues. This potential has yet to be fully exploited.

Artificial
intelligence

3 The decision aid: Rapid growth in the fields of artificial intelligence and "expert" systems would strongly suggest that computers could have active involvement in the decision-making processes of primary care. Given the great diversity of problems presenting in primary care and the delicate nature of the patient-doctor relationship, this may not occur until well into the future for all but certain specified common conditions.

GLOSSARY

AAHP: American Association of Hospital Pharmacists.

Backup: A means of storing a copy of important files and programs, usually on floppy disks or magnetic tape. Keep in a fireproof cabinet.

Byte: A character representation or a functional grouping of bits (binary digits). Early models had 8 bits to the byte; now, 16 or 32 bits to the byte are the norm.

CPU: The central processing unit (CPU) is the brain of the computer, the particular arrangement of circuits where the data are actually manipulated.

Disk: Soft or floppy disks are flexible, flat, plastic storage devices, commonly with a diameter of 5.25 or 8 in; newer ones are smaller. Hard or Winchester disks are rigid flat devices, often stacked on each other and sealed from the elements. Both are used for data storage. Hard disks hold 10 to 100 times the information stored on floppy disks.

File: Analogous to a medical record—a collection of specific pieces of information, usually with a particular relationship, stored in a particular place.

Hardware: Physical equipment in a system.

ICD 9: International Classification of Disease, Version 9.

ICHPPC-2: International Classification of Health Problems in Primary Care, Version 2.

ICPC Process: International Classification of Primary Care, Process code.

Interface: The connections between physical pieces of equipment.

Memory: The amount of information stored by the computer without having to refer to the storage device.

Modem: A piece of equipment that translates computer signals into a form that can be transmitted or received via a telephone line.

Operating system: The specific programs designed to manage the whole spectrum of operations of the computer.

OXMIS: Oxford Medical Information System Code.

RCGP: Royal College of General Practitioners (U.K.) Code.

Software: The programs that tell the computer to perform the required operations in a specific sequence.

VDU: Video display unit, the televisionlike screen, usually with a keyboard, a small pointing device (mouse), or a special touch-screen, for data entry.

REFERENCES

1 D. Levinson, "Information, Computers and Clinical Practice," *Journal of the American Medical Association,* **249:**607, 1983.

2 G. Schmittling, "Computer Use by Family Physicians in the United States," *Journal of Family Practice,* **19**(1):93, 1984.

3 R. MacLachlan, "Practising with a Computer," *Nova Scotia Medical Bulletin,* **62:**145, 1983.

4 J. Rodnick, "Evaluating Feasibility and Selection of Computers in Family Medicine," *Journal of Family Practice,* **19**(1):86, 1984.

5 M. Salkind, "General Practice: Hardware and Software," *British Medical Journal,* **287:**106, 1983.

6 M. Petreman, "Introducing the Computer to Family Practice," *Canadian Family Physician,* **30:**847, 1984.

7 D. Shires, "Can a Computer Save You Money in Your Practice?" *Canadian Family Physician,* **30:**859, 1984.

8 "Working with Video Display Terminals: A Preliminary Health Risk Evaluation," *Morbidity and Mortality Weekly Review,* June 27, 1980, pp. 307–308.

9 M. Salkind, "Implementing a System in General Practice," *British Medical Journal,* **287:**199, 1983.

10 L. Ritchie, "Computers in General Practice: A Review of the Current Situation," *Health Bulletin,* **40**(5):248, 1982.

11 H. Janson, "Will Computers Dehumanize Medical Care and Education?" *Journal of Family Practice,* **18**(4):525, 1984.

12 D. Metcalfe, "The Computer in General Practice," *Journal of Medical Engineering and Technology,* **8**(2):53, 1984.

SUGGESTED FURTHER READING

Bear, J., *Computer Wimp,* Hutchinson & Co., London, 1984. Excellent reading for the skeptical computer neophyte.

Canadian Family Physician, April 30, 1984. Majority of issue is devoted to computers in family practice.

Computers in Primary Care, Occasional Paper 13, Royal College of General Practitioners, 1982.

Journal of Family Practice, **19**(1), 1984. Entire issue is devoted to computers in family practice.

Ritchie, L., *Computers in Primary Care,* William Heineman Medical Books, London, 1984.

Part Eight

The Complete Approach

Chapter 50

Ethics and Issues

S. Sherwin, Ph.D.

Moral and ethical questions present daily problems for the family physician. How might the family physician approach such problems? Principles and models for guidance exist to assist the physician in recognizing and clarifying the ethical components of care.

This chapter attempts to identify the ethical principles applicable to family practice. Practical clinical examples and theoretical models provide family physicians with insights to help them make choices among competing values.

Medical ethics is concerned with the questions of moral value that arise in medical practice; questions of moral value are those involving such terms as "right," "wrong," "good," "bad," and "ought." Sometimes a situation creates a conflict between moral values, so that one value must be pursued at the expense of another; for example, a professional desire to use the most medically effective techniques may occasionally be incompatible with a desire to deal honestly with a patient who resists such treatment. The purpose of medical ethics is to develop a framework for resolving such problems as they arise in medical contexts.

Some clinical examples will help make these definitions more meaningful.

Using medical ethics

Clinical Example 1: An 84-year-old man with advanced lung cancer arrives at your clinic from a remote and isolated community. He has never been away from his home community before and is worried about his wife, home, garden, and the chickens he cares for.

The best medical treatment would appear to be chemotherapy given at regular intervals with close monitoring, but for that he would have to stay in the hospital area, away from his family. He prefers to go home without treatment. As the resident in charge, what should you do?

Clinical Example 2: A 28-year-old woman arrives at the hospital in the early evening with a compound fracture of the arm and various lacerations that resulted from a vicious beating by her husband. The arm is set by Dr. Jones, who prescribes a nonnarcotic painkiller. At 3:30 a.m. the patient regains consciousness. She is howling with pain and the nurse has summoned you as the resident in charge.

You have potent painkillers at your disposal, but you know Dr. Jones strongly opposes the use of narcotics as a dangerous crutch, likely to do patients more harm than good in the long run. Also, you suspect that the patient's emotional trauma might make her particularly susceptible to developing a drug dependency. Still, she is suffering greatly and pleads with you to help reduce the pain. What ought you to do?

Clinical Example 3: A young couple arrives at your office with their 3-year-old son, their only offspring, who is suffering from fever and respiratory infection. The child is very uncomfortable and quite irritable. The parents, who are worried and rather irritable themselves, demand a prescription for an antibiotic. You are certain the disease is a result of a virus and that an antibiotic will have no pharmacological benefit; however, it may help reduce the parents' anxiety. The parents are very insistent. What should you do?

Clinical Example 4: The 15-year-old son of a family you have been treating for 7 years has been suffering from chronic renal failure for the last year and a half. He tolerates dialysis poorly. A transplant was performed with the kidney of his older sister, but the kidney failed within a month. The family is under a great deal of stress. The mother has developed hypertension, and the sister who donated the kidney is suffering from depression that seems tied to a sense of guilt for the kidney's failure. The three younger children are being somewhat neglected and are frightened by the anxiety they perceive in the older members of the family. The patient is a very mature, reflective teenager. He and his parents have discussed his poor prognosis and the misery each day brings, and together they have decided to stop dialysis. The dialysis unit staff is horrified and have called upon you to use your influence to convince the family to continue treatment. You know that the boy's chances of recovery are remote. What should you do?

All these cases are examples of ethical dilemmas in medicine. They require that decisions be made by trained physicians on the basis of technical medical facts. But they also involve an appeal to *values* and hence require a different sort of expertise as well. The physician involved must choose between alternative courses of action, and the final choice must reflect not only knowledge of facts but also a certain ordering of values.

Value
judgment

In example 1, a choice must be made between (*a*) allowing the patient to return home as he prefers and (*b*) trying to keep him in the hospital for chemotherapy in the hope of lengthening his life span by several months. The former would be the choice of one who values the individual's freedom and believes that the quality of the remaining time is more important than the quantity; the latter would be the choice of one who values extending life whenever possible. It is, of course, possible that other, less drastic options exist. A more limited program of chemotherapy might be manageable if visiting nursing care could be arranged or the patient's wife could be persuaded to move to the city for the duration of the treatment. The desirability of any of these options has to be determined by a choice between the values which each one represents. The "best" choice is the one that is most nearly consistent with the most significant of the competing values (length of life, quality of life, freedom) or with some combination of those values.

The dilemma
of choice

In example 2, if you prescribe a powerful narcotic, you do so presumably because you feel that it is right to relieve suffering when medicine provides the means to do so and because you are convinced that the use of addictive drugs in crisis situations need not result in serious addiction problems. If, on the other hand, you are inclined not to use a more powerful drug, you probably share Dr. Jones's worry about the dangers of such drugs and you may believe that the risks in such cases outweigh the benefits. Presumably, you believe that it is better to suffer a specific pain over a clearly limited time than to risk the potentially uncontrolled suffering that a drug dependency could unleash. These alternatives are based on competing values.

Competing
commitments

It is also possible that you might prefer not to change the medication because you believe that such decisions should be made by the physician in charge of the case and that one should overrule a colleague's order only in life-threatening situations. If this is the case, the operative value is a commitment to a certain norm of medical practice, a belief that medicine can best fulfill its purpose by allowing individual physicians the greatest autonomy in deciding on treatment for their patients. You might also refrain from changing the prescription because you believe that a policy which allows physicians to undermine one another's decisions by changing prescriptions when the patient's life or long-term health is not in dan-

Acting for
another
physician

ger would be less effective than a policy that prohibited such interference. This viewpoint represents a commitment to the value of effective health care delivery.

Freedom or what is best

Understanding of the patient

In examples 3 and 4, you must choose between allowing the patient (or the patient's representatives, i.e., the parents) to choose the treatment, and hence the ultimate result, and reserving the decision for yourself. The choice is between the parents' freedom to decide what is to happen to their child and your conviction about what is best for the patient's health. There are, however, some important differences between the two cases. Clearly, they differ in the severity of the consequences; but also there is a difference in the validity of the decision-making process. In example 3, the parents are deciding in ignorance and on the basis of mistaken beliefs. Their choice is not compatible with their own overall values (the child's health) because they misunderstand the facts and are ignorant about the effects of antibiotics. In example 4, the family have the information necessary for making a responsible decision. They know that discontinuing dialysis will result in the boy's death. Moreover, the patient himself is also involved in the decision making. In this case, there is a genuine difference in values, not knowledge, between the family and the health professionals: the staff think any life is better than none; the family finds death preferable to the quality of life available to the boy.

In all of these cases, and in a great many other clinical situations, physicians are called on to make decisions that involve values as well as facts. Whenever a decision appeals to what is good or bad (or right or wrong, or to what should or should not be done), it is an ethical as well as a medical decision. A strategy for resolving ethical dilemmas is included in Table 50-1.

What ought to happen

Ethics (also known as *moral theory*) is the study of how people *ought* to behave. It is concerned with identifying principles for action (norms) that will guide a person's behavior in accordance with those matters held to be of most fundamental value. The discipline of ethics differs, then, from the social sciences, which investigate how people do in fact behave, and from the law, which determines how people are permitted to behave in particular circumstances.

Table 50-1   Strategy for Resolving Ethical Dilemmas

1   Consider the possible courses of action.
2   Try to determine the outcome of each, and the likelihood of each possible outcome.
3   Consider what values each option meets and what values each conflicts with.
4   Choose the option most desirable in terms of values maintained.

Ethicists (moral theorists) are interested in understanding what we value most fundamentally and how our value scheme can best be put into practice. Ultimately, ethical studies are concerned with determining the values that *should* be preserved, promoted, or encouraged by a particular society (e.g., happiness).

Although we make ethical value judgments all the time, we are often unaware of it, since most of our judgments pose no conflict. For instance, we recognize intuitively that it is wrong to keep slaves or to hurt someone gratuitously, and that it is wrong to murder and right to be truthful. When faced with a choice between keeping and breaking a promise, we believe that we should keep it. When our moral obligations are clear to us, we feel that we should act in accordance with them. In most ordinary situations, we find that we do not need to spend time in ethical analysis.

Most moral decisions are straightforward

There are, however, some circumstances in which we are not certain what we are morally required to do; that is, we do not know what is the right thing to do. Sometimes one's own moral principles are in conflict. Consider, for instance, the following case:

Conflicts between principles

> *Clinical Example 5:* Sam Brown, 53, has been home for 3 weeks, recovering from extensive abdominal surgery. After the surgery, he complained steadily of pain, and morphine was prescribed in the hospital; he was given additional medication when he left the hospital. Dr. Green has been his physician for several years, and she knows that he tends to worry excessively about discomfort. He is now asking her for more painkillers and some agent to help him sleep. The doctor is worried about his developing a drug dependency and thinks there is no longer a clear physiological need for medication. But she also knows him well enough to predict that he will be unhappy and even frantic if not given a prescription. She is inclined to prescribe a very mild anxiolytic, which she expects to be useful primarily for its placebo effect.

In this case, the physician is torn between two moral values. She is inclined to prescribe the placebo because she thinks it is the least dangerous method of relieving Mr. Brown's suffering and she believes she should always try to relieve suffering when this can be done without harm. However, in prescribing the placebo, she is not being fully honest with Mr. Brown, since she is encouraging him to believe that he is receiving a powerful chemical agent that can control his distressing symptoms. In our society, there is a moral imperative against acting deceitfully. Dr. Green has to make a choice between the conflicting principles of reducing suffering, on the one hand, and behaving honestly, on the other, and it seems that at least one principle must be violated. Which value takes priority in such a case? How are such issues to be resolved?

Priority of values

To answer these ethical questions, we must consider what fundamental values underlie our various concerns and competing moral principles. We will be able to choose between conflicting values only if we can determine how these are organized and ordered, which are basic and which derivative, and which have the highest priority. From such an analysis we can develop a procedure for making moral choices in the complex cases in which our intuition fails us.

THE NATURE OF A MORAL JUDGMENT

Approaching complex moral decisions

One can judge the validity of any set of moral guidelines only by appeal to ethical theory, just as one can judge the appropriateness of treatment of a disease only by appeal to physiological theory. An understanding of underlying principles and values will help to settle doubtful cases. Moral theory is important to ethical behavior in much the same way as immunologic theory is important to the practice of medicine or statistical theory to the study of science.

The Need for a Theoretical Approach

It is necessary to emphasize that a theoretical approach to ethics is required, i.e., an approach that involves a comprehensive and consistent set of ethical principles according to which all kinds of ethical problems can be evaluated. Only by such an approach can we deal consistently with specific problems and reduce the probability of reliance on subjective judgments.

Generalizing

We must first consider how we are to characterize a moral theory, i.e., what criteria it must meet to be acceptable. Moral duties and rights are derived from general principles that can be applied uniformly. For example, if it is wrong to lie, it is wrong for anyone to lie, however strongly one wishes to do so. According to this universal criterion, an action is right only if it would be right for anyone to perform it under the same conditions, and wrong only if it would be wrong for anyone to perform it under the same conditions.

Treat Similar Cases Similarly

Exception to rule

Exceptions to moral rules must also be *universal.* Thus we arrive at the basic ethical tenet to *treat similar cases similarly.* Whenever we decide we ought to override an ethical principle because we recognize that an exception to the rule is called for in a particular case, we must do so in terms of the special features of that case that we consider to be ethically relevant, features which in themselves will be grounds for exception in other cases. We may, for instance, believe that we are obliged to obtain informed consent from patients

Table 50-2   Definition of a Moral Theory

A moral theory is a comprehensive set of principles explaining and guiding our specific moral views. The principles in any moral theory should ensure:

1 Universality (appropriate for everyone)
2 Ability to reflect relevant similarities and differences
3 Consistency (not involving contradictory directions)
4 Completeness

before treating them, and yet feel that this requirement should be overlooked in dealing with irrational patients. This view can be defended by an argument showing that informed consent is only meaningful when obtained from rational agents. It would then be valid to conclude that exceptions to the informed consent requirements are always appropriate under conditions of irrationality. Hence, we must also be willing to give up our own right to provide informed consent in circumstances when we ourselves are judged to be irrational. This standard of generality or universality is often taken to constitute the moral point of view, since it requires us to evaluate actions from an objective position of fairness rather than from one of self-interest.

Consistency and Completeness

A moral theory must also be *consistent*. (For a definition of a moral theory, see Table 50-2.) If a theory contains principles that might prescribe contradictory actions under some circumstances, then it should probably also contain a principle deciding which action takes priority in such cases.

Ideally, the theory should also be *complete*; that is, it should provide direction for every sort of ethical problem that might arise. No satisfactory moral theory has been developed that is complete, so we cannot insist on this requirement. We can, however, reject a theory as too narrow if it cannot handle a major proportion of ethical problems.

Consistency

Completeness

SOME MORALLY SIGNIFICANT VALUES

For practical purposes, most moral theorists specify what is of fundamental value and then guide moral decisions by weighing the value of the outcomes of the various options and also taking account of the probability of each outcome. Theories of morals are distinguished by differences in their proposals of what is of value or worth. Claims of superiority cannot be substantiated by empirical methods, since any such test would presuppose that some ordering of the values has already been made. Each person, as a

Significance

moral agent, must finally decide on his or her own value scheme. This decision requires reflection on many complex kinds of situations, evaluating the consequences of different alternatives. Fortunately, upon reflection most people agree on what values are most important and differ only in their order of priority, so that the task of choosing a value scheme is not altogether idiosyncratic.

Examples of various moral theories will help clarify and organize one's own value scheme. Very briefly, five major theories exist, which take account of the most commonly held values.

Human well-being

1 A prominent theory, that of *utilitarianism*, considers *human well-being* to be the primary value. Although it is difficult to define "human well-being" precisely, utilitarians focus on such factors as happiness and pleasure and pain. They are concerned with what is good for a person, i.e., what is in each person's best interest, but not to the exclusion of the good of others. The basic moral principle of utilitarianism is that one should try to determine how one's actions will affect all concerned and, in the light of such deliberations, one should pick the action that will result in the most happiness and least overall suffering.

Freedom

2 For most moral theorists *freedom* is an important value to be considered in any case where it is at stake. Theories that rank freedom ahead of all other values are called *libertarian*.

Fairness

3 *Fairness* is another important moral value. Fairness, or respecting an individual's right to be treated as an equal, is important in theories concerned with questions of justice as the matter of prime importance. Such theories are generally known as *egalitarian*.

Respect for the individual

4 Many theorists argue that the ultimate concern is *respect for the individual*. To treat persons with respect requires that they are not treated as things; their interests must be considered in any interaction. This principle is sometimes formulated as an obligation never to treat persons merely as means or objects to be used in pursuit of someone else's goals, but always as ends in themselves, valuable in their own right, and with interests and goals of their own. Those who hold that persons are of fundamental value strongly oppose the use of people as experimental subjects without their fully voluntary, informed consent; they feel that using people without consent, even for a very noble purpose, is treating them as mere means.

Sanctity of life

5 *Sanctity of life* or sanctity of *human* life is often cited as a key value. Although sanctity of life is often viewed as an absolute value, few people who make this claim are consistent about it. Everyone recognizes the need to take life continually. Some people object to the killing of "higher" forms of life, especially mammals, but no one opposes all killing of plants, fungi, bacteria, etc. We are not therefore committed to sustaining all life for its own sake. Rather, it seems, we believe *human* life is particularly valuable. But such a conclusion calls for further analysis. What sense of "human" is significant—the biological, genetic, behavioral, or moral? Is it really human *life* we value, or is it the *person* whose life is at stake? If the latter, perhaps the fourth value (the individual) would suffice. If the former, which value takes priority—the person's life or his or her interests—if he or she chooses to discontinue lifesaving treatment?

It is always appropriate to investigate the foundations on which any value rests. If any of the values cited can be seen to derive from some other value, understanding this can help us resolve apparent conflicts between them.

Other commonly held values such as health, honesty, privacy, and altruism can be shown to be desirable in terms of one or more of the fundamental values on our list. As derivative values, they can be reduced to their more fundamental components for guidance in situations of conflict.

Other standard ethical values

These, then, are the fundamental values that underlie the moral view of most reflective people and help to guide our decisions in particular situations, such as those illustrated in the clinical examples above. To resolve particular dilemmas, it is usually best to list one's options, try to determine the likely outcomes of each, and consider which option produces an outcome most compatible with one's overall value scheme.

AVOIDING PATERNALISM

An understanding of ethical theory helps in understanding the moral difficulty with the common medical habit of paternalism. *Paternalism* is the term ethicists use for the practice of making decisions and taking actions on another person's behalf but without that person's consent. The freedom of the person affected is lost in such cases, and that is undesirable from a moral point of view even though the paternalistic agent is concerned with the other person's welfare. Paternalism is also objectionable because people sometimes have conceptions of their own interests that differ from those held by others; thus paternalism may result in reduced well-being from the affected party's point of view. Let's look at some dramatic cases.

Paternalism deprives the patient of consent

> *Clinical Example 6:* A Jehovah's Witness is thought to be very likely to die without a blood transfusion. The patient presumably does not want to die, but blood transfusions are prohibited by his religion. If the physician does not share this religious belief, she will think it in the patient's best interest to be transfused and to live. But the patient, though he wants to live, thinks it even more important to follow his religious scruples.

Rational patient's judgment should prevail

Patient and physician weigh the two competing goods differently in this instance, and the final evaluation as to which is the best outcome requires a value judgment. If the patient is generally rational (or was when he made the decision to resist transfusion at all cost), there is no ground for assuming that one judgment is necessarily more "right" than another. Thus, even though it runs counter to her estimation of the patient's welfare, if freedom is highly valued, then the physician ought to respect the patient's judgment and allow him the freedom to make his own choice.

> *Clinical Example 7:* A patient is diagnosed as having breast cancer. Her physician thinks radical mastectomy is the most reliable treatment for the type of tumor she has, but the patient has a genuine horror of mutilation. She has read of promising results with radiation treatments for tumors like hers and would prefer such treatment to surgery.

Helping the patient choose well

Who is to decide? A choice must be made between the alternatives, and it must reflect a balance between the success rates of the surgery and its potentially negative effects. The severity of such effects should be weighed according to the patient's values. Some people consider mutilation a much more serious evil than others. Some are seriously troubled by the effects of radiation and general sense of illness, while others prefer the constant feeling of sickness to the terrifying drama of surgery. Many things can affect a person's estimate of what is the lesser evil. Respect for personal autonomy directs us to leave the choice to the patient. The physician's role is to help the patient to choose well according to the patient's own values.

Paternalism is condescending

A paternalistic physician would administer the transfusion to the first patient and insist that the second patient receive radical surgery in the well-meaning belief that those treatments are in the patients' best interests. Indeed a sensitive person who shared the physician's evaluation of the facts might be tempted to do likewise. But paternalism is generally wrong because it ignores the importance of individual autonomy and does not treat people with the respect they deserve. Assuming oneself to be a better judge of a person's values (not health) than he or she is leads to condescending behavior which does not grant a person full human dignity. Furthermore, paternalism is usually a poor way to maximize the well-being of the individual patient. People differ in their estimation of what is valuable to them, and when they are allowed to make their own decisions in matters that primarily affect themselves, the most overall satisfaction is achieved. Hence, the first four moral theories we reviewed tend to reject paternalism in most circumstances.

Paternalism is not always wrong, however. It is wrong when it violates autonomy, but individuals are not always capable of autonomy. Autonomy implies the ability to make choices, which in turn requires a measure of rationality. Young children, severely retarded persons, seriously senile adults, and others suffering from various afflictions are virtually incapable of making rational decisions. Older children, the moderately retarded, many persons dubbed "mentally ill" but still functioning, and others are capable of making important decisions in some areas but probably not all. Some measure of paternalism is not only permissible but obligatory in dealing with such individuals. The degree of paternalism appropriate will vary with the degree of autonomy the patient is able to exercise.

Sometimes paternalism is necessary

Thus paternalism, while generally ill-advised, is sometimes in order. When we decide to exercise it, we are morally required to justify our action. We must show either that it is not a restriction on autonomy or that it is respecting a higher level of autonomy. For example, individuals may foresee that their powers will be limited at some point and request that their wishes be ignored under the anticipated circumstances (perhaps under the influence of a mood-affecting drug). Such consensual paternalism is acceptable. Paternalism is also justifiable when an individual is *unreasonably* risking life or capacity under some *temporary* influence and we seek to protect that individual from an unreasonable and dangerous action.

Paternalism must be justified

In determining whether or not paternalism is justified in particular circumstances, one must ask whether any reasonably rational individual would consent to relinquishing self-determination if affected by those circumstances. Paternalistic action is justifiable only if we ourselves would consent to relinquishing autonomy under similar circumstances. Note that the circumstances are to be similar and not necessarily identical: in the Jehovah's Witness example, we need not imagine ourselves in need of a blood transfusion, but in a position of being forced to do something very much against our religious beliefs.

General rule for paternalism

There are two aspects of paternalism that ought to be kept distinct; the first is *deciding* what is in another person's best interest, and the second is *acting* against that person's will on the basis of that decision. It is only when we are acting against a person's will that we may be violating that person's autonomy and acting wrongly. We cannot avoid making judgments about what is in a person's interests. But we should consider the individual's personal circumstances and values in making those judgments, recognizing that reasonable people disagree about questions of value.

Deciding is not acting

If we suspect that a patient might benefit from discussing a subject which he or she has not voluntarily raised, e.g., sex, death,

Table 50-3   Paternalism

Paternalism is acting from one's own evaluation of another person's interests without that person's consent. It is *wrong, unless* there is good evidence to believe that:

1   The person is incapable of judging his or her own interests adequately at the time.
2   If the person were able to do so, he or she would agree with the decision taken.

or progressive physical disability, it is not being paternalistic to suggest or invite such discussion. It would be paternalistic, however, to force the patient to listen to long lectures on the topic if the patient insisted that he or she did not wish to discuss it. It would also be paternalistic to decide that such a conversation could only harm the patient and effectively ignore all the openings he or she might offer. (Many doctors are skillful at ensuring that unpleasant subjects like death never come up, even with terminally ill patients.) Compassion requires us to be sensitive and responsive to a patient's needs whether the patient states them or not, while respect for autonomy requires us to watch that we do not force any action on a resolutely unwilling patient. (See Table 50-3.)

INFORMED CONSENT

A guarantee of the patient's autonomy

It is for reasons of autonomy that *informed consent* is such a significant procedure in medical contexts. The legal requirement of a signed official consent form is intended as a tool for ensuring respect for patient autonomy. The contractual model tells us that patients are to be given control over significant decisions affecting their own lives. Obtaining informed consent is an important guarantee that patients are being allowed that control. Unfortunately, since it is often viewed merely as a legal procedure, informed consent is not always effective in achieving its ethically motivated purpose; many patients sign informed consent forms without understanding them, and others, when presented with a legal-looking document, suddenly hesitate and waste valuable time questioning a procedure they have already agreed to. Informed consent is intended to protect the patient's right to decide important questions concerning his or her case. It is therefore the best way to protect the general values of autonomy, well-being, and probably even justice.

Informed consent does not apply to all aspects of decision making. Patients are not usually asked for their consent on matters of technical detail, such as the kind and amount of anesthetic to be used or the length and placement of an incision, but they are entitled to decide whether they want surgery at all. They have a right to decide, for instance, if they prefer the pain of natural childbirth to the diminished awareness and possible risk involved in an anesthetized delivery. Informed consent ought to ensure the patient's control over aspects of the case which he or she considers significant.

Uses of informed consent

Many doctors discount the value of informed consent by pointing out that most patients do not have the medical background to make an informed choice. Strictly speaking, this is correct. Most people do not fully understand the workings of chemical agents or the routine risks of radiation therapy. However, they can be helped to understand how those various procedures might ultimately affect them, and they are likely to prefer to make their choice in light of such factors.

Help patients to understand

What information is needed for consent to be considered informed? It is the information that is relevant to the patient's value structure and that is likely to be significant in the decision-making process. The doctor's task is to determine what information is relevant and to provide it in a comprehensible way. Even when this has been done, the doctor will still have a great many decisions to make. Patients tend to relinquish responsibility for detailed decisions to their physicians because most of the technical details are not relevant to them.

It is important to be realistic in assessing the patient's need for information. It is easy to fall into implicit paternalism here and sincerely assure the patient that the procedure in question is the best one for the condition when that is your judgment as the attending physician. But we have already noted that "best" is an ambiguous term that varies with one's value scheme, and in many cases a physician is not justified in assuming that the patient shares his or her value scheme.

What is "best"?

Determining what the patient needs to know in order to give informed consent and providing that information (and perhaps repeating it or explaining it differently) is a time-consuming task, and physicians may feel that this is not the most valuable use of their time. In many cases this is a valid position; the doctor's expertise may be needed for more urgent matters. The solution, though, is not to sacrifice informed consent, but to have another qualified health professional take charge of that area of patient care. For example, most prenatal classes offered by maternity hospitals now perform this function for future patients. (See Table 50-4.)

Physicians may delegate the explanations

Table 50-4　Informed Consent

Informed consent is important to preserve freedom and guard against
unjustified paternalism. Informed consent should be:

1　Offered voluntarily.
2　Decided on the basis of all information relevant to the patient.

OTHER MORAL PROBLEMS

When and What to Tell the Patient

Communi-
cation
problems

Among the many other moral problems that arise in the communication between patient and physician is the amount and kind of
information to convey to patients. This can only be decided by attention to one's values. Often there seem to be ethical grounds for
providing less information than is necessary to obtain fully informed consent. For instance, sometimes a physician makes a diagnosis that might only cause harm if shared with the patient; for
example, a doctor may suspect retardation in a newborn infant but
fear that if the parents are told immediately, they will reject the
child and not form the important initial bonding on which the
child's future well-being could depend. There have been several
well-publicized cases of children born with Down's syndrome and
duodenal atresia in which the parents refused permission for surgery. Presumably, if the parents had not been told of the Down's
syndrome, they would have permitted the surgery and the lives of
those children could have been saved. But does a physician who
would have preferred that outcome have the right to impose his or
her value system on such parents?

Patients' Right to Know

To tell at all?

A different problem is exemplified by a teenager experiencing facial tics who is diagnosed as having multiple sclerosis. The physician believes that this patient may never have further symptoms
but that because of his personality he would expect the worst if told
the diagnosis. Again, the decision of what the patient (and family)
should be told must be based on the recognition that the patient
has the right to make important value decisions about his or her
life. The problem is that often the physician fears that the patient
will use the information to make inappropriate decisions. The patient may needlessly limit his activities and goals even though there
is a good chance that the disease will cause him very little trouble.
Withholding information in such a case could be justified by most
of the theories we reviewed.

Here the physician shares a patient's values but fears that the patient will misinterpret or improperly weigh the information even if it is presented carefully and explicitly. In this case, paternalism may be justified if it can be shown that not allowing the patient to have the diagnostic information needed to make a serious decision does not take away the patient's overall autonomy. But remember that *paternalism must always be justified*; the burden of proof lies with the physician, who must establish the special character of the particular case.

Paternalism may be justified

When Value Schemes Differ

Another possibility is that physician and patient may have different value schemes, and information that is deemed crucial by one may be considered irrelevant by the other. For example, a physician who is unaware of the Jehovah's Witness prohibition against blood transfusions may not think it worth mentioning that elective surgery may involve blood transfusions, while to a Jehovah's Witness this will be a crucial piece of information. Or a physician may believe in the sanctity of human life and think nothing warrants its deliberate destruction, but may also be convinced that a particular patient prefers not to undergo a lingering and painful death and will commit suicide if told he or she is suffering from untreatable bone cancer. In such a case, the physician withholding information from the patient would be unjustifiably imposing personal values on the patient, who has the right to make the decision of how to deal with the prognosis.

Crucial information

Parents as Decision Makers

The case cited earlier of the infant with birth defects has its own special complications. The law gives parents the right to make decisions for their child, but they are not properly the patient. One may reasonably question whether they ought to have the exclusive right to decide for their children, especially if they cannot be clearly shown to have the child's best interests at heart. Obviously, someone must make decisions for an infant, but it is a moral, social, and political question whether that power should always lie with the parents. As long as it does, however, parents have a right to all relevant information unless there are overriding circumstances.

Deciding for children

Distinguishing between Facts and Values

Patients, or their guardians if they are not rational agents, ought to be given whatever information is likely to be relevant to them in making value decisions about their own lives; in addition to facts, such information may include the physician's advice and opinions

The doctor may reveal his or her values

on matters of value. It is not wrong for a physician to offer a considered opinion on the value issues, but the physician should be clear about what information is derived from facts and what is a result of an evaluation based on a personal value scheme.

What the
family
physician
should explain

Conversely, when the physician seeks information from patients, he or she should make clear to them what the significance of such information might be. A family physician who believes that all aspects of a patient's life are potentially relevant to that patient's health ought to explain to the patient that he or she holds such a belief. If this approach to family medicine is explained in the initial contacts with a patient, the patient will be better able to understand the nature of the doctor's concerns. Patients will then understand the nonreciprocal probing into their private lives and will be more apt to respond sincerely rather than politely.

Problematic Concepts

Ethical
ambiguities
remain

Clinical
ambiguities

Ethical problems that arise in medical contexts, particularly in the patient-physician relationship, have been discussed to show how they may be resolved by considering one's fundamental values. However, many ethical problems in medicine cannot be resolved simply by weighing values, since their resolution requires analysis of problematic concepts such as personhood, death, or health. Considerable ambiguity is associated with all these concepts, and many debates about them can be found in the literature of bioethics. As long as the ambiguity remains, we are bound to run into difficult ethical problems in trying to settle questions posed in these terms. The concept of personhood, for example, is sufficiently ambiguous to prevent us from trying to argue that abortion is wrong just because the fetus is a person, since it may not be a person in the morally relevant sense. Nor can we defend the involuntary commitment of a depressed patient by claiming that it is being done for the sake of that person's health as long as it is not clear either that depression is an illness or that institutionalization will cure it. The concepts must be more clearly defined before they can be invoked as moral arguments.

Scarce Resources

Other moral problems arise because the resources available to the individual physician and the financial and social services provided by society will influence the kind of care that can be offered. If a patient needs only home care but has medical coverage only for hospital care, the physician may have to resort to hospitalization even if it is wasteful and psychologically bad for the patient. If the patient requires an organ transplant or dialysis, the physician will have to compete with other physicians acting on behalf of their patients for the limited resources available. The physician may also have to decide who is the more worthy recipient—a decision that clearly extends beyond any medical training.

Problems in the Industrial Setting

Physicians involved in industry may find themselves engaged in political disputes if the industry involves dangerous activity. Those who work for commercial employers, insurance companies, state institutions, schools, or health maintenance organizations (HMOs) will sometimes find there is a conflict between their obligations to patients and to employers. For example, a company physician may detect a slight heart problem in an employee 2 months before the employee is eligible for retirement. In such a case, it would be in the company's interest to terminate the patient immediately, but the patient may feel that it is in his or her interest to continue working for 2 more months. Whose interests should the physician serve?

Other Problem Areas

Physicians will sometimes be given information in confidence that it could be dangerous to conceal. For example, a psychiatrist may learn that her patient is an arsonist. There will then be a conflict between the physician's duty to society and her professional duty to maintain confidentiality. Those who are involved in research must worry about the many ethical problems involved in experimenting with human subjects. Physicians dealing with adolescents will have difficulty determining when the patient should be treated as a responsible decision maker and when confidentiality must be breached and parental consent sought. Value decisions will also have to be made about when to use genetic screening techniques and what procedure to recommend to patients at some risk of bearing diseased children.

Confidentiality

Research

Adolescents

SUMMARY

The ethical problems that arise in medical practice are endless, and with further breakthroughs in knowledge and technology, new problems will crop up. It has been suggested that the best way to handle difficult ethical problems is to reflect on the options available and compare the relative values of the outcomes expected from each possible course of action. Ultimately, ethical decisions are choices between values; hence it is necessary to set priorities for the competing values. Careful attention to abstract issues will provide guidance in concrete situations.

Chapter 51

The Whole-Person Doctor

B. K. Hennen, M.D.

"The individual isolated from the surrounding environment is not and cannot be whole. He, indeed, takes his individuality in part from it. But neither can the individual who is focused entirely on past and present [be whole]. Just as there is no wholeness without society, there is no wholeness without the future."[1]

What of the immediate future? Is it possible for a single physician—a generalist providing primary care to the whole family—to consider the health of each individual in a holistic way? We believe not only that this is possible but also that it may be the most cost-effective and efficient way of providing holistic care, at least within the health care requirements of western society.

THE PHYSICIAN AS CLINICIAN

The family physician must be an alert clinician who reacts to subtle clues and is capable of finding quick and practical solutions.

Interviewing is a basic skill

In our opinion, interviewing and history-taking techniques are important basic skills. These skills require an understanding of human behavior and family dynamics and an awareness of the community aspects of health. They are difficult, if not impossible, to learn indirectly by emulating others; that is, they cannot be acquired merely through apprenticeship or training without a thorough understanding of the principles on which they are based.

In contrast, the minor technical skills demanded of most family practitioners can be learned within the context of the expectations and needs of the community. For example, when a new physician moves to a community, he immediately becomes aware of whether or not he should be doing closed reductions of Colles's fractures. If this skill is usually expected, it is one that can be learned with the help of a cooperative expert, supervised practice, and extra reading concerning complications. It is not so easy for new practitioners to develop the complex interviewing, history-taking, family therapy, and community types of skills required of good family physicians. These skills should already have been acquired.

Interviewing is difficult to learn on the job

Because of his or her "front line" availability, the family physician must be a clinician who is alert to very subtle clinical changes. These are often easier to detect or interpret when the physician is familiar with the particular characteristics of the patient and with the family and community context in which the patient's problem is presented. These clinical skills must be constantly emphasized as absolutely essential to any family physician.

Alert to subtle clues

SERVING THE PATIENT'S NEEDS

Serving the needs of the patient should be the basic objective of every family physician and health professional. Sometimes the needs are obvious only to the patient, sometimes only to the physician, sometimes to both. Sometimes the needs are obvious to neither patient nor physician, but are identified by someone else close to the patient: a family member, friend, teacher, or employer. At times the needs can be anticipated only by an awareness of the risks the patient runs because of age, sex, social circumstances, personal habits, inherited susceptibilities, or as a result of the health professional's experience and skill in foreseeing illness.

Identifying the patient's needs

It is therefore important to understand illness behavior and to make anticipatory guidance and health risk appraisal a part of the regular office routine. (See the chapters on illness behavior, the family life cycle and anticipatory guidance, and a prospective approach to health maintenance.)

Family Resources

An overall general task for the family practitioner is to make sure that the people in his or her practice make the best use of available health care resources, including, and in particular, the resources of their own families.

Selecting problems for doctors to solve

This involves prevention, health education, high-risk identification, awareness of why people present with their problems, the application of self-care, and the best use of family for health maintenance and illness management.

In the case of prevention and high-risk identification, the challenge is to reach out to patients, making the most of opportunities that present themselves during office visits to carry out preventive and screening activities.

If we understand why people present to physicians with their health problems, we can educate them to handle on their own the problems which they can deal with, and to bring to us those for which we can give them guidance, direction, and possibly even cure.

Self-care whenever possible

When evaluating self-care, we should realize that if it is at least as good as the care we can provide, it is a more desirable alternative. Self-care is less costly and also more personal when it takes place in the home and family environment. New approaches to home care are badly needed, in particular for care of the chronically ill and the elderly and for palliative care of the dying patient, especially in North America, where "excellence in health care" is too often viewed as synonymous with "hospital care."

Most families can make a tremendous contribution to care, serving as an information source, a motivating source for seeking care, and a therapeutic source in terms of reaching (with our help) all the above goals of prevention, education, and appropriate use of the health care system, and use of family resources. In the case of families that are too dysfunctional to provide or learn how to provide such resources, we can substitute community services and health professional expertise.

Continuity of Care

The challenge

All the special skills discussed above extend beyond good clinical medicine and depend on a continuous relationship with patient and family. To ensure that holistic care is available for patients wherever they live, after they move away, or whenever individuals are separated from their family is a challenge to all who practice family medicine. The challenge also exists for those who control the organization and financing of health care—the medical profession and the government.

THE ROLE OF PATIENT ADVOCATE

An honorable role

We often hear a family doctor talk in a self-deprecating way about making "social" or "clerical" visits to patients. This is especially common in major centers where care (often in hospitals) is provided by teams of physicians and other health professionals. Instead of being played down, the role of patient advocate should be looked on as a legitimate and honorable function of family practitioners. A family physician is a link between the advance technological resources for health care and the personal idiosyncracies and characteristics of the individual patient and family. Most consultants and specialists acknowledge the need for this role, and most patients appreciate it and understand it. It is up to the complete family physician to ensure that he or she becomes expert at the advocacy role and accepts it as an integral part of family practice.

AREAS OF SPECIAL CONCERN

A threat to the renewed emphasis on holistic care provided by specifically trained family physicians lies in the tendency for areas of special interest to develop once again, leading to narrow and limited practice pursuits. We believe that many of these special interests can be built upon basic family medicine training. This training provides a broad approach which will make the ultimate pursuit of the special interest more effective and satisfying for both patient and physician. Among such interests are geriatrics, obstetrics, emergency medicine, occupational medicine, and sports medicine. In all these areas we believe it necessary for the family physician to maintain the generalist concept that is basic to family medicine.

Family medicine is the foundation

Geriatrics

Most geriatric services are provided through family physicians, although geriatricians may be required as consultants for complex individual problems and for advice on the organization of scarce resources for elderly patients.

Obstetrics

Every family physician should have sufficient training in obstetrics to be able to provide good prenatal care and to recognize high-risk pregnancies. He or she should also be trained to attend an uncomplicated obstetric delivery. Special training other than in the use of outlet forceps is required for such complicated deliveries as a cesarean section and those requiring the interpretation of the records of monitors. Involvement in these activities depends also on available resources, transport facilities, patient needs, etc. Guidelines are required by hospitals in peripheral communities that do not have complete obstetric services. An example of such a guideline is profided by Black, who says:

At present there is no adequate means of identifying obstetric patients who are liable to require emergency operative intervention. In the absence of valid selection criteria it is not practical for the small hospital to plan to do only "normal" obstetrics. Any hospital practicing obstetrics should be prepared to manage complications. It is suggested that a unit with fewer than 100 deliveries per year cannot maintain the ability to manage complications and hence should discontinue all obstetric practice. Similarly, at small hospitals that continue obstetric practice elective cesarian section should be done so that the staff can maintain their ability to do emergency cesarian sections. . . .[2]

Emergency Medicine

Most emergency room problems are basically primary care problems and family practice–oriented (capable of management in a family practice) and are not emergencies. The best physician for the job is a complete family physician who has the extra training needed to deal with the small number of acute emergencies.

Occupational Medicine

Occupational medicine requires an understanding of family and community, as well as the workplace, and once again family medicine is good basic training. For example, in identifying in a family those health risks related to the occupations of family members, the physician has to deal with concerns such as toxicology, accident proneness, "workaholic syndrome," and alcoholism.

Sports Medicine

At first glance, sports medicine would seem to be a more individualized kind of trauma medicine, but one only has to take the example of community involvement in amateur athletics to realize that the family physician has a considerable role to play. Amateur athletics brings up concerns about proper fitness and injury prevention and involves problems such as inappropriate parental intervention and the emulation of professional-sports violence.

We do not deny that to work in any of these areas, the family physician needs extra training. We merely emphasize that the basis on which this training should be built is a thorough knowledge of family medicine.

SUMMARY

The theme that runs through all of family medicine is continuous care of individuals in the context of their families and their communities. This is not to say the family physician is the sole provider of good health care. Like that of the patient, the role of the family physician must be seen in the context of society as a whole. The family physician must depend on consulting colleagues and community resources and must be prepared for a lifetime of education in order to be able to respond to society's changing needs and expectations. The family physician depends for his or her wholeness on a dynamic attitude toward the future.

REFERENCES

1 I. H. Buchen, "Humanism and Futurism: Enemies or Allies?" in Alvin Toffler (ed.), *Learning for Tomorrow: The Role of the Future in Education,* Vintage Books, New York, February 1974, p 143.
2 D. P. Black and S. Gick, "Management of Obstetric Complications at a Small Rural Hospital," *Canadian Medical Association Journal,* **120:**31–37, January 6, 1979.

Chapter 52

The Future of Family Medicine

D. I. Rice, M.D.

Family medicine is meeting a need for people-oriented and health-oriented medical care. As an ambulatory based discipline, it offers experience in alternative methods of care and increasing cost benefits. The combination of the primary care family physician and the consultant specialist working cooperatively in the health system provides the preferred model of efficient care.

The relative acceptance of family medicine as a distinct and creditable academic discipline is the result of it having met the legitimate and previously unmet needs of particular groups and individuals within our society.

Patients want personal holistic care

Family medicine is meeting the needs of an increasing number of perceptive *patients* who express concern that the rapid and extensive development of the specialties has resulted in the practice of medicine becoming increasingly fragmented, depersonalized, disease-oriented, hospital-based, and expensive. In responding to these needs, those responsible for the training of family physicians emphasize the importance of the *holistic* approach to patient care—total care of the whole patient within the context of the patient's changing environment. Family physicians are being trained to be people-oriented and health-oriented as well as disease-oriented.

Medical students have expressed concern that the absence of family medicine as a part of the undergraduate medical curriculum and the lack of exposure to family physicians as teachers preclude the opportunity for students to place family practice and specialty practice in proper perspective vis-à-vis the selection of a preferred professional career.

Students request exposure to family practice

The development of university departments of family medicine and the presence of family physicians as teachers at both the undergraduate and graduate levels of medical education now provide all medical students with the opportunity to observe the base of family medicine and the specialities in proper perspective—in terms of total patient care. The result of meeting this need of medical students, is the growing number of young physicians who are choosing family medicine as a professional career.

Two decades ago, *general practitioners* voiced concern that the experience of an undergraduate period of training combined with a one-year clinical internship was inadequate preparation for the responsibilities of community practice. Lacking the availability of additional training in family medicine, one of two alternatives resulted—graduate training in a traditional specialty or the acceptance of a limited general practice that in many instances lacked professional satisfaction. While the opportunity for residency training in family medicine has continued to be limited even where the family physician is acknowledged as the central figure in the health care delivery system, those physicians who have had the benefit of this additional training express satisfaction with the appropriateness of their training, remain in family practice, and acknowledge a much higher level of professional satisfaction.

Family practitioners initiated more adequate training

Health planners in both the private and public sectors have observed the rapidly escalating costs of a health care system that is unduly influenced by technology that results from specialization and subspecialization, and where hospitalization and extensive investigations make a major contribution to these increasing costs. Family medicine—with its orientation toward ambulatory or out-of-hospital care, preventive medicine and health maintenance, the selective use of diagnostic investigative procedures, and the greater control of drugs and therapeutics—has been welcomed by health planners as one substantial means of controlling health care costs while preserving and enhancing the quality of patient care.

Planners recognize an efficient system

The future of family medicine is assured, primarily because these needs will continue and will have to be fulfilled. The ongoing challenge to medical educators will be to constantly monitor these changing needs and to make the necessary changes in educational programs to respond to these needs.

While there is no international consensus respecting an appropriate name (the general practitioner, family physician, primary care physician, or generalist), the value to society of properly qualified physicians trained to provide primary, continuing, and comprehensive care, working as part of a team with consulting specialists and other health professionals, is being increasingly acknowledged by health planners throughout the world as providing the most efficient and effective health care system at a controlled cost.

While the problems that serve as deterrents to the orderly development of an increasing number of qualified family physicians vary from country to country, certain problems are common. These include the following:

A generalist and consulting specialist model works

There needs to be wider acceptance, particularly within the established medical profession, of the primary care–consulting care relationship between physicians. Family physicians should be trained as primary care physicians, specialists as consulting physicians. This relationship should continue in the practice setting.

While the relative roles of family physicians and consulting specialists will vary—depending upon the distribution of the general population and other factors—manpower projections must be more precise and be based on these relative and accepted roles, rather than on existing and at times questionable considerations.

Resources are necessary for the education of family physicians

Present resources for the training of physicians in many instances need to be reallocated, and where necessary, additional resources provided, to ensure that the proper number of family physicians in the appropriate ratio to specialists is being maintained, if society's total needs for medical care are to be met.

In summary, family medicine is being accepted as a new and necessary academic discipline because the family physician—the end product of the educational objectives on which training programs are based—is meeting a major need of society for improved patient care, and at the same time is enjoying the degree of professional satisfaction that is necessary if continuing generations of physicians are to be attracted to this discipline.

To ensure the future of family medicine, health planners and health educators must be more sensitive to the changing needs of society for total health care and make the necessary resources available that are required to train family physicians and other health professionals in appropriate numbers to meet these needs.

Family physician educators must accept the opportunity to respond to the legitimate concerns of critics who support the need for formal training programs in family medicine, but who question its relative lack of appropriate research and of the body of literature that by tradition is expected and required as the basis of all legitimate academic disciplines.

This textbook, *Family Medicine: A Guidebook for Practitioners of the Art,* is intended as a contribution toward ensuring the future of family medicine.

Index